Carers, Professionals and Alzheimer's Disease

Editor
Desmond O'Neill BA, MB, MRCPI

Lecturer
Department of Care of the Elderly
University of Bristol and Frenchay Hospital, Bristol

Former Chairman
Scientific Committee
Alzheimer Society of Ireland

John Libbey

JL

LONDON PARIS ROME

British Library Cataloguing in Publication Data

Carers, Professionals and Alzheimer's Disease
1. Man. Brain. Alzheimer's disease
I. O'Neill, Desmond

616.831

ISBN 0 86196 298 2

Published by

John Libbey & Company Ltd
13 Smiths Yard, Summerley Street, London SW18 4HR, England.
Tel: +44 (0) 81 947 2777
John Libbey Eurotext Ltd, 6 rue Blanche, 92120 Montrouge, France.
John Libbey - C.I.C. s.r.l., via L. Spallanzani 11, 00161 Rome, Italy.

Contents

Foreword

On 17 November 1899 an Irish psychiatrist, Dr Connolly Norman, read a paper on Senile Dementia[1] to the Medical Section of the Royal Academy of Medicine in Dublin. At the beginning of a remarkably wide-ranging lecture on the condition, he told his audience that "in spite of the ease with which its broad features may often be recognised, and of its hopeless prognosis, this affection presents certain points of interest often overlooked." Connolly Norman's lecture fell on deaf ears and it is only now, almost a century later, that the condition is beginning to attract the attention it deserves.

Much of the impetus for this new-found interest comes from the Alzheimer's societies which are being established throughout the world. Indeed, great credit is due to the Alzheimer Society of Ireland for organizing the special international conference in Dublin in 1989, the proceedings of which form the basis of this book. The conference was special because it brought together both carers and scientists of international repute to discuss Alzheimer's disease in a very broad context. This book, which has been carefully edited by Dr Desmond O'Neill, captures the flavour of this unique meeting.

The book gives us a comprehensive picture of the progress which has been made in the diagnosis, treatment and care of patients with Alzheimer's disease. There are many examples of lateral thinking throughout the book and many new and exciting approaches are described. There is a fascinating section on architecture relating to Alzheimer's disease, an area which has been very neglected in the past.

It is obvious from the book that the former *ad hoc* approach towards the care and treatment of patients with Alzheimer's disease is gradually being replaced by a much more structured approach. The book should prove invaluable for those who are already in the field and who wish to keep up-to-date with the most recent advances. It is also an ideal book for those who are approaching this very challenging subject for the first time covering, as it does, the condition from the perspective of both carer and professional.

Professor Davis Coakley, MD FRCPI
Director
Mercer's Institute for Research on Ageing
St James's Hospital, Dublin 8

1. Norman C. Remarks on Senile Dementia. *The Dublin Journal of Medical Science* 1900, CX, **346**, 250-265.

Acknowledgements

The production of this book would not have been possible without the effort and energy of Michael F Coote FMII, chairman of the Alzheimer's Society of Ireland who led the team organizing the 5th Alzheimer's Disease International Conference in Dublin. Thanks are also due to the organizing committee members: Winifred Bligh, Vivienne Bradley, Janet Convery, Eithne Grealy, Mary Higgins, Joe Rowe and Ronan Smith. Particular gratitude is due to Nuala Dunphy, whose organizational flair and efficiency eased the task of arranging the conference. Typing help came from Gaye O'Kennedy, Breda Martin and Mary Boyle. I am indebted to Ronald Haynes of the University of Bristol for technical advice. Support for production of the book came from Sandoz and the Alzheimer Society of Ireland.

Finally, I should like to thank my wife for her patience, good humour and support during the preparation of this book.

D O'Neill
Bristol
November 1990

SECTION 1
Alzheimer's Disease
into the 90's

Carers, Professionals and Alzheimer's Disease. D O'Neill ed © 1991 John Libbey & Company Ltd

Chapter 1

ALZHEIMER'S DISEASE INTO THE 1990's

RN Butler *MD, Chairman and Brookdale Professor, Ritter Department of Geriatrics and Adult Development, Mount Sinai Medical Center, 1 Gustave Levy Place, Box 1070, New York, New York 10029, USA*

We continue to engage in a variety of research projects, yet we are unable to identify a clear diagnostic marker for Alzheimer's disease. While we may have some hopeful messages from trials of THA, we are still a long way from a cure for Alzheimer's disease. It may not be a curable disease, but this does not mean that it is not treatable. We continue to make progress in a variety of scientific fields, working as individuals and in interdisciplinary groups, not only in trying to understand the basic underlying mechanisms of Alzheimer's disease but also in investigating appropriate means of intervention.

I thought that I would forego a review of the contemporary research and instead challenge you all to think of certain very painful topics, perhaps they might be called the unmentionables, that are extremely important to the constituency which we represent – the community of patients with Alzheimer's disease and their families. I would like to suggest some action that we might take in response to these topics. In all instances I am guided by one inner thought, and that is to provide and maintain autonomy and choice for the Alzheimer patient to the maximum degree possible. After all, autonomy and choice constitute the meaning of that oft-used word dignity.

Action points

These are the concerns I would like to discuss:

(i) *The continuing inadequacy of nursing-home conditions, and the continuing denial of patient rights, including the over-use and misuse of physical and chemical restraint.*

3

(ii) Care-giver burden and burn-out, which is an assault upon the independence, economic security and health of women, who make up some 80 per cent of the care-givers and whose long-term survival after the death of the patient is little-noted.

(iii) The marital deterioration that occurs often among older people, with or without Alzheimer's disease, but is often made worse in cases where Alzheimer's disease exists.

(iv) Elder abuse, or the battered old-person syndrome where the confused, demented Alzheimer's patient is made a victim at home, in the street or in a nursing home. Abuse may occur in both directions: i.e. the assault of an Alzheimer patient upon a family member.

(v) The rising rate of suicide among the old, at least in the United States since 1981, which may be associated with the depression seen frequently in Alzheimer's disease and other dementias. The anticipation of a sense of helplessness or the anticipation of dreaded institutionalization may predispose to the suicidal act.

(vi) The increasing public discussion of, and even calls for, physician-assisted suicide or active euthanasia, moving us beyond the threshold of passive euthanasia. I would argue that this constitutes the excesses of the "right to die" movement which can become all too attractive a movement to cost-cutting governmental and other budgeteers.

(vii) The inadequate concern for the inner life of Alzheimer patients, whether or not they are in nursing homes. Often besieged with memories of the past, including a resurgence of conflicts, they too require an opportunity to review their lives. Our failure to be attentive to the inner psychological life of all such patients is distressing.

(viii) The alleged rising competition for resources between Alzheimer patients and patients with AIDS.

(ix) The still incomplete development of a major "philosophy of longevity and ageing". Such a philosophy is not very visible in the broad landscape of Western thought.

Before I enlarge on the discussion of these nine matters, I must acknowledge first that I rely mainly on the American experience, and that although Alzheimer's disease may afflict people long before they reach the stage of life that is normally recognized as old age, for the purposes of this paper I must stress that the predominant age of incidence for Alzheimer's disease is old age.

Nursing homes and restraint

Despite the superb report of the United States National Academy of Science, Institute of Medicine, the results of a Committee (ably chaired by Sidney Katz, which recommended major nursing home reforms in the United States), the recommendations have not been implemented and therefore not enforced in American nursing homes. I cannot speak for many countries, but I know that few have the widespread use of physical and chemical restraint found in the United States where half a million people are estimated to be under these restraints in nursing homes. Therein may be a lesson, a possible model, and we in the USA could profit from studying other countries in this regard.

Eighty to ninety per cent of nursing home care is provided by nurse's aides, people with very good intentions, but often hired off the streets without any pre-service education, or even later in-service training and with as high as a 150 per cent rate of annual turnover. They work with minimum pay and very little career opportunities and options. To save money, nursing-home administrations attempt to minimize staff numbers and provide little education to implement alternative forms of management of behaviour, leading to the minimization or elimination of restraint. Most American nursing homes do not provide or represent prosthetic environments to protect the patient, from a fall out of bed for example.

It is obvious that society has to be educated not only to appreciate the necessity at times for nursing-home-type care, but also to appreciate the need for reforms, and have the willingness to pay for them. It is not enough to be periodically upset when some fresh nursing-home scandal arises. Rather it is essential to create high quality institutions in the first place, with adequate staff levels with first rate training. In doing so, we could avoid inappropriate use of physical or chemical restraint. Instead of, for example, the restraining of individuals by the use of psychoactive medications, the staff could become acquainted with a variety of techniques for coping with agitation and restlessness. Relieving pain and suffering through socialization, enhancing the quality and frequency of visitation of family, friends and acquaintances and providing occupational therapy, touch, music and massage could be used in lieu of the automatic and all too frequent over-use of medications.

The care-giver's burden

When we talk about the care-givers' burden, we must recognize that it is the family, mostly women, who bear that burden. Women are also the poorly-paid care-givers in institutions and home-health care agencies subject to burn-out and, indeed, to exploitation. In the government policy debate in which I play a part in Washington DC, it is often said that if we move towards entitlements the family (meaning women) would abandon its care-giving responsibilities towards its older members and seek governmental help instead. This is referred to as the "wood-work effect": meaning that once these entitlements are available, people will "come out of the woodwork" to take advantage of them, leading to more governmental expenditures. What is the evidence for this governmental anxiety? Has it happened in other countries when they have provided more services? Here is an opportunity for trans-cultural comparison.

The economic security of our families in almost all developed nations continues to depend on the two-pay-cheque household. Therefore we need to value more the

5

work of women, for example by awarding social security credits and constant-at-tendance allowances for the care not only of older persons and the disabled persons with Alzheimer's disease, but also of other disabled persons and children. True pay equity for men and women is essential. Also required are changes in the expectations placed on men at work and the transformation of men's behaviour so that they may participate more actively in care-giving. I do realize that some 15 per cent of the care-givers are men, but I would note that frequently we men are able to hire help and not provide the direct care ourselves. In the United States an important book was recently published. *The Second Shift,* by Arli Hochschild, a distinguished University of California, Berkeley sociologist, which demon-strates that feminism has not reduced women's work and has not transformed men to a new height of domesticity.

I would challenge the women's movement in our various countries to move beyond their legitimate concerns with economic equality and reproductive rights and to concentrate also on the problems of older women, their own future selves. In part because of living longer than men, women have a greater chance of economic destitution (60 per cent of American women on widowhood) and a greater chance of being trapped by burdens of care, first of others and, eventually, of themselves. We know that there is a very high incidence of depression among care-givers. The National Institute on Aging recently concluded a study counting the cost of the care of Alzheimer patients by families. A very conservative methodology of estimation produced a total of 88 billion dollars, a significant part of which is reflected in the productivity lost as a result of the burden of care-giving.

Marital deterioration and elder abuse

In studies which we carried out at the National Institutes for Health in the 1950's and 1960's, we were shocked to learn that up to one third of marriages between healthy community-living elderly people went through a deterioration. In my practice as a clinician, I am often struck by the further impact of various diseases, particularly dementing illnesses, on marital relationships. We must alert the caring professions and institutions, in particular psychology, psychiatry and family agencies to be much more attentive to this fact and much more supportive.

With regard to elder abuse, we need hot-lines and other methods of crisis intervention to help the older people who, often out of embarrassment or of fear, do not make those calls. Furthermore, services must be available to help deal with the root causes of the tension that led to the abuse.

Suicide

It is amazing how little there is in the Medline database on the relationship between suicide and Alzheimer's disease. We could only find one citation which dealt jointly with homicide and suicide. There is a high rate of suicide among older persons throughout the industrialized world. In the United States, older persons have accounted for some 20 per cent of suicides for many years. Old age suicide is found predominantly in the male population. Men in their eighties commit suicide twelve and a half times more frequently than women in their eighties. How much is suicide a function of an anticipation of helplessness? Some of us remember Nietzche's comment that "the thought of suicide is a great consolation. By means of it one gets successfully through many a bad night". The thought of suicide may give an individual the feeling that he or she has some control over life after all.

However, whatever its rationale, suicide in a family has profound effects on the survivors. It echoes throughout the lives of these families to the children and the grandchildren. Whether bluntly or subtly, suicide erodes the meaning and value of life itself. When an older person decides to commit suicide, he or she is frequently successful. There are some actions that we can take to help prevent this eventuality. We must press suicide-prevention centres to develop special preventive services for Alzheimer's disease patients and their families, as well as for other older people. We need studies, which we in the United States call a "psychological autopsy", when a suicide is committed, to better understand how and why it happened. As a preventive measure, we must have mental health services available to Alzheimer's disease patients and care-givers. We must be able to diagnose "chronic suicide". Although it may appear to be a contradiction in terms, "chronic suicide" refers to the action of those who decide not to eat or not to take life-sustaining medication. They are also committing suicide, a suicide that is not taken into account by any of our national centres for health statistics.

The growing cause for euthanasia

Undoubtedly, the psychological importance of control is one of the reasons why the concept of physician-assisted suicide has arisen as a possibility or even a reality and in some countries perhaps as a cause, for example in the Netherlands. In the United States and the UK, there are significant memberships for the Hemlock Society which advocates physician-assisted suicide. I affirm, or reaffirm, the importance to individuals of having autonomy and control over their own dying and death. Nevertheless, autonomy over one's self during one's life cannot be and is not a total desideratum. Society certainly has some rights as expressed and represented by the state. I worry a lot that the state, particularly the United States, with its preoccupation on costs and cost-containment, could find it extremely attractive to avert its eyes at the prospect or reality of subtle forms of euthanasia. This also includes reduced care and triage, a concept that was originally provided for times of emergency or of war. It seems to me that we see triage at work in peace-time conditions, usually perpetrated against the poor and the vulnerable, and if you live long enough and have Alzheimer's disease you are likely to be both. We must be careful that "Do not resuscitate" orders do not become "Do not treat" orders. Let us be sure that social coercion, depression and personal feelings of being a burden do not hasten the wish for death of someone who might otherwise enjoy further opportunities for family and interpersonal relationships, such as surviving to see a favourite grand-daughter graduate from

7

college, a grand-daughter whose college education the individual might have helped to finance.

I think that we should worry a lot about physicians participating actively in euthanasia. We might come to that day when we would wonder if that syringe coming towards us is the lethal dose or the therapeutic dose. Physicians have been acculturated by tradition to serve on the side of life. To condemn them for their continued allegiance to maintenance of life as a supreme value would be socially unwise. Every home-nursing agency, every nursing home, every hospital, senior centre, every element of the health and caring spectrum should have an ethics committee, composed of lawyers, ethicists, physicians, nurses and lay people. But ethical decisions should not be the equivalent of economic decisions. I grew up believing that certain verities were eternal and did not depend on the particular economic status in a given situation.

Technology – use or abuse?

Many organizations of the aged and many older persons themselves have been concerned about the excessive use, or misuse, of technology. There has been an active "right to die with dignity" movement in the United States. The living will has been adopted in forty states and the District of Columbia in the United States. However, I would warn that we should not let social pressures coerce us into feeling that we have a duty to die when we reach a certain age or health status. Some people believe that everyone with cancer has untreatable or uncontrollable pain. This is not so: hardly more than one-third of cancer patients fit that description. Similarly, not all patients with Alzheimer's disease are in the end stages of that disease, or in a coma. For many patients there is still so much life to be enjoyed.

Alzheimer's disease is not the only illness targeted in discussions of euthanasia. Other populations with significant mental impairment, such as those with Down's syndrome, could easily be made the target in any resurgence of movement towards active euthanasia. Our own United States Alzheimer's Disease Association is on record as follows: " it recognizes and affirms the taking of another's life, whether premeditated or not, is against the law and cannot be condoned." This was restated at the time of the Roswell–Gilbert case, a celebrated case in the United States, where a husband killed his wife who had Alzheimer's disease and who would have had to be committed to a nursing home. The Alzheimer's Association also agrees that when a person's wishes have been made known in the case of an incurable illness, it is permissible for the physician to withhold treatment that would serve mainly to prolong the dying process. This includes withholding nutrition and hydration artificially administered by vein or gastric tube if the patient rejects food and water, but not spoon-feeding, which should be continued for purposes of comfort.

As persons grow older or prematurely older and sense the proximity of death, I believe that they experience a life review, that is reminiscence and a resurgence of conflicts. These can be therapeutic and comforting: they can also be depressing and painful. In the presence of Alzheimer's disease, one's ability to make this review is affected, the ability to process information is fragmented. At this point, they need all the help that they can get to get to grips with and resolve some of the issues of their lives.

The growing competition for resources between AIDS and Alzheimer's disease communities

Both groups require greater resources for the discovery of new knowledge, and people with either AIDS or Alzheimer's disease require some of the same treatment and therapy resources, day-care centres, home care and hospice care. But note that every step of improvement through new medications or new interventions, whether for AIDS or Alzheimer's disease, is actually likely to lead to greater social cost until the time arrives when effective treatment or prevention is available. It is time for these two communities to make common cause. Perhaps it is because the United States has developed the least strengthened long-term care programme among industrialized communities that we may be more sensitive to this problem than are some other nations.

A philosophy of longevity and ageing

On an individual level such a philosophy may in part translate into developing our own "letter of instruction" in an effort to establish a degree of autonomy and mastery into the last days of our lives. But later life is an expanding period and also a very vital one: the life of the vast majority of elder persons is one of vigour, health and challenge. We must understand that this new longevity provides an extraordinary opportunity for us.

As one looks back into Western civilization, we find references to old age in Ecclesiastes, Job, Plato, Socrates and Cicero's remarkable essay *De Senectute*. Some further thoughts on ageing and how one might conduct one's self in one's later years are found in the essays of Montaigne, and references to stages of life are found in Shakespeare and Rousseau. Goethe expressed some ideas on the subject, and we have some very interesting thoughts from Metchnikoff, who introduced the word and concept of gerontology in 1906. There are the five linked plays by George Bernard Shaw in *Back to Methuselah*, and more recently we have the wonderful novel *Love in the Time of Cholera* by Gabriel Marcia Marquez, a supreme love story of old age. These works aside, there is precious little in Western thought by way of sign posts or guidelines to help us understand this new territory that is the new longevity. I suspect that in Eastern philosophy there might be more in terms of life cycle as a natural process. It would be fascinating to have a seminar on the comparative philosophy of longevity and old age, bringing together philosophers from China, Japan and the Western world. If there were ever diseases that demanded a philosophy from us, they are the dementias, since they so tragically destroy our ability to relate to our loved ones and to maintain meaning in our life.

9

Final thoughts

Because the aged are growing in numbers relative to other age groups, they will have growing power. Within this growing number of elderly people comes a minority who are disabled physically and mentally, and we have to use our power strongly and wisely to help them. We know that small steps, no matter how useful, are not going to solve the problem, because the demographic or longevity revolution is unprecedented – an additional 25 years of life-expectancy in this century alone – and overwhelming. What will the longevity revolution demand of us in the 21st century? It will require a new and fresh biomedical research agenda, and new pressure to understand the role of the biology of ageing in disease and disability, as in the expression and interweaving of environmental and genetic factors in the genesis of disease.

The longevity revolution demands a transformed system of education of health providers. In the United States today it is nearly impossible to teach medical students the natural history of the course of disease because we have so contracted the amount of time that individuals remain in hospitals that the luxury that I remember enjoying as a medical student of seeing the unfolding of an illness is not available to them. Therefore we must redistribute the way in which we educate. Medical students must be seen in nursing homes, and day-care centres, in day hospitals and in home-care situations to appreciate the character and natural history of disease and disability. In a sense we need not just the traditional teaching in hospital but also the teaching of the nursing home, the teaching of the adult day-care centre and in home-care programmes. The demographic or longevity revolution also demands that we build a very different sort of social organization of the way in which we deliver care, including the key elements of geriatric assessment and management of patient care.

All of us have the power to carry our voices to our respective political institutions: as long as we live in social democracies, we can effect change. Why should a 79-year-old who has had a heart attack in the United States be able to be ensured care and financial support when a 79-year-old patient who has a "brain attack" does not have such care? We should not accept special prejudices and discrimination based upon particular diseases.

Conclusion

As George Bernard Shaw has said, "even our oldest men do not live long enough: they are, for all the purposes of high civilization, mere children when they die". We have this new longevity, and if Shaw had his way we would have even more in order to have a mature civilization. This longevity revolution was not a biological event but a great social achievement already enjoyed by many of us. But how much better will we enjoy it when we are liberated from the dementias, and we will be! We now see some extraordinary changes in the world, with reconciliation and accommodation between the two great super-powers, a setting aside of great investments in armaments, the rising movement of environmentalism. We note the continuing process of the new biology, and the advances (since the unravelling of DNA) in cell biology, giving us still more power over health and disease. But each of us must become a powerful advocate for our constituency, the Alzheimer patient and his/her family. We must assure them autonomy, respect and dignity through attention to some of the rarely mentioned and controversial matters which I have outlined in this paper. And certainly we must all press for enhancement of funds to search for new knowledge, and apply that new knowledge for better care and treatment.

Further reading

Butler R. *Why survive? – Being old in America.* New York, Harper and Row, 1975.

Carers, Professionals and Alzheimer's Disease. D O'Neill ed © 1991 John Libbey & Company Ltd

Chapter 2

THE SILENT EPIDEMIC – WHO CARES?

Nori Graham *FRCPsych, Chairman, Alzheimer's Disease Society of England, Wales and Northern Ireland, 158-160 Balham High Rd, London SW12 9BN, UK*

This paper gives me a unique opportunity to describe the work of our society, the Alzheimer's Disease Society, as we are on the threshold of making a real impact on the public awareness of this disease. The Alzheimer's Disease Society is an organization which aims to support the carers of people with Alzheimer's disease and other related dementias. This very fundamental aim arises because it is firmly believed in our country that there is a limit to what the family can tolerate or should tolerate. Most of us now live in two-generational families, and often these two generations are dispersed for reasons of work or housing. Most men and over half of our working women go out to work, so cannot be expected to endlessly support their elderly relatives. It is, therefore, against this background that we have formed this society over the last ten years, specifically to do all we can to support the carers of those affected by this tragic disease.

Origins of the Alzheimer's Disease Society

I should perhaps start by describing how our society was originally founded. Our founder member is Cora Phillips, who is now a retired nurse and one of our vice-presidents. She cared for her husband with Alzheimer's disease until he died in 1978. In 1979 she heard Professor Alan Davison, professor at the Institute of Neurology in England, give a broadcast on his research into Alzheimer's disease and she wrote to him suggesting the formation of a society. At around the same time another carer of a younger sufferer, Morella Fisher, also one of our vice-presidents, wrote an article in one of our national Sunday newspapers entitled the "Sad, Silent Epidemic". She received many hundreds of letters as a result of this article: one of these letters came from Cora, asking her to join with her to form a society to support other carers. These two ladies, together with Professor Wilcock, a contributor to this symposium, who was and still is involved with research into this disease, along with many other founder members founded the Alzheimer's Disease Society. Professor Wilcock became the chairman and remained so for many years. Anne Brown, our vice-chairman, and one of the vice-presidents of the Alzheimer's Society of Ireland, was also one of the founder members.

The society has gradually grown over the last ten years: I have been chairman for two years. I am a full-time psychiatrist working in London and I specialize in seeing people over the age of 65 with mental illness. Half of my work is concerned with the assessment and management of people with dementia, and I support the carers of my patients, whether they be family members or professionals, either in their own homes or in institutions. The specialty of old-age psychiatry is, I believe, fairly uncommon in other countries. However in the United Kingdom it has been in existence for over twenty years and has undoubtedly encouraged assessment and care for people with dementia, and support for their carers. I also believe that this specialty has highlighted the problems of this particular disadvantaged group of people, and has helped to raise their status. In addition to my clinical work I have been involved with several research studies looking at the prevalence of dementia, both in the community and in residential care, as well as looking at the problems of families looking after people with dementia at home.

Research directions

A good deal is now known about Alzheimer's disease and its prevalence, but it is only in recent years that the social aspects of the disease have been investigated. Most of the interest in these social factors lies in the impact of the disease rather than in its aetiology, as there is no evidence that psychological intervention or improvement of social circumstances can do anything to prevent the condition occurring or have any impact on the rate of deterioration. Undoubtedly the best data on the impact of dementia on carers in the United Kingdom comes from the very extensive study carried out by Enid Levin and her co-workers from the National Institute of Social Work in London. I was one of the two psychiatrists involved in the study, and our findings were published in book form[1] in 1989. I believe that this represents a very authoritative work on the subject: I will summarize the findings of the study, and then describe the role of the Alzheimer's Disease Society in mitigating the impact on carers of this tragic disease.

However, before doing so, I have to emphasize that the long-term goal must be to identify the genetic cause of this disease: it seems clear to me that a gene for Alzheimer's disease will be found. Already a gene for a very rare familial early-onset form of dementia has been discovered. Identification of the gene may take many years, and if and when it is found, the implications for prevention will need further extensive research. So in my view, possible solutions to this disease are one to two decades away: meanwhile in the United Kingdom by the end of this century there will be one million people suffering from dementia, and many more carers than that. It is our responsibility to become as knowledgeable as possible and as efficient as possible in understanding the problems of the carers, and to do something about them in as practicable a way as possible. It is in this connection that Enid Levin's supporters study is very relevant, and came about because it became obvious that the policy of government and professionals in the United Kingdom was to keep people with dementia in their own homes. Not only was this the policy, but families wanted it that way. However, it was clear that this placed a great stress on carers. There had been no systematic study of the problem until 1979 when the government funded the the National Institute of Social Work to carry out this study with the specific aim of looking at the problems of families caring for people with dementia at home.

Carers and patients study

We looked at 150 families looking after 150 elderly people with confusion, virtually in all cases due to dementia. The families were either living with the elderly person or living close by. The families and supporters were interviewed with a very extensive semi-structured interview schedule, and the sufferers themselves were interviewed by two psychiatrists. They were looked at in 1979–1980, and again one year later. The average age of the elderly people was 79, and 80 per cent of them were suffering from a dementia: in half of these cases the dementia was classified as severe. The illness had been present according to relatives for an average of five years, and in some instances for up to twenty years. Half of the elderly people were suffering from a severe physical illness, and falls, incontinence and pain were particularly associated with severity of dementia.

Of the supporters, half were spouses and half were children. They had been living with the elderly person for an average of 36 years – a very long time. Their own average age was 61, i.e. near retirement age; two-thirds of them were in poor physical health, and a large number of them had a physical disability. Three-quarters of them suffered from stress, and a third of them indicated psychiatric morbidity on a well recognized scale: this is twice the prevalence one would expect from a similar age-group not looking after a relative with dementia.

One year later, one fifth of the elderly population was dead, which might have been expected, and a further third were in institutions. We were very interested to find out what it was that seemed to precipitate admission to institutions. The higher the stress in the supporters, the more likely it was that their elderly relative would be in an institution one year later. Although this would appear to be a matter of common sense, it is very important that this should be proven by study. Either death or admission to an institution was associated with reduced stress one year later. A very important finding was that the more help accorded to the relatives, the less likely was it that the relative would be institutionalized one year later. The sort of help was either home-help, which in the United Kingdom is a person who helps with shopping, washing, cooking and physical help around the house, as well as any sort of nursing care or day-care. These things were associated with a reduction of stress in the supporter, and much lower likelihood that institutions would be used one year later.

The problems of supporters were associated with 6 main factors:

15

(i)   the behaviour of the elderly person

(ii) difference in relationship with the elderly person

(iii) restriction of social life

(iv) the unrelieved physical labour of caring

(v)   physical ill health

(vi) the severity of the illness

Basic requirements

We concluded that carers had some basic requirements. The first and foremost is identification of the problem of dementia, accurate assessment and prompt referral to specialists. Back-up and review are needed until the end of life as is medical treatment for any physical problems that occur and not a dismissal of them, just because someone is suffering from this dreadful disease. Information about the disease is vital: a single explanation is not enough. Carers need to be told over and over again so that they can really understand. Advice and support are required for coping with the carers' own feelings as well as advice on dementia. Practical help in the house is needed. Breaks are very important, whether for an hour daily, or for a holiday. Financial help is equally important, as well as information on where financial help may be obtained: many carers do not avail themselves fully of their entitlements as they are unaware of them. Last, but not least, we need high-quality residential care for when carers can no longer cope, or when sufferers have no family.

All of us involved with the study, having spent many hours with the carers and the sufferers, were left in no doubt about the distressing effects of the dementing illnesses, the needs of the supporters and the key role that carers play in keeping people at home. Our conclusions were that there are a large number of people who do want to keep their elderly people at home, but they need support to do so. In the United Kingdom we do have a pattern of services, benefits and care-givers that the carers value and of which much is good. We have shown clearly that these can reduce the build-up of stress and can postpone or prevent admission to an institution. We also found that there are many professional workers who are really committed to supporting the carers: what we really need to do is to build on these strengths. We know the range of resources that people need, and don't need to invent new ones: but we do need to ensure that carers are aware of resources that are available to them and that there is proper information about them. We also need to ensure that services are as effective and as high-quality as possible and that carers get what they need from the range of possibilities.

A voluntary society can meet all of these needs and I have come to realize that we are in a unique position in the voluntary sector in providing some of them and in giving guidance on others. In the voluntary sector we can be flexible and innovative; our money comes from many different sources, and above all we have the experience of the membership of the society to help with planning and to raising public awareness.

Responding to needs

I wish now to illustrate how our society is trying to met some of the needs that Enid Levin and her co-workers have shown to be key requirements. The provision of information is one important area: the hunger for information is shown by the hundreds of enquiries that the national office receives every week. The enquiries range from wanting to know more about the disease, to financial and legal matters, details about nursing-homes, looking for a shoulder to weep on, "shall I throw away my aluminium saucepans?", and so on. Over the last two years our national office has become highly efficient, with a cohesive, cheerful, enthusiastic team of paid workers, led by our very dynamic executive director, Noreen Siba. We have a splendid open-plan office in south-west London which is fully computerized, and we publish an excellent information-packed monthly newsletter which is sent to all our members. In addition we have an ever-growing collection of fact-sheets and advice sheets in response to the commonest enquiries and written by professionals. There is a growing number of publications and we are building up a library of books, videos and papers, again to meet demand. Provision of information is one of the key requirements for carers: being in possession of all the possible facts is a source of psychological strength.

We have made a conscious decision to be a membership society, because we feel that for many carers this is what they want. Caring for someone with dementia can be a very isolating experience, and the knowledge that there are others around who understand your problems, and who you can contact, can be very reassuring. Our membership now numbers several thousand, but we are a long way from being able to contact all possible carers. One of the important opportunities that carers have by becoming members is to meet one another in self-help groups or in other sorts of meetings. Self-help groups facilitate discussion, the sharing of problems, and of course, the sharing of information. We now have many small groups and larger branches all over the country developing at a very fast rate, so much so that we have an increasing number of paid development workers, supported by a coordinating officer based in the national office.

Training and services

Another area of paramount importance is the area of training. Often the quality of care is good, but so often it is poor or uninformed. Care-assistants in long-term care institutions often have no background training in the work that they are supposed to be carrying out, nor are they given any information about the illness or the behavioural problems of the people that they are caring for, or any sort of guidance as how best to do their work. We feel very strongly that there is an urgent need for material to demonstrate to carers, both in their own homes and in institutions, on how to cope with the various problems that arise as dementia progresses. In addition there is a need for material of a more visual kind to present this information. As a result of this necessity, we are currently producing a series of videos which have been scripted for us by two experts in the field, with literature attached. These will be completed soon, and I think that we will have material which will be of very wide-spread benefit. Better informed and better trained carers is the key to ensuring that our elderly people are looked after in the best possible way.

We are well aware of the services needed for the carers to carry on the support: these include home-care services, day-care, sitting services and residential care, providing for the all-important need for respite care and often permanent care. Research work has shown that these resources are the over-riding resources that carers need access to, although each carer may have a different requirement. Finding the right solution can reduce the stress on carers and, as we have seen above, may reduce the rate of institutionalization. However the problem remains that an individual carer's needs often cannot be met, because resources are so patchy, non-existent or just ineffective. It is, therefore, an important task for the society to recommend criteria of good care for services, to be able to help carers to make choices and to provide models of good practice. We are indifferent whether these criteria are best met by the public, private or voluntary sector, despite the tradition in the United Kingdom of looking to the public sector only. In fact, it is certainly beginning to appear that a more hopeful solution may be emerging from the private sector.

We have produced some criteria on residential care and what to look for when one is choosing a home for a relative. In the area of day care, with a recent generous grant from industry, we are going to set up some day-care initiatives around the country: we hope to monitor and evaluate them and from this information draw up some simple guidelines as to what good day-care should consist of.

Public awareness

All the areas I have considered inevitably increase public awareness of Alzheimer's disease and other dementias. Television, radio and press all show a good deal more about the disease and I feel that we owe this publicity to the hard work done by workers all over the country, to all the researchers. In particular our society owes special thanks to our president, Dr Jonathan Miller, who has a real genius for communication, and has been one of the leading lights on many of the programmes on television about dementia seen in the United Kingdom in recent years. Many of us spend time lobbying politicians and other professionals on many issues, and I believe that there is a greater concern amongst the general public. We have to make links with both the politicians and the professionals to make sure that Alzheimer's disease is seen as the priority area of concern that the numbers absolutely justify. But harnessing these interests and turning them to the society's benefit, bearing in mind that we are not the most glamorous of organizations and have to compete with many other calls on the public purse, is a highly professional task. Happily, we have tackled publicity and money-raising recently with some success: it is a tribute to our treasurer that we have tripled our income over the last two years.

Research support

All this is for the here and now, and is a progress report which most charitable organizations would be proud to be able to give; but the long-term interest, about which we are persistently questioned, is the issue of research, and how to support those who are looking for cause and cure. I believe that research in Alzheimer's disease is at a particularly exciting point with all the developments in the molecular biology area. Our society regards it as very important to keep the membership as up-to-date as possible and we have a very prestigious medical and scientific committee, chaired by Professor Wilcock, to support this side of our work. Much of our money goes to provide the sort of support which I have outlined above: but we do have to look further ahead and, in this context, we are concerned to fund some more basic research. We have recently funded some scientific studentships, as well as some research on the social side.

In addition, we provided some money for a brain bank and we hope to research our own membership more extensively as well as evaluating some of the work that we are doing. Money must be encouraged to support research to find a cure. There are a number of organizations funding research in the United Kingdom, the most notable ones being the Medical Research Council, the Wellcome Trust and the Mental Health Foundation. Funding research is very important, but we also have to acknowledge that there is no other organization so specifically involved with the carers of Alzheimer's disease as we are. Finding an appropriate vehicle for research in dementia which gives us some assurance that results will be forthcoming on a manageable realistic time-scale together with the risks involved is a task which will face us continuously over the next few years.

Fund-raising

Inevitably we are constantly needing to raise funds to pursue all these aims. The government gives us a grant for which we are grateful, for it shows that they are fully supportive of all that we are doing. However the major amount of our funding comes from individuals, from trusts, from industry and there are signs that public awareness is really on the increase by the steady increase in our funds. Having enough money is important but equally important is how to use the money as efficiently as possible with careful budgeting along prepared activity lines. This is, in itself, a skill which few people possess. Our society is very fortunate in having such guidance from our treasurer, George Cyriax, whose background in business, finance and publishing has given us immense help and expertise in this direction. On looking back on my own professional experience, I have no doubt that the fusion of personal experience, business experience and professional experience, difficult though it may be to accept, is of primary importance to both sides. Our society, and those of all nations, face a daunting array of tasks. We have to raise awareness as the basis for everything. We have to improve the quality of care in line with compelling demographic trends. We must not be insensitive to the quality of care-giving, people and their commitments but, above all, as carer societies we have to give support in a meaningful way to the front-line people coping with Alzheimer's disease – the carers. In the United Kingdom, we feel that we are beginning to get to grips with this problem. I am both optimistic and excited; if I am right, then this is an epidemic which needs neither to be sad nor silent

Reference

(1) Levin E, Sinclair I, Gorbach P. *Families, services and confusion in old age.* London, Avebury, 1989.

Carers, Professionals and Alzheimer's Disease. D O'Neill ed © 1991 John Libbey & Company Ltd

Chapter 3

INTERNATIONAL PERSPECTIVES IN ALZHEIMER'S DISEASE

F Baro *MD, Department of Brain and Behaviour Research, Faculty of Medicine, Katholieke Universiteit, Leuven, Belgium*

Many national Alzheimer's organizations pose the question as to what are the benefits of an international organization. It is an appropriate question, for there is so much work to be done in the native country that there must be compelling reasons to "go international". I consider that there are four principal goals of national organizations: (i) the need for mutual support, (ii) the need for information and education, (iii) public awareness and influence on government policy, and (iv) the need to instigate and support research. These are national objectives: can we strive for international objectives with Alzheimer's Disease International? These national movements are now present world-wide: the international perspective may represent an as yet unfinished phase of the development of the movement.

If we try to define international objectives, we can gain some help from the points outlined at the United Nations Assembly on Ageing in 1982, a very historical meeting, the Vienna International Plan on Ageing. I arrange them in a somewhat altered order, but the four straight-forward objectives are identical to the objectives of the national self-help groups. This is not surprising as the United Nations had to build up these solutions to the problems in the same way as self-help groups. Alzheimer's Disease International is considered by the United Nations and other international agencies as a non-governmental organization.

Mutual support

To look at these four objectives in turn: when we consider mutual support, an example could be the case of Mexico, where the 1990 Alzheimer's Disease

International meeting was held. This illustrates the interaction between Alzheimer's disease and related diseases and the national development of a developing country. Although we should not lump all developing countries under one heading, United Nations figures show that 72 per cent of people over the age of 60 and 60 per cent of the over-80 age group will live in the developing countries, rather than in the relatively prosperous Western hemisphere, by the year 2025. The absolute numbers will increase dramatically, especially for women, because in developing countries the difference in longevity between men and women tends to be more pronounced. The economies of these developing countries might improve, but the vulnerability of the economies means that formal support for carers will be uncertain: nobody knows how much money will be available for its innovation. The informal support structure is reducing in all of these countries, although it is difficult to quantify this decline. Therefore, the more developed countries will have to provide mutual support for carer organizations in developing countries. In November 1988, I was invited to Spain to advise on the founding of the Spanish Alzheimer's disease association, and I was amazed to see the potent influence of the presence and experiences of the Alzheimer's Disease International representatives at this gathering. The queen of Spain, Queen Sophia, who was attending a meeting on self-help for Alzheimer's disease, took time after the meeting to ask for more information and decided on the spot to become a patron of the fledgeling Spanish Alzheimer's disease association. This will be a very great support for the Spanish people, and I certainly hope that the Alzheimer's Society of Ireland has experienced this feeling of mutual support after the presence of so many nations at the 5th Alzheimer's Disease International meeting in Dublin in 1989.

Information and education

Information and education is the second objective. A very important role for the Alzheimer's Disease International will be to act as a clearing network for information and education. This is important because there are many successful approaches to Alzheimer's disease which are not used because of lack of information transfer between different countries. For example, the ADA of Canada has produced a leadership training guide for Alzheimer's disease support groups, an excellent production which would save a lot of time and effort for other groups if they were aware of its existence. The clearing network should not confine itself to simple methods but can take advantage of advances in communications technology such as electronic mail and fax machines: computer-based material could be sent to member groups and could be of great help in assessing resources, setting up newsletters, organizing meetings and finding training opportunities for young professionals. The Alzheimer's Disease International should do this in collaboration with other agencies such as the National Institute of Aging in Washington, an education centre that produces a lot of excellent material in conjunction with the Alzheimer's Disease and Related Disorders Association, or the International Psychogeriatric Association, or indeed many other international bodies.

An example of an approach to care that a clearing centre might diffuse comes from the Geriatric Unit at Ter Kersalaere in Belgium. In the past few years they have experimented with sheltered housing. Ter Kersalaere has ten housing units associated with the Geriatric Unit, but which are open to the community at large. The most amazing feature of the sheltered housing is that it caters for an elderly couple where one of the couple is very dependent on skilled nursing care: if it were not for this facility, they would be separated, with the dependent spouse going to a geriatric centre. Evaluation after one year showed numerous gains, such as preservation of married life, improvement in the quality of care and quality of life and also a saving of money for the family and the community! This example shows that saving of money is achieved because home care would be too expensive. The family saves money due to the fact that a social trust rents the houses at a lower rate than the family's previous rent. A properly evaluated scheme that is efficient in human and economic terms is worth sharing with other national organizations.

Advocacy

The third element is that of advocacy: an example of a topic that needs advocacy is informal care. Seventy per cent of the elderly in the US have only informal support, and 27 per cent have a mixture of formal and informal care. The majority of this care is given by women, and these figures are very relevant for the advocacy programme developed by the Alzheimer's disease association in the US. They put forward a National Programme to Conquer Alzheimer's Disease in 1989, an advocacy programme. Another example is that of Alzheimer's disease care in Belgium. As 80 per cent of Alzheimer's disease patients live at home, this puts a large burden on the family: support programmes for the informal care-givers are practically non-existent. However the Belgian government is very keen to promote a more intensive programme of home-care than exists already. Although relatively little is known about the carers, the most important issue of the advocacy programme is to inform and influence policy-makers when they are reallocating resources at times of economic restraint. The Alzheimer's Disease International can take a broad outlook and can start international advocacy on issues such as home-care. The World Health Organization conference at Alma Ata in 1978 (which gave us the slogan "Health for all by the year 2000") started this process politically when the ministers for health agreed to totally reverse the pyramid of health-care, with less emphasis on expensive tertiary hospital and nursing-home care and expensive secondary care such as specialists, and more emphasis on primary care. They also added a fourth dimension of care, that of lay-care, and this was noted to be the most important and broadest level of care. This was a rediscovery of a phenomenon which predated Alma Ata by a long time and which continues to grow in importance. It is important, too, that Alzheimer's Disease International will make its presence felt in 1992, the year of the opening of Europe's frontiers. A conference will be organized by all European Community members in Brussels that year on home-care and support for the informal care-giver: this topic needs appropriate political recognition. The Alzheimer's Disease International should work in conjunction with such bodies as Eurolink-

Age, a lobby in the European Community for the problems of the elderly, and other groups.

Research

The final objective is initiating and participating in research. There are a lot of unanswered questions of international importance where the Alzheimer's Disease International might play a role. For example, Japan has a much greater incidence of vascular dementia than Alzheimer's disease: what is the underlying cause? In China, Katzmann has found that people with a very poor level of education tend to have an increased risk of Alzheimer's disease. This could be a methodological problem, perhaps due to using psychological tests that were too "Western" in nature, which would disadvantage poorly educated people. But Chinese researchers claim that they tried to avoid this bias, and indeed it may be true that more poorly educated people are at a higher risk of Alzheimer's disease. Professor Ozuntukum of Nigeria thinks that he has never seen Alzheimer's disease in the black population of Nigeria: if this is true, then the finding is of major significance. However other researchers doubt these findings, pointing to a possible lack of perception of Alzheimer's as a disease by these African families.

All these topics point to a great need for cross-national and international research, and this research can take two forms. Either the data can be pooled, or the data may be compared in order to try to appreciate risk-factors or protective factors. For instance, diseased brains can be collected into a brain-bank, or migrant populations such as people in Detroit of Flemish origin can be compared with the native population from whence they came, i.e. Flemish people in Flanders, Belgium. The discovery of either significant differences or lack of differences would help us to gain insight into the nature of Alzheimer's disease.

Cross-cultural studies

There are very major difficulties in cross-cultural studies, and the presence of concerned families who will help researchers with conceptual issues, such as what the families understand by the dementing process, will be of great use. This understanding will vary greatly from country to country and only families can help professionals and researchers to understand more about the problem. One good approach is demonstrated by an agreement between the World Health Organization and the National Institute of Aging in Washington, where the two agencies assembled a Special Research Programme on Ageing covering four topics put together by a distinguished scientific advisory board in Geneva: one of these topics was that of age-related dementia. Although this programme is just starting, we hope that it will be productive. Another example is the programme of the Mental Health section of the World Health Organization in Geneva to classify and diagnose dementing illnesses. When the World Health Organization carries out a research programme in a country, it will always strengthen the national capabilities for research, and this is a big step forward: a small group of researchers participating in such a programme will enable research in that country to make a big advance.

Finally, I should like to comment on a body that the Alzheimer's Disease International started in Mexico in 1990, the International Medical and Scientific Advisory Board. The objectives of this body parallel those of a national Alzheimer's association or of the Alzheimer's Disease International: scientists and professionals as well as families have to give each other mutual support. This board will also digest and diffuse current news relevant to dementing illnesses in science. It will help in advocacy to influence scientific policies internationally. It should propose specific studies of importance to the Alzheimer's Disease International. These issues will not only be biomedical, but should also include psychosocial, philosophical, ethical, legal and other topics.

Conclusion

It is as important for the Alzheimer's Disease International to be successful internationally as it is for national societies to be successful on a national basis, and there will surely be a positive interaction between the national and international organisations. The Alzheimer's Disease International and the Alzheimer's disease associations may be likened to a locomotive that causes a train to move with increasing speed. The train represents many problems besides those of Alzheimer's disease, but the Alzheimer's Disease International and the Alzheimer's disease associations are pioneers and the outcome will be important not only for Alzheimer's disease sufferers but for many other people as well.

SECTION 2
The Social Implications of Dementia

Carers, Professionals and Alzheimer's Disease. D O'Neill ed © 1991 John Libbey & Company Ltd

Chapter 4

ECONOMIC CONSEQUENCES OF ALZHEIMER'S DISEASE

MA Creedon *DSW, President of The Creedon Group, Clinical Professor Gerontologist, The University of Bridgeport, Ct, USA*

Introduction

This paper approaches the causes that account for the costs of Alzheimer's disease from three angles. The first angle looks at the individual costs of Alzheimer's disease, the second examines the overall social costs, and finally the cost of dementing illness in the work place and to workers is assessed. This latter subject has not enjoyed prominence in the Alzheimer's literature to date. The data I will present is all specific to the United States, but a good deal of it will have obvious applications elsewhere.

Catastrophic health initiative

In the United States there was a huge upheaval in 1989 about the catastrophic health initiative, approved by congress under the presidency of Ronald Reagan. This most recent major extension of public support for health care of the elderly was an extension of Medicare, intended to provide coverage for people who had extensive hospital stays. It was intended to provide support for people after they had covered several thousand dollars of expenses themselves. Thereafter, all further costs would be taken care of. However, it was to be paid for by the elderly themselves, almost like an income tax. It was an income transfer programme, in that richer elderly people would pay more and the poorer elderly would pay less. It has just gone into place in the past year and the richer elderly discovered that they were paying $800 a year in additional taxes, rising up to a possible $2,000 within a few years. The middle class elderly of America have been very exercised and have protested vociferously. The catastrophic health programme legislation was repealed in late Fall 1989.

Unfortunately, this will suffocate all initiatives for increased long-term care coverage for the next four or five years in the United States. It was unfortunate that the U.S. government decided to start with the catastrophic health initiative, because the long-term care costs and needs for the elderly are a much more pressing problem for a broad array of older people with health-care problems than are the needs of the few for heart transplants and other high-tech surgery. So, the pressure on families to cover the cost of long-term care for the Alzheimer's victim will become increasingly oppressive. The cost estimates are fairly staggering and I will refer to them later on.

Individual costs

First of all, the cost to individuals of overall health care is large and growing. The overall health-care cost for individuals in the United States in 1987 over the age of 65 was $1,600 per year, representing 15 per cent of income. The mean by 1990 will be $2,083 per person over age 65, representing 19 per cent of income. The Office of Technology study in 1987 suggests that the mean for those aged over 85 currently equals 41.7 per cent of income, and the mean for health care for all those over 85 is approaching 50 per cent of income. These figures convey an idea of the overall costs of health to the elderly as a group.[1]

Looking more specifically at examples of care, such as nursing-home care, the cost to the individual over 65 years of age who goes into a nursing home is best stated by the fact that he/she would be impoverished within thirteen weeks of admission to a nursing home. This information is based on the amount of people transferring from private payment of nursing-home fees to Medicaid, which is governmental health insurance for the low-income elderly: within thirteen weeks, 63 per cent will transfer to Medicaid. The situation for couples where one party in the couple goes into a nursing home is also grim: 37 per cent of couples are impoverished within thirteen weeks after placement of the spouse.[2] In order to be eligible for Medicaid, the person is forced to spend their assets until they reach the poverty level. There have been judgements in courts, particularly in New York City, in which the judge has over-ruled the requirement that the spouse must also become impoverished, so that the spouse can retain some assets. Some middle-class people, and wealthy people also, transfer their assets after age 65, especially if they think they are becoming frail, so that the government can not get at those assets to cover the cost of care. Home care can be equally burdensome financially, since many home services may have to be paid for out of pocket.

Private and public care

In the United States, approximately 50 per cent of the older population are highly dependent on social security income and other public sector programmes to support themselves. Therefore, more than half of our elderly are highly vulnerable to any cuts in public programmes. They have marginal incomes of approximately 130 per cent of the poverty level, so a significant number become impoverished as soon as they have to care for a spouse full-time. If we look at Alzheimer's patients cared for by their spouse in their own home, 16 per cent are impoverished after thirteen weeks, and this figure rises to 46 per cent after one year.[3] These figures give an idea of the financial and social vulnerability of American families when they are providing care to their older relatives, particularly those who are taking care of Alzheimer's victims.

An estimate of the total cost of care for a typical eight-year course of Alzheimer's disease is approximately $148,000: although many Alzheimer's victims exceed the normal prognosis (some recent studies in the United States suggested that the average life-span was 4.7 years after diagnosis). Nursing and community care is not a cheap option: the average cost of one year of community care is $11,700, which actually approximates the average income of people aged over 65, while the mean cost of one year of nursing-home care is $23,000. In the United States, 75 per cent of long-term nursing home care is provided by for-profit facilities. Increasingly, these for-profit facilities are taking only private patients who can afford to pay higher rates than the public re-imbursement rate. Nursing homes with more than 50 per cent of patients paid for under Medicaid are under tremendous stress to maintain a balanced budget. So, there is a pre-occupation with keeping a healthy mix of public and private patients. Those in the North-Eastern metropolitan areas are very likely to be paying far more than $22,000 a year for nursing-home care. Alice Day in her study on Family Care of the Elderly in the United States has noted that the share of costs paid by the elderly are estimated to increase more than twice as fast as their incomes over the next ten years.[4]

So the cost of care for the Alzheimer's patient, including diagnostic and treatment costs not covered in the figures above, is accelerating exponentially. At the same time the Federal Government is highly unlikely to provide any major increases in public re-imbursement. Individual states are responsible for 50 per cent of Medicaid, which is the primary source of payment for long-term care. This is less of a burden for a state such as Connecticut, which has the highest per capita income in the United States, than for a state like West Virginia, with the lowest per capita income in the United States. In many states the fastest growing element of the state budget is the cost of Medicaid, and they are responding to this in a whole variety of ways. One of the most common and popular ways is to freeze the licensing of nursing-home beds. If there is no bed available, the state cannot be held responsible to pay for it. As a result, in many states increasingly long lines of people are waiting for admission to nursing homes.

One of the greatest crises in providing long-term care for the elderly will be this huge liability, and the ability or inability of states to cover the cost. Despite the Federal Government providing the other half of the cost of Medicaid, individual states regulate the providers and by using licensing rights they have some control over their costs. This way of fighting costs simply means that those needing long-term care who have private resources will have better access to care.

31

Costs to society

Any discussion of societal costs must incorporate estimates of disease prevalence. In 1989 Evans *et al* published the results of an in-depth study of persons over 65 in East Boston, Massachusetts.[5] They found that some 10.3 per cent had probable Alzheimer's disease (3 per cent of those aged 65–74 years; 18.7 per cent of those aged 75-84 years; 47.2 per cent of those aged greater than 85 years). While further studies are needed before one can generalize with comfort to the U.S. population at large, they report a significantly higher incidence of the disease than prior research had suggested. Their findings imply that the costs to America will grow rapidly along with the growth in our oldest age groups.

The cost to society is less widely researched, and is quite an emotive subject. The Irish electorate in 1989 spoke out loudly on the issues of access to health care, with some resulting improvement in health care support: perhaps this will also happen in the U.S. The societal cost of Alzheimer's disease has been studied in the Office of Technological Assessment Study of 1987, called *Losing a Million Minds*.[1] It is probably the best summary of the costs and related issues of dementing illness in the United States. They estimated the costs to society, both direct and indirect, of all dementia at $40 billion in 1987. Direct costs are the costs of nursing-home care, hospital care, medications, physician services and community services. Indirect costs are more difficult to quantify and include such things as the cost of taking somebody to the physician for treatment, the cost of visits to the nursing home and the cost of foregone economic activity by the person becoming ill.

The studies that I have looked at in preparation for this paper did not include the cost to care-givers who have to cut back on their work schedules to provide care. So, some of those costs to families do not wind up in the complete picture. Hay and Ernst in 1987 estimated costs and suggested that the estimated cost was between 27.9 and 31.2 million dollars for Alzheimer's disease cases diagnosed in 1983, which they estimated at 337,000 cases.[6] Estimated costs in the United States with a population of 250 million people is a tricky business: particularly as there is great variability in our estimates of the actual incidence of the problem. The conjectures of the number of people affected by severe Alzheimer's disease range from 1 to 2 million, a 100 per cent difference. Cost estimates should, therefore, be approached with caution, as they are sometimes based on assumptions of uncertain reliability (partly because the diagnostic assumptions are uncertain and partly because we do not have the empirical data).

One of the better studies of the total cost of illness estimate is that of Hu, Huang, and Cartwright.[7] This group has been to the forefront of research into the economics of Alzheimer's disease. Even so, these estimates should be treated with caution. They estimate the cost of Alzheimer's disease and multi-infarct dementia at 102 billion dollars for patients aged over 65 years. The cost of the dementia alone, apart from the diagnostic work-up, is estimated at $77 billion. Direct costs, meaning the cost of the actual care-giver or professionals, are estimated at $61 billion. The total indirect cost is $40 billion. This latter estimate may not include all indirect costs: visits to nursing homes, for example, are costed at one million dollars which is probably far too low. The cost of foregone income is estimated at $38.9 million: the assumptions they are working on are less than certain, as they are only working with people over the age of 65 years. The cost of foregone income for somebody getting Alzheimer's at 45, 50 or 55 will obviously be far higher and would have to be included in any total societal cost for Alzheimer's disease.

Costs at the workplace

Perhaps less widely recognized is the impact of elder care on the workplace. Estimates of this effect in the United States are now based on a whole variety of studies, including some that I have been involved with personally. These suggest that 25 per cent of employees in an average workplace have some elder care responsibilities.[8] At the University of Bridgeport we got involved in the first University based research on this issue with several major corporations. We found that 25 per cent of the employees over age 40 at Pitney Bowes Manufacturing Company and People's Bank of Connecticut had elder care responsibility. The highest rate was in the bank with about 30 per cent, mostly women employees, caring for elderly relatives. In our university study of 33 companies, we found that 23.6 per cent of employees had eldercare responsibilities. IBM have just completed a study of their employees: of 250,000 employees in the U.S., 30 per cent had some eldercare concern. For half of those, the elderly relative lived more than one hundred miles away from the care-giver. We have a much greater problem of long distance care-giving than that experienced in the British Isles or in Western Europe, as we have a continental society where people are very often hundreds or thousands of miles away from their family of origin.

The results from this care burden are various and considerable. In one study by Elaine Brodie in the Philadelphia area, 28 per cent of a group of women who were taking care of older relatives had given up their job.[9] A national survey found that 11 per cent of care-givers had quit work, and in a study with brain damaged adults, The Family Survival Project in San Francisco studied 2,000 families and found that 12 per cent had left work to provide care.[10] This is obviously a major economic cost to those families, but it is also a significant cost to the workplace. In the United States, the cost of recruiting and training a new employee is estimated at approximately 50 per cent a year's salary. So, the loss of a secretary earning $15,000 a year implies a recruitment and replacement cost of approximately $7,500. As this is the lower end of the salary scale in the United States, the cost to the work place of care-giving for elderly relatives and Alzheimer's victims is a very significant one.

A further factor is the low unemployment rate in the United States: in the Washington, DC, area we have a 2.5 per cent unemployment rate. This means that employee recruitment is very difficult. The cost of replacement becomes more extreme in a high employment society. In countries with higher unemployment, the replacement costs are lower, but training costs are still significant. Apart from the cost of losing workers who resign to care for elderly relatives, working spouses with elder care responsibilities tend to reduce their work commitment: 30 per cent work fewer hours, 35 per cent change their schedules, and 20 per cent take time off without pay. The average age of care-givers for elderly people with various disabilities in the United States was 47 years in a study in 1989 by AARP of American households.[11] In our study at the University of Bridgeport of three corporations in Connecticut, we found the most frequent age for employees providing elder care/parent care was 40 to 45 years.[8]

In terms of the workplace, this means that the impact of eldercare is heaviest among the peak-productivity age groups. The largest group affected by taking care of older parents and relatives is not just people who are about to retire, but is mid-career employees who are very valuable to their companies. They are the ones who have the heaviest burden of care and we are seeing a very significant growth in what we call Dual Dependency. This is typified by an Oregon study where 41 per cent of those who had elder care responsibility also had childcare responsibility.[12] Hence, the average age of our workforce is going to be 39 years by the year 2000 as the baby boom generation in America moves into mid life and this is likely to be a very heavily oppressed group, particularly the female spouses who are going to be coping with children, older adults, their own career, their spouse's career, commuting to work, etc. A typical scenario might be the woman who has three children at various stages of pre-school, and with a mother who is an Alzheimer's victim and attending Adult Day Care during the work day and otherwise living with the adult daughter and her family.

Responding to the challenge

What are the workplace responses that we are experiencing? Family Leave policies are now becoming very prevalent in America. Champion started a six-month leave of absence policy in 1987 for any family care issue. IBM in 1988 established a one to three-year leave of absence policy. These breaks are without pay, but the job is guaranteed on return. AT&T in the summer of 1989 negotiated the first major union contract that specifically included elder care in the contract. This corporation, which has 330,000 employees, made an agreement with the Communication Workers of America to provide $3 million of support for childcare and elder care and $5 million of that would be dedicated to community services. About $4 million would be for direct elder care support services for their employees. IBM this year also installed a nationwide toll-free number for elder care referrals. Employees who are having a crisis problem with elder care call and get a professional who will then within a day get back to them with the precise name and phone number of the service agencies and the name of the person who will best help them with the care of their elderly relative. This is becoming a common policy in American corporations. The IBM contract is worth $3 million, so if you just take 300 American corporations with contracts like this, the corporate commitment to eldercare support for employees is probably now close to $100 million and is growing quite rapidly. So, the workplace cost of eldercare is an issue that is only beginning to be explored in the U.S. and the work responses are just being developed in this decade.

Conclusion

The costs of care for Alzheimer's disease in the United States are undoubtedly the highest in the world. This is due in part to our very costly health care system and perhaps also the high mobility of the American family – it is hard to provide family care from great distances. Such factors as the growing patterns of dual-career families also affect the family's ability to provide care. The tight labour market in the U.S.A. and the high cost of housing add significant economic pressures pushing the traditional care-givers into the formal workforce. The positive aspect of the current situation is the growth of corporate programmes to help working care-givers cope with work and family care of older relatives.

Besides the costs to family and to the public sector, this article has attempted to delineate some of the workplace costs related to society's care of its members who have Alzheimer's disease – these costs are significant and must be considered in any reckoning of the total societal expenditure for care. In the future we may see a three-way support system in industrialized societies: the family, the public sector, and the corporate sector.

References

(1) US Congress, Office of Technology Assessment. *Losing a Million Minds: Confronting the Tragedy of Alzheimer's Disease and Other Dementias.* Washington DC, Government Printing Office, Publication OTABA-323, 1987.

(2) National Institute on Aging, Task Force. Senility reconsidered: treatment possibilities for mental impairment in the elderly. *Journal of the American Medical Association* 1988, **244** (3).

(3) Max W, Lindeman D, Segura T, Benjamin AE. *Estimating the utilization and costs of formal and informal care provided to brain-impaired adults: a briefing paper.* University of California, San Francisco, Institute for Health and Aging, 1986.

(4) Day AT. *Who cares? Demographic trends challenge family care for the elderly.* Washington DC, Population Reference Bureau Inc, 1985.

(5) Evans DA. Prevalence of Alzheimer's Disease in a community population of older persons. *Journal of the American Medical Association* 1989, **262** (10).

(6) Hay JW, Ernst RL. The economic costs of Alzheimer's Disease. *American Journal of Public Health* 1987, 77.

(7) Hu T, Huang L, Cartwright WS. Evaluation of the costs of caring for the senile demented elderly: a pilot study. *The Gerontologist* 1986, **26** (2).

(8) Creedon M. *Issues for an Aging America: Employees and Eldercare.* Washington DC, The National Council on the Aging, 1987.

(9) Brody E. Work status and parent care: a comparison of four groups of women. *The Gerontologist* 1987, **27**(2), 12.

(10) Enright RB, Friss L. *Employed Caregivers of Brain-Impaired Adults: An Assessment of the Dual Role.* San Francisco, Family Survival Project, 1987.

(11) American Association of Retired Persons. *Working Caregivers Report.* Washington, DC, American Association of Retired Persons, 1989.

(12) Ingersoll-Dayton B, Chapman N, Neal M. Programs for caregivers in the workplace. *The Gerontologist* 1990, **30** (1).

Chapter 5

CARE-GIVER CONSIDERATIONS IN INSTITUTIONALIZING DEMENTIA PATIENTS

S Cahill *M Soc Science,* L Rosenman *MSW, PhD Social Work,*
University of Queensland, St Lucia 4072, Brisbane

Introduction

With the ageing of the Australian population, dementia is fast emerging as a major public health problem.[1] This has serious implications for policy, practice, and social expenditures in health, long-term care and social services. Because of the nature of the illness, institutionalization may become a necessary care option for many families. Yet little is known in Australia about the processes which lead to this decision to institutionalize, a decision referred to as the "nadir" of life[2] and often arrived at with much reluctance, only after all other alternative care options have been exhausted.

This paper is a first attempt to examine the processes involved in the decision to institutionalize a dementia patient in the Australian context. It is based on in-depth interviews with a sample of 45 primary care-givers recruited in the Brisbane metropolitan area and selected from both community and institutional settings. The study has two points of central focus. The first is the patient and the second is the primary carer. In addition, the research reports on carers' own reasons for opting for institutional care and the part played by health professionals in assisting them reaching this decision.

Patient characteristics

Most people assume that it is the deterioration in a patient's condition that leads to the need for permanent institutional care. In other words, as a patient becomes more confused, then institutional care is more inevitable. However, as Table 1 shows, although the majority of the patients involved in this study were either moderately or severely demented, the extent of memory loss did not determine the type of care received.

Table 1.Type of placement vs severity of disease

	MILD	MODERATE	SEVERE	TOTAL
Community	7% (3)	24% (11)	18% (8)	22
Institution	2% (1)	24% (11)	24% (11)	23
TOTAL	4	22	19	45

The table also shows that for all those with a moderately severe diagnosis, there were as many patients being cared for in the community as there were in institutions. For those in the severe category, there was a slight difference, but this was not statistically significant, and merely suggests a trend. In other words the severity of the diagnosis did not appear to be the key factor determining the type of care received.

Associated with dementia there are a number of disturbing behavioural patterns which can be quite disruptive to the primary carer and have been referred to in the literature as factors positively associated with institutionalization.[3] We asked our care-givers to report on the type of problems that they were experiencing and we also asked them to report on the problems they found most difficult to manage. Although relational and personality problems, such as aggressive and demanding behaviour were the most frequently reported-on problems, they were not the considered the most difficult behavioural problems to manage. Wandering for the community-based care-giver and paranoia and delusions for those who had chosen institutional care were the most difficult problems to manage at home (Table 2).

When the two major items, i.e. paranoia and delusions, were compared against all other behavioural problems collectively, no statistically significant difference was found. This may well be due to the relatively small sample size.

Characteristics

The primary carers in the study were predominantly spouses of the dementia sufferer (52 per cent) or alternatively adult children, generally daughters (38 per cent). A small proportion were either siblings (4 per cent) or more distant relations or friends (6 per cent). We looked at the relationship that the primary carer had with the patient in relation to the type of care the patient was receiving (Figure 1). In general, spouse carers were much more likely to be providing community care compared with non-spouse carers. In contrast, non-spouses were more likely to choose institutional care for the patient.

Table 2: Carer's perception of the most difficult problems to manage by residence of patient

TYPE OF PROBLEM	COMMUNITY	INSTITUTION
Wandering	5 (29%)	3 (16%)
Paranoia and delusions	3 (18%)	8 (42%)
Incontinence	3 (18%)	2 (10.5%)
Sleep disturbance	2 (12%)	1 (5%)
Aggressive behaviour	2 (12%)	2 (10.5%)
Talking difficulties	1 (6%)	0
Demanding behaviour	1 (6%)	3 (16%)
TOTAL	17 (100%)	19 (100%)

This difference between the two groups in relation to the type of care given was statistically significant. Although the reasons for this difference must be hypothetical, at this point in time, they rest on two probabilities. One is that non-spouses were younger and had competing demands on their time, including employment and looking after their own family and spouse. On the other hand, the majority of spouse care-givers were themselves retired so they had more

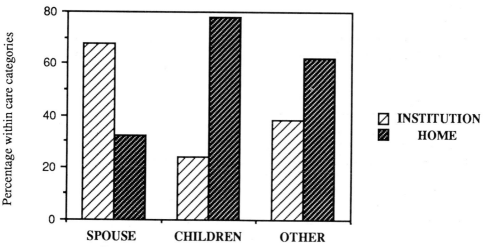

Fig. 1. Relationship of carer to the type of care given.

limited alternative use of their time. An additional but less easily measured difference may be the degree of emotional commitment to the patient that a spouse partner has compared with an adult son or daughter. Whilst spouses are expected to care for each other in sickness and in later years of life, children are reared to become independent of their parents. This may account for the variability, and may explain why carers who are children can make the decision to institutionalize more speedily, and at a different point in time compared with spouses.

Stress

Researchers have indicated that high stress levels among care-givers make it increasingly more difficult for them to continue maintaining a dementia patient at home[4,5] and that "care-giver burden" is a factor positively associated with the need for institutional care. In this study, carers self-reported stress was measured using a three point scale of mild, moderate and severe stress categories. The results, however, also showed that carers who opted for institutional care continue to experience stress long after placement has taken place. As many as 40 per cent of that category reported severe stress even after the patient has been institutionalized. In addition to the stress of regular visiting, meeting expenses and monitoring care, many of these care-givers reported feeling guilty about the decision a long time after it had been taken.

Reasons for institutionalization

Finally, why did care-givers opt for institutional care and what part was played

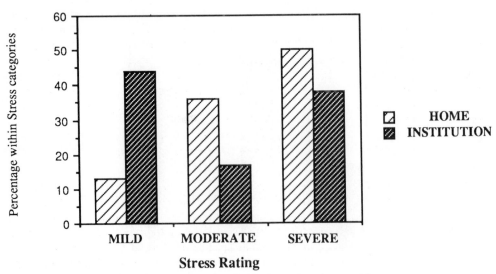

Fig.2. Self-reported stress and place of patient residence.

by health-service professionals in helping families make this decision? Amongst the twenty-three men and women who had chosen institutional care, twelve said that they could no longer cope physically or emotionally with caring demands and that caring had become dangerous. There were four people who gave reasons of their own ill health and in three cases the patient made the decision voluntarily. Four others discontinued community care because of the patient's delusions and paranoia.

The decision to institutionalise a relative was a great source of stress to care-givers who had been through it and was identified as a future stressful decision for those who had not. In most cases, care-givers made the decision to institutionalize in consultation with other family members but not in consultation with health-service professionals. There were five cases where doctors had advised the family to consider institutionalization and four where nursing staff recommended it. The role of respite care as an entrance to permanent institutional care was also examined. This was of some interest because in Australia respite care is offered as a type of emergency service allowing the carer a break. It is considered a service which may help delay institutionalization. But in our sample it seemed that the reverse occurred and that using respite care made professional carers aware of the high level of care required. In fourteen out of the twenty-three cases long-term placement was facilitated by use of respite care and an immediate admission from respite care was organized. In some cases this was because the respite admission alerted professional health-care staff to the high level of dependency of the patient, and thus facilitated long-term admission.

Conclusions and implications

The results from this research suggest that the relationship between the primary carer and the patient may be a significant determinant of home versus institutional care. Therefore, in making decisions about care options, professionals need to evaluate not only the patient's medical status but also his psycho-social situation and that of the carer. Secondly, the decision to institutionalize a patient is extremely stressful to the primary carer and findings suggest that this stress continues long after the placement has taken place. The results would point towards the need for health professionals to be more actively involved in this decision-making process and thereby share with the family some of the responsibility involved in institutionalising a patient. Such involvement might well help to reduce some of the guilt and sense of failure frequently associated with the decision.

Findings also point towards the needs for spouse care-givers, many of whom are elderly and are themselves heavy users of health care services. Programmes which help to maintain a dementia patient at home but at such high costs that the carer's own physical and mental health is at risk need now to be re-evaluated. Administrators, in planning community care services, need to consider not only the patient's quality of life but also that of the carer and his/her family. Finally, care-givers should be helped to realize that family care may not necessarily be the most preferable care option. Institutionalization may represent a more balanced sharing of the caring task and may best suit both care-giver's and patient's needs.

References

(1) Henderson S, Jorm AF. *The Problem of Dementia in Australia.* Canberra, Australian Government Publishing Service, 1986.

(2) Cath SH. The geriatric patient and his family: the institutionalization of a parent – a nadir of life. *J Geriatric Psychiatry* 1972, **5,** 25-46.

(3) Chenoweth B, Spencer B. Dementia: the experience of family care-givers. *The Gerontologist* 1986, **26,** 267-278.

(4) Morycz R. Caregiving strain and the desire to institutionalize family members with Alzheimer's disease: possible predictors and model development. *Research on Ageing 1985,* **7** (3), 329-361.

(5) Zarit S, Todd P, Zarit J. Subjective burden of husband and wives as care-givers: a longitudinal study. *The Gerontologist* 1986, **26,** 260-266.

Carers, Professionals and Alzheimer's Disease. D O'Neill ed © 1991 John Libbey & Company Ltd

Chapter 6

ALZHEIMER'S DISEASE IN MEXICO

Lila Mendoza *AMAES (Mexican Association of Alzheimer's Disease & Related Disorders), Irlanda 124, Col. Parque San Andres, Coyacan, Mexico 21, D. F. 04040*

Mexico is a country of 80 million people, of whom 6 million are over 60 years old. It is a developing country with few resources. Social resources are mainly directed at the younger generation: half of the population are younger than 25. We have typical third-world diseases affecting children and adults. The elderly have not been, and are not, a priority. Over 35 per cent of the elderly are illiterate. The worst possible combination in Mexico is to be old, poor and ill (especially with Alzheimer's disease). I would like to describe in this paper how I personally became acquainted with Alzheimer's disease, how the Alzheimer's disease association came into being and to outline the problems in developing an Alzheimer's disease association in a large developing country.

Personal experience

My mother was a victim of Alzheimer's disease and died in 1987. She had been diagnosed with Alzheimer's disease in April 1986 after a hospital admission with a fractured hip. Fortunately, there was a geriatric unit with expertise in Alzheimer's disease in the hospital. I now realize that she may have had the disease in a very mild form since 1979: she would often complain about "forgetting things". It was very difficult to appreciate the first signs of the disease because she was so well in all other respects. Her memory loss progressed to misplacing items such as keys, money and bankbooks around the house. Gradually further problems appeared: inability to handle money, getting lost, asking the same questions over and over again. She became anxious and depressed, lost interest in daily activities and slept a good deal during the day. Despite her mental impairment she struggled to remain independent, making it very difficult for me to provide assistance or supervision. Disturbing features of her illness were the paranoid

43

symptoms: accusing her grand-daughter, housekeeper and daughter of stealing her money, etc. Finally the neighbours reported that she was forgetting to turn off the stove and was not answering the phone or the door. Her god-daughter moved in with her and found that my mother was also forgetting to eat. Eventually I was forced to come back from Sweden to take care of my mother. Both she and the entire family found the circumstances very trying.

I wish that I had the knowledge about Alzheimer's disease then which I now possess. After discharge from the hospital, instead of mother or a person, I took home a "human package": incontinent, not walking and not eating. So I had to teach her everything from the very beginning, and took care of her and her rehabilitation. She began to walk again. Probably just like many others, I was "mothering" her until the end. In a sense she became my 80-year-old daughter. Despite working very hard with mother's rehabilitation, she suffered several small strokes and the rehabilitation had to start from the beginning again. Due to my exhaustion the doctors recommended that I should place her in a nursing home. However she recovered to a certain extent and was able to walk again. Since then I have been working on a volunteer basis with the geriatric team to set up an Alzheimer's Association in Mexico city. It was horrible and devastating but at the same time I was forced to learn and to develop creativity and common sense to solve everyday problems. It still hurts: I have been sharing my experience with others and trying to help them get through similar painful situations.

Two sources of information for me at the time were LS Powell's book on Alzheimer's disease which I read and later translated into Spanish (in press) and *The 36 Hour Day*. I learnt of the latter in March of 1987 when I heard that the *36 Hour Day* had been translated into Spanish. After contacting the publisher in Mexico city, Dr Rosalia Rodriguez (head of department of a geriatric unit) and I were invited to review the translation. We were happy to do this and wrote down our comments: both books are available in Spanish.

First meeting of the Alzheimer's Association

In October 1987 Dr Gaitz from Houston gave a lecture in Mexico city on Alzheimer's disease. After the lecture there was a question and answer session. The first question was: "Who can train us in Mexico?". We felt that this was the time to make the first public announcement that a multidisciplinary group working at Lopez Mateos Hospital had been discussing the possibility of setting up a National Organization with the following goals:

(i)   to set up support groups for care-givers;

(ii)   to educate health-care professionals about dementing illnesses;

(iii) to draw up a list of informed and reliable professionals who understand and are interested in dementing illness;

(iv)   to heighten public awareness of Alzheimer's disease, and to ensure more dignified and understanding care for Alzheimer's patients.

The meeting produced an overwhelming response from care-givers and professionals, including physicians, psychologists, social workers and geriatric nurses. Our first public meeting was at the hospital in November 1987, and was attended by twenty professionals and ten care-givers. Dr Rodriguez talked about the geriatric unit, the dementia clinic and an Alzheimer's project. I presented a paper on "Social consequences of memory loss", and outlined the four goals of our national organization. After questions, answers and comments, we elected a board of directors. A week later we had the first meeting of the support group and since then we have had weekly meetings. Valuable support for our national group came from the Lopez Mateos Hospital, the National Institute of Neurology and Sandoz, who are interested in producing our first brochure about Alzheimer's disease and the Mexican Alzheimer's Association. The members of the support group now attend meetings twice a month, and use the translations of *The 36 Hour Day* and *Alzheimer's Disease – a Guide for Families* as guides.

Further development

The following January we initiated planning meetings to develop strategies for tackling the problems of dementia in Mexico, based on the four principles outlined above. Education of the public was, and is, a major priority because Alzheimer's disease in Mexico is still a silent epidemic. The publication of the first Mexican editions of books on the care of Alzheimer's disease will provide a focal point for a media campaign. This will give us the chance to reach more care-givers who will have the opportunity to share their experiences and ventilate their problems in the support groups. Our first broadcast of a 40-minute radio programme elicited a deluge of phone calls from the audience. As a result we have many new members in our support group.

Training of health-care professionals is also a priority as the diagnosis of Alzheimer's disease is still extremely rare: many patients with Alzheimer's disease have been wrongly diagnosed as having organic brain syndrome, arteriosclerosis, cerebral vascular accident or stroke. It is encouraging that we have been requested to arrange a course on Alzheimer's disease at one of the clinics of the Social Security Institute. This was an 8 hour introductory course over four days and was attended by 25 physicians.

A further major problem is that we do not yet know the prevalence of Alzheimer's disease in Mexico. We presume that it is a highly prevalent disease representing a large social and medical burden, as has already been established in the Western world, but we do not have the data to verify this. This will be our first research project, once we can find the necessary funds. As a preliminary step I undertook a visit to the United States to learn more about Alzheimer's disease. As well as attending support group meetings, I also visited geriatric units, day-care centres and nursing homes.

Research and scientific activities

The scientific committee started by classifying all scientific articles and papers

45

on Alzheimer's disease available in Mexico. They held monthly medical meetings to which they invited other health-care professionals. Our first research group enlisted researchers who have been working on projects into basic, clinical and psychosocial aspects of Alzheimer's disease. This research involves the following institutions in Mexico city: the Advanced Research Centre at the National Polytechnic Institute, the National Institute of Neurology and Neurosurgery, the Lopez Mateos Hospital, the Social Security Institute for government employees, and the Mexican Association of Alzheimer's Disease and Related Disorders (AMAES). These workers were joined by the Biomedical Research Institute from the West Medical Centre, Social Security Institute, Guadalajara and a private day-care centre for Alzheimer's disease patients in Guadalajara.

We have presented papers about Alzheimer's disease in two different congresses: Dr Rosalia Rodriguez spoke about "General management of the Alzheimer's disease patient, therapeutic alternatives – a multidisciplinary approach" at the International Congress of Biological Psychiatry and Dr Lilia Mendoza presented "Home care of the Alzheimer's disease patient" at the Annual Congress of the Mexican Association of Geriatrics and Gerontology.

Developing outside the capital

To outline some of the distances that must be covered in the developing Alzheimer's disease groups in Mexico, I visited Monterrey (a city located 596 miles north of Mexico city) where the family of an Alzheimer's disease patient who is a 47-year-old lawyer were interested in starting a support group. They and I investigated services available in that city and undertook to start the group . On a second visit to Monterrey we helped to organize the 12-family support group and broadcast a 30-minute TV programme.

Guadalajara is over 470 miles from Mexico city. I visited it after the daughter of a carer had made informal contact with the AMAES national office. Her mother, a lady of 82, was diagnosed as suffering from Alzheimer's disease two years previously by a psychogeriatrician who has a day-centre for Alzheimer's disease patients in Guadalajara. He and I broadcast a 25-minute radio programme on Alzheimer's disease and the Mexican Alzheimer's Association. This resulted in many enquiries from the audience. Some of them were interested in the support group, but above all they wanted information in Spanish about Alzheimer's disease. On my second visit to Guadalajara we helped to organize the 20-family support group, and set up a meeting with the research group at the Biomedical Research Institute at the West Medical Centre.

There are over 350,000 Alzheimer's sufferers in Mexico. We have support groups in Mexico City, Guadalajara, Monterrey, Puebla, Cuernavaca and Queretaro attending approximately 400 families. Two books already been translated and published in Spanish are *The 36 Hour Day* by Nancy Mace and Peter Rabins, and *Alzheimer's Disease, a Guide for Families* by Lenore S. Powell.

The Mexican Alzheimer's Association has been working on a volunteer basis and now we are trying to raise funds in order to promote and advance our cause.

International links

Mexico was accepted as a member of the Alzheimer's Disease International (ADI) during the fourth international meeting of the ADI in Brisbane, Australia. The presidents of the various national associations welcomed the newly founded organization with great enthusiasm and warmth. An arrangement was effected between Mexico and the other members to exchange relevant literature and audiovisual programmes. Many countries will provide brochures and books for Spanish translation to the Mexican Alzheimer's Association, which will be returned to the countries of origin for the benefit of their Hispanic populations. As a result of this agreement, brochures produced by the Australian Alzheimer's Society will be made available in 17 different languages! Mexico city hosted the sixth International Meeting of the ADI in 1990.

A representative attends the annual meeting of the ADRDA in the USA. This is a valuable experience as it provides the opportunity not only to increase our knowledge of Alzheimer's disease, but also to make connections with leading members of the American Association, to exchange experiences and to arrange for translations of Alzheimer's disease literature for Spanish speaking people. The staff of the National Office of the ADRDA have provided us with valuable information, advice and practical tips.

The fact that the Mexican Alzheimer's Association (AMAES) organized the VI meeting of the ADI in 1990 provides us with important publicity, and draws attention to the problems of organizing Alzheimer's societies in developing countries. It is urgent to make the public, the professionals and the government aware of this devastating disease, which must be fought with the aid of international cooperation. With more countries actively involved in searching for the cause, the cure and the treatment of Alzheimer's disease, our efforts to care and share in this endeavour will be multiplied, our immense burden will be lighter and the task ahead easier.

Chapter 7

EASING THE BURDEN OF ALZHEIMER'S DISEASE:

The Medical and Community Connection

MA Curti[1] *RN MS,* K McGuinness[2] *BS, Department of Psychiatry & Behavioural Science*[1]*, Health Sciences Center, State University of New York at Stony Brook, StonyBrook, New York 11794-8101; Senior Day Care at St James*[2]*, PO Box 3, St James, New York 11780, USA*

In this paper we would like to present the services of the Long Island Alzheimer's Disease Assistance Centre, (LI-ADAC) and the Geriatric Evaluation Service (GES) which is located at University Hospital, StonyBrook, New York. This paper will include a discussion on the integration of services between LI-ADAC and the St. James Adult Community Day Care Programme. The collaborative efforts between these two agencies have helped to ease the burden of care for families of patients with Alzheimer's disease.

As an introduction it is worth reviewing the demographics of the population aged 65 and older on Long Island. Present projections indicate that this age group is increasing at triple the rate for New York State. Of the 2.7 million people who live on Long Island, approximately 256,000 are over age 65 and have medical and social needs which are increasing relative to their increasing numbers. Dementia is a major concern in this adult population: 38,000 Long Island residents have a diagnosis of dementia and 19,150 of these have a diagnosis of probable Alzheimer's disease. In order to adequately service this population, a centralized area providing comprehensive and coordinated services is essential. In 1988, LI-ADAC was established through a grant from the New York State Department of Health. Presently, there are 8 ADAC's throughout the New York State region which are currently funded and managed by the New York State Department of Health Bureau of Adult and Gerontological Services.

Psychological and social intervention

Alzheimer's disease is a progressive irreversible brain disorder which affects

49

cognition, memory and behaviour. It destroys not only its victims but devastates family members as well. A plan of care consisting of multiple interventions is needed to address the varied components of this illness. Psychologist Robert L. Kahn notes that dementia has been described as a "bio-psycho-social phenomenon": since the biological aspects are not currently treatable, the psychological and social are often amenable to intervention.[1] Thus, while medical intervention is an essential factor, the primary treatment aim must focus on the quality of care that the dementia patient receives as well as the resulting burden on families.

This goal is currently being met through the following spectrum of services provided by LI-ADAC and GES's multidisciplinary team.

(i) Diagnosis and assessment of needs. The main thrust of this assessment is aimed at differentiating irreversible dementia from treatable dementias. This is done through psychiatric evaluation, neurological examination, neuropsychological studies, laboratory tests and neuroradiology. Multi-disciplinary referral is arranged and follow-up evaluation and reassessment is organized.

(ii) Patient intervention – care planning and care co-ordination. The goals of our patient intervention programme are to capitalize on the patient's strengths by identifying and assessing community options for care, to support and assist the family with various carer decisions, and to utilize community interventions as social supports to help alleviate stress.

(iii) Education. LI-ADAC provides didactic sessions on Alzheimer's disease for formal and informal care-givers. We help family members cope with the physical, emotional and behavioural patterns symptomatic of the disease through a Care-givers Practical Help Course. We sponsor professional conferences which address the medical, legal, financial and legislative issues relating to Alzheimer's disease. Case conferences and seminars for university physicians and staff are conducted with a focus on the recognition and treatment of dementia, as well as on issues in follow-up and management.

Referral and evaluation

Referrals to LI-ADAC come from community physicians, ADRDA support groups, community day-care programmes for the elderly, programmes for Alzheimer's disease patients and residential communities. Other sources include community care companions, county officer for the ageing and university hospital sources, as well as patients and care-givers. We use the following criteria for evaluation of patients at LI-ADAC. Patients are accepted for investigation of gradual memory loss, decline in ability to perform routine tasks, increasingly impaired judgement, increasing disorientation in time and place, personality change, loss of language skills and increasing social isolation.

Since its inception in April, 1988, LI-ADAC/GES has maintained a case load of approximately 200 patients with a total of 1,696 clinic visits over an eighteen-month period. Fifty to sixty per cent of the patients evaluated had a diagnosis of dementia. Consistent with the multi-disciplinary basis for care in our unit, 33 patients were referred for neuropsychological testing and 43 were referred to community adult day programmes. LI-ADAC maintains that the multi-faceted problems of both patient and family will best be met by coordinating and accessing key community support services such as those provided by the St. James's Adult Day-Care Programme.

Adult Day-Care Programme

The second half of this paper is from the point of view of the Geriatric Social Worker at the Senior Day Care-Centre at St. James, a former carer, and co-founder and Vice-President of the Nassau-Suffolk Counties chapter of the Alzheimer's Association. This account is based on experiences and observations of people in both the family support group setting and in the adult day-care centre.

The Senior Day-Care Centre at St. James is a social model adult care programme. We care for 46 clients with an age-range from 60 to 98. Approximately 90 per cent of clients suffer from dementia and about 70–80 per cent have a diagnosis of probable Alzheimer's disease. Of the 43 clients referred by LI-ADAC to the community adult day programmes in the period from April 1988 to September 1989, one- third were accepted for admission to the St. James's Senior Day- Care Programme. Adult day-care brings services to older people who are socially isolated and provides opportunities for social contact, particularly for those who do not have family care- givers and who cannot function in their community without assistance and resources.

Clients

Since Alzheimer's disease may have a prolonged course, a person who enters day-care in the fourth stage of the Reisberg Global Deterioration Scale[2] can participate in the programme for a possible 2 to 3 years, or even longer. While adult day-care offers opportunities for respite hours for both the Alzheimer's disease client and his/her care-giver, this is not the sole aim of the programme. Therapeutic interventions include reality orientation, reminiscence therapy and socializing with peers. These activities are designed to improve the psychological and physical well-being of the client.

Adult day-care also serves as a monitoring mechanism for changes in the client's personality, mood, cognition and behaviour. The changes in the client's activities of daily living that we note specifically are toiletting, eating and grooming. If the client wanders, family members are encouraged to get Medi-Alert bracelets for their family members and we refer the client to the Nassau-Suffolk County's Wandering Adult Programme. We also look for medication side effects, including extra-pyramidal symptoms, akathisia and increased confusion. In addition, adult day-care can be an important means of monitoring the client who may live alone in the community and is in need of full-time companionship and supervision

Carers

Carer stress is periodically evaluated and vigilance is maintained about the sensitive issue of elder abuse. This service is augmented by the consulting services of the visiting LI-ADAC psychiatrist and by comprehensive case management with staff and the social worker. Day-care utilization has provided respite to 16 care-givers and enabled 11 care-givers to maintain employment. Twelve care-givers participated in a carer support group and seven families were referred back to LI-ADAC's educational series on dementia.

As Alzheimer's disease progresses so, too, does the dependency of clients on the carer. Over time, care-givers have been observed to develop many needs, such as education and information, referral, support and long-term care planning. Usually they want advice on the myriad everyday issues that are associated with Alzheimer's disease: diagnosis, incontinence, catastrophic reactions, perception problems, delusions and hallucinations, safe home environment, communication problems, social isolation, role-reversal, sundown syndrome, sleeping disturbances in both the client and the care-giver, feelings of grief, guilt, anger and resentment associated with the loss of their companion. Other queries include change in living arrangements – Mom and Dad have now moved in with the adult child, early retirement for both the client or the care-giver, driving, financial planning, applying for government entitlement programmes, possible hospitalization, home-health care (both short- and long-term), companionship, planning for institutionalization and the sensitive issue of autopsy. Establishing a long-term care plan for the client is an absolute necessity, and health-care professionals must utilize the expertise of the family care-giver. When the care-giver is viewed as an integral component of the multi-disciplinary team approach, the care-giver will generally experience a sense of empowerment over their struggle and will often escape the role of victim. The St James's Adult Day-Care Programme affords care-givers the opportunity to build a goal-orientated plan and encourages them to act as their own advocates whenever possible.

Conclusion

The integration of services and co-operative interdependence between LI-ADAC, a large medical facility, and the senior day-care centre at St. James, a small community programme, affords the Alzheimer's care-giver and care-receiver the following: (i) A comprehensive plan of care, (ii) improved quality of life, and (iii) the necessary supports to help ease the burden of Alzheimer's disease.

References

(1) Zarit SH, Orry NK, Zarit JM. *The Hidden Victims of Alzheimer's Disease: Families under Stress.* New York, New York University Press, 1985, 2.

(2) Reisberg B, Ferris SH, de Leon MJ, Crook T. Global Deterioration Scale (GDS) for age-associated cognitive decline and Alzheimer's disease. *Am J Psychiatry* 1982, **139**, 136-1139

Carers, Professionals and Alzheimer's Disease. D O'Neill ed © 1991 John Libbey & Company Ltd

Chapter 8

THE FAMILY AND DEMENTIA

G du Faur *MBE BHSc, Vice-President, Alzheimer's Disease and Related Disorders Society, PO Box 2808, Christchurch, New Zealand*

I come from New Zealand, a country with three and half million people with health concerns which are very similar to those in other developed countries except that we seem to have the highest ratio of cot deaths (and asthma occurrence) in the world. As far as we know, the incidence of dementing illness is much the same as it is in Western Europe or North America. This means that there are approximately 26,000 cases of Alzheimer-type dementia in our community, and that one-fifth of those over 80 will suffer from cognitive impairment.

It follows that in areas with large numbers of elderly people there will be many sufferers of dementing illnesses. The Bay of Plenty, where I live, has delightful physical features and a clement climate, attracting residents who want to spend retirement in pleasant surroundings. Among the health problems affecting elderly people, it is predictable that there will be a proportion of dementias with all the associated difficulties of care.

The national organisation, the Alzheimer's Disease and Related Disorders Society (ADARDS) was organised in 1986, and now there are fifty support groups throughout the country. I work with the ADARDS (Tauranga) in a district of 90,000 people. Our observations and practices may be useful to others

The family

Chronic illness in the elderly always affects the family, but there is no disorder which requires so much adjustment to family functioning as dementia. This condition in one person causes stress to the other family members in their attempts to care for the afflicted person. There are strains in their relationship with the sufferer and with one another. Everyone is a loser – the patient loses social skills and the ability to communicate normally, the spouse loses a companion and a confidante, sons and daughters no longer have the support of a parent, and grand-children cannot understand what has happened to a special friend. Spouses, siblings, sons and daughters and grand-children are likely to experience a wide range of reactions at various stages of their caring. These can be sadness, pity and guilt, shame, fear, anxiety and loneliness, feelings of helplessness and nearly always abiding grief. Bobby Glaze Custer, one of the founders of ADRDA in USA, described her feelings as like "being at a funeral which never ends". In these circumstances, it is understandable that constant support for care-givers is essential if the families' emotional bonds are to remain intact. There must be a balance between serving the patient and meeting the needs of the care-giving family.

The majority of patients with senile dementia of the Alzheimer type remain in the community with their spouses or their children, so families bear the burden of care. The multiplicity of problems strain the physical and emotional resources of the carers and support is needed to give assistance with the decision making and comfort when they are weary and laden with care.

Assessing the impact

It is important to determine what the illness means to the family. Can they accept that the changes are irreversible and that the impairment of the brain has caused a major personality and behaviour alteration? Can they accept that the individual is no longer the spouse, the brother, the sister, the father, the mother or the grand parent they knew? The quality of care is often determined by the strength and warmth of previous relationships: obviously a former trusting and loving relationship provides a better basis for understanding than one where there has been distrust and hostility. However, even in the best of earlier circumstances, the unresponsiveness of the patient and the frustrations experienced change the attitudes of the carer.

ADARDS volunteers aim to provide a level of support which enables the care-givers to cope with their own emotions, to meet and resolve difficulties, and most of all to understand what has happened to the person they once knew. A simple account of the irreversible changes in the brain can often bring an explanation as to why simple tasks which could be performed yesterday can not be done today without supervision. Success one day does not mean that the same process will be remembered and done correctly the next day – or even one hour later – and failure on the part of the patient is not an act of deliberate defiance.

Ideally ADARDS volunteers should be in contact with the family from the earliest stages of the patient's illness: but Alzheimer-type diseases are of slow onset and the recognition of the illness and its confirmation by a physician often takes place long after the family members have been driven to distraction by the behaviour of a dementing person. Early referral to an ADARDS counsellor gives an opportunity to learn about the illness, it's nature and it's prognosis. The caring family needs to come to terms with the knowledge that the condition may persist for years and require more and more resources. The counsellor's role is to assist care-givers in coping with emotional responses and poorly-defined fears. Sometimes negative reactions of carers can direct family conflict and expressions of anger towards the patient. Assistance can help in the development of caring skills and the adjustments which are necessary in dealing with social and business situations.

Remembering the patient

In the concentration of efforts to support the carer, the patient is not forgotten. We realise that in the early stages of dementia, the patient is well aware that "something is wrong". There are often fears of brain tumours, insanity and impending incapacity. Often there is depression and paranoia complicating the major condition. There can be increasing demands towards retaining a secure position in a known place with the constant company and support of the spouse or other companion. Frustrations develop easily and there can be false suspicions about the deeds of others – for example, blame for stealing money is laid against innocent relatives or friends, devoted spouses may be accused of infidelity and plotting. At this stage, the patient needs constant reassurance and friendship. Social contacts outside the family and activities which use the remaining skills can divert and entertain the patient and give respite to the carer.

As the disease progresses, there is a gradual loss of faculties. Impairment of the ability to express thoughts and words and speak intelligently become apparent. Reading, writing and cognitive skills disappear and the patient may not be able to recognise his wife, his family or his friends. Often there is socially unacceptable behaviour which further isolates the carer and the patient.

At all stages of the illness, patients are able to feel pleasure and pain: reaction to the displeasure can be anger, non-cooperation and sometimes violence. Where unhappy responses are experienced, it is helpful to discuss these events with a counsellor and to try to identify the causes so that the intensity or occurrence of similar episodes can be avoided. As an example of a pleasurable event, I quote the comment of one patient after he had enjoyed an outing. He said "I do not know where I have been – but I know it was good and I was very happy." If the sufferer is feeling comfortable and alert, care-giving is easier and can be rewarding. Living with a spouse or parent through the period of five of ten years of observing and coping with physical and mental deterioration is very stressful. No one can eliminate entirely the worry, sadness and devastation caused by dementia, but there are coping skills which can be learnt with the help of counsellors, which can help individuals to reduce tension between the carers and the patient.

It is essential that the main care-giver be encouraged to have time off from caring and to maintain some activities which give personal satisfaction. Advice may be needed about a number of social and management issues.

Family and social factors

Relatives and friends of the family may find the patient's behaviour so strange that visiting or social contact is avoided. The carer sometimes ceases to participate in social activities and withdraws to give attention to the patient. Both patient and carer are thus denied the variety of company which can stimulate and retain interest, even if only for a short period. The isolation imposed by this situation is compounded if sons, daughters and grand-children are unable to face even brief contact with the person who does not recognise them and talks nonsense. This rejection may not be noticed by the patient but is very hurtful to the primary carer.

Volunteer visitors can visit the whole family, assuring them that the new patterns of behaviour are not deliberate, making it easy for them to discuss their concerns and fears, especially the fear that they or their children may develop a dementing illness. Encouragement can be given about retaining contact and sharing caring. Suggestions can be made about expressing feelings with friends and explaining the sufferer's unusual deeds. Friends are often relieved to be involved in open discussion and can share conversation in a relaxed manner.

Grand-children can be especially sensitive: usually perplexed, sometimes silent about the changes they see, sometimes wondering whether they had a part in causing the illness. There is often resentment that so much time is spent with the grand-parent and dismiss their rejection of the patient saying: "What is the use? Grandpa does not know me anymore." Young people need the assurance that it is realised that the situation is tough on them, and that their needs will be recognised. If properly approached, they can make a valuable contribution to family care and their efforts will be appreciated. Discussion can give grand-children confidence about explaining their grand-parent's illness to their peers.

Dementia in one family member changes the circumstances and life style of the entire family. Male spouses who never managed a kitchen now have to do so. Wives who know little about money have to learn about it. Sons and daughters and their partners find themselves in reverse roles giving parental care to their fathers and mothers, and grand-children become important contributors to the comfort of their grand-parents.

Legal and financial aspects

Any long-term illness can bring financial stress. The requirement for years of care of dementia patients uses savings and other resources to pay for respite care and other services. The person with the dementing illness will reach a situation where he is not able to make reasoned decisions or manage even simple business transactions. An important role of the counsellor is to ensure that the care-giving family has access to information about legal and financial matters which must pass from the control of the patient. The prospect of a long and costly period of care is a concern to everyone: to individuals as they contemplate their budget for an indeterminate time, to providers of the public health system for the increasing numbers of brain-impaired elderly.

In New Zealand, no one has assessed the cost of care to the state and individuals, but studies in the USA estimate the total sum used in the care of dementia patients to approach $40 billion. Wherever people live, the burden is unfair. Often the financial as well as the emotional resources of an elderly spouse are destroyed and there is no opportunity to recoup. One of the important functions of ADARDS counsellors is to collate information so that the society can act as an advocate to improve provisions and devise a fairer system. Governments in every part of the world will know about Alzheimer's societies!

Environment and support services

At some time before the patient becomes immobile, the carer and family will want to review the suitability of the existing residence and either arrange a complete change or adapt facilities to remove potential hazards. If the carer is usually alone with the patient, or if the patient lives alone, availability of local support services and helpful neighbours should be explored. Eligibility for supplementary financial help should be discussed and recorded so that there is easy recall of information. Often the carer is strongly independent and reluctant to use resources. Sometimes the carer says "I am managing." ADARDS workers look for signs that the carer really is not managing or is managing at great personal cost. In these incidences, tactful discussion accompanied by gentle persuasion often achieves acceptance of assistance.

Care planning

Many books are available to give advice about caring for Alzheimer-type patients. However, there is no substitute for personal discussion with a professional advisor or an experienced counsellor. Family members should be assured that counselling and practical aid are accessible for the whole extended time of the illness and afterwards.

In the first stages of counselling, carers are often encouraged to express their anger and their guilt, being assured that these are quite acceptable and should not be suppressed. Carers are encouraged to plan time off, to participate in functions that interest them and to value their own health by admitting feelings of frustration and exhaustion before a crisis is precipitated. Some behaviours which worry carers need special advice. They do not all happen at the same time and therefore can be discussed as they arise. Situations which seem to be most trying are well known to all of us: wandering, sleep disturbance and incontinence, all of which can be managed. We know that some dementia patients are depressed and paranoid. For these and some other conditions, there must be attention, advice and, if possible, relief to enable care to continue.

The final stages

In the final stages of the illness, family care often becomes impossible and there must be transfer to full 24-hour care. The decision to make the change from home to hospital or other institution is traumatic: the carer can suffer a renewed sense of failure and loss. At this period the support of family members for one another and the assurance of friends and professionals is especially important.

When death finally releases the load, the counsellor remains available to help the carer to participate in a different world and in a life of a different pattern. We recognise the aptness of the comment of Dr. Elizabeth Kubler-Ross who said "When anger, resentment and guilt can be worked through, the family has a period of preparatory grief. The more this grief can be expressed before death, the less unbearable it becomes afterwards." To express the aims and the hopes of family counselling in dementia cases, I should like to borrow the words of Dr L Feldman-Brun of West Germany: "Some care-givers succeed in turning their eyes from the past to the present through loving their patients not only for what they have been but for what they are now. The stranger can turn into a different but well-known person whose signals can not only be decoded but also accepted. None of us began by expecting that the heavy burden of caring could change to a new affectionate relationship which is rewarding for both patient and care-giver."

Conclusion

It is the aim of ADARDS workers to encourage personal growth and development of family members in an atmosphere of understanding, interest and open-mindedness so that they can arrive at solutions and decisions appropriate to their individual situations. In this field and all others concerned with the Alzheimer's type illness, we are reminded of a nursery rhyme which begins: "Monday's child is fair of face". In the field of Alzheimer's disease we are like Thursday's child: We have far to go but it is to be hoped that in the meantime those who work with carers and patients can try to be like Friday's child – loving and giving.

> *Monday's child is fair of face,*
> *Tuesday's child is full of grace,*
> *Wednesday's child is full of woe,*
> *Thursday's child has far to go,*
> *Friday's child is loving and giving,*
> *Saturday's child works hard for a living,*
> *But the child that is born on the Sabbath day*
> *Is fair and wise and good and gay.*

Chapter 9

SOCIAL IMPACT ON ALZHEIMER'S DISEASE FAMILIES CO-OPERATING IN A SCIENTIFIC RESEARCH PROGRAMME

G De Winter,[1,3] *social worker*, A. Vandenberghe[1] *PhD*,
J Gheuens[2] *MD*, JJ Martin[2] *MD*, C Van Broeckhoven[1] *PhD*
[1]*Dept. of Biochemistry, and* [2]*Dept. of Medicine, Born-Bunge
Foundation, University of Antwerp (UIA), Universiteitsplein 1, B 2610
Antwerpen,* [3]*Innogenetics Inc., Industriepark Zwijnaarde 7, Box 4,
B-9710 Gent, Belgium*

This paper attempts to explore what it means for a family to be involved in a scientific research programme. The research programme aims to find the defective gene which causes the hereditary form of Alzheimer's disease. For this purpose it is essential to get in touch with large families where as many members as possible are willing to give blood samples. It is essential that not only patients, but also all members of one family co-operate, in order to find differences in their hereditary material, i.e. DNA. It is my task to contact families and to find other members of this family through research in registers in order to elucidate the full pedigree. I also have to try to motivate as many family members as possible to co-operate.

It is my experience that family members contacted are relatively unconcerned about the technical aspects of the research. Their concern is more of a psychological and social order. Their experience and our responsibility towards the co-oper-

59

ating persons, is the subject of my paper which is divided into three parts. The first part will outline the family structure. The second part will describe the procedure we follow in contacting the family-members. Finally, the implications of involvement in a scientific research programme for a family will be discussed, and I would like to give some suggestions about the role of the social worker.

Family dynamics

This paper describes work with a family which was brought to our attention by Prof. Dr. J. Gheuens of the Department of Medicine, Born-Bunge-Foundation, University of Antwerp. The family has been the subject of research since 1940. Alzheimer's disease occurs in this family at the very young age of 35 years. The patients typically die between the age of 40 to 50 years. In an attempt to elicit possible genetic factors, the family was contacted again.

When we contacted the family three years ago, there was only one surviving patient, who died in 1989. After contacting other family members we discovered two young patients in the at-risk generation. The older generation is very aware of the fact that there is a genetic disease in their family. The patients' widows and widowers had coped with the disease in different ways. In most cases the patients were taken into institutional care, some very soon, but others later in the course of their disease. In one case the wife looked after her affected husband until he died. Due to lack of information, unaffected family members were apprehensive about acquiring the disease. In some cases they severed contact with their brothers and sisters-in-law because they could not cope with their problems. In other cases, they felt these problems were so terrifying that the stress caused great conflict with their in-laws. In this generation Alzheimer's disease often led to alienation and family break-up.

The younger generation was not always aware of the genetic disease in their family. The oldest children were often involved in caring for parents with the disease and often had to take great responsibilities at a very young age. They sometimes were very conscious of the intellectual and behavioural deterioration of their parent. The younger children have only vague memories about what happened to one of their parents. Some children were too young or were brought up in children's homes. Overall, this generation was not aware of the genetic nature of Alzheimer's disease in their family.

Research approach

Our approach to the family members was to contact each person individually by phone or letter and to ask for permission to pay them a visit at home. The purpose of this visit was to inform them about the research programme and to collect data about the course of the disease of their relatives. We also asked for their cooperation in giving a blood sample. The older generation – widows and widowers of patients – were contacted first. This was felt to be important not only to generate trust and cooperation in this generation but also to canvass them about our project to contact their adult children. Although we did not need formal approval of the parent to approach their adult children, we thought it was very important that they gave their view. Their feelings and experiences were indeed an important help in approaching the younger generation.

Our approach and any scientific research in this domain means confronting the family with the problems associated with the disease itself and its unpleasant nature. The reactions varied from person to person and from generation to generation. In the older generation I experienced reawakening of old grief when talking about the course of the disease of their partner or relative. I experienced anger, sometimes aggression towards their parents, parents-in-law, or towards the doctors who they felt had kept them ignorant of the nature of the disease. There was also anxiety about the recurrence of dementia in their children and grand-children. However they expressed enthusiasm and hope for the future when they realized that Alzheimer's disease was a research topic. Their concern about how their children were going to react to our demand sometimes led to an initial refusal of permission to talk with the younger generation. It is likely that feelings of guilt, suspicion and fear about the outcome of this research caused this behaviour.

The younger generation

In the younger generation, we were confronted with reactions of fear and uncertainty towards their health, their relationships, their children and their future. They were confronted with all the problems of being an at-risk person or of sharing life with an at-risk person. This situation is very stressful, provoking very strong feelings and is the biggest problem that they confront. We also found relief that the taboos around the disease in the family were broken. In some cases our research request seemed to have initiated an open discussion among family members about this matter. As a result of this new frankness, the younger generation had the opportunity to talk and share their experience of the disease when they were children with other family members: they also discussed their strategies for coping with the problem at present. They also got answers to a lot of questions that they had been harbouring silently for many years. This was most pronounced for the very young children who lacked memories of their deceased mother or father.

The role of the social worker

It is impossible to talk about the function of the social worker without talking about the function of the family in the whole project. The co-operation of the family is a *conditio sine qua non:* therefore they are treated as respected collaborators in the programme. The success of a scientific research programme depends not only on the capability of the project leader and of all the collaborators but also on the ability of the collaborators to work together as a team. Every scientific research programme needs a permanent evaluation. In the case this evaluation should not only concern its scientific meaning, but also the psychological and social repercussions on the co-operating family in particular, and on society in general. In this evaluation the contribution of the family is of great importance.

The role of the social worker should, therefore, be defined as broadly as possible in order to take care of the psychological and social problems resulting from integrating families in a scientific research programme. The social worker takes care of the individual follow-up concerning the problems arising from our request to co-operate. It is necessary for the social worker to have regular contact to exchange information in both directions, to be permanently approachable and to mobilize help from outside bodies such as the Alzheimer's association. The social worker is also the mouth-piece for the experiences and the discoveries of the family members co-operating with the research group.

Because the co-operating family members are collaborators, their discoveries need the same attention as those of the researchers. They need to be integrated in the whole concept of the research goals. In my opinion this integration is the most important prerequisite to justify research in this domain. This approach guarantees to both the families and society that the scientific research is carried out with a human face, and that the motivation of the researchers consists not only of scientific curiosity but also reflects social responsibility.

In the light of the professional orientation of social work, the social worker will almost certainly identify more closely with the cooperating persons than with the research programme in which he/she is involved. This is not necessarily a problem! Everything depends on the interest and the frankness of the whole team in this matter: they decide whether the social worker will behave as a colleague or as a watch-dog.

SECTION 3
Alzheimer's Disease and the Public

Carers, Professionals and Alzheimer's Disease. D O'Neill ed © 1991 John Libbey & Company Ltd

Chapter 10

GETTING YOUR MESSAGE ACROSS

B Moss *BHA AASA AHA, Executive Director, Moorfields Community for Adult Care, Honorary Secretary, Alzheimer's Disease International, PO Box 470, Hawthorn, Victoria 3122, Australia*

Introduction

Since the beginning of time, people have been attempting to communicate with others. A variety of methods have been used through the ages. We have moved from the simple grunt to complex language structures; from crude signals to complete, precise images from the other side of the world.

What an era we live in when it comes to getting the message across! Apart from meetings such as the 5th Alzheimer's Disease International, we have seminars, forums, conferences, lectures, study tours, symposiums, creative teaching methods, interpersonal communication, and the competing interests of the print and electronic media in all its forms.

In this generation we have moved from the industrial revolution into the information revolution. We have moved from delayed communication to instant communication.

Are we getting the message across?

But even given the enormity and speed of change which we have seen in communication methods the question still remains: "Are we getting the message across?". Some individuals are obviously better communicators than others. Some organisations seem to get their message over more effectively than others. Some "causes" have received greater prominence than others. Is this simply an accident or are there reasons why this should be?

In addressing this question, there is one important point to bear in mind. This is not a period in history for the strong, silent type. We live in an era when our message can easily get lost in the communication barrage. Our audience is under attack from all sides. Today, more than ever before, an enormous range of competing interests and a multitude of groups are trying to get their message across. Those groups which are effective in getting their message across are those which have an unequivocal and professional commitment to good communication.

Four key considerations

I would also like to state that any expertise I may have in this area, is an expertise born out of personal experience. In this paper I intend to share my understanding of "how to get the message across" based on my personal experience over many years. There are, I would like to suggest, four key considerations when it comes to getting the message across and I will address each in turn.

Know what it is that you want to say

The first is to know what it is that you want to say. We have all heard people say: ".... ah what am I trying to say" – particularly in the middle of a heated discussion. Unfortunately, many groups, organisations and individuals place themselves in exactly the same situation over and over again. They are not really sure what they are trying to say.

Let me illustrate: during 1988 a national representative body in my country was lobbying our Government on changes in Nursing Home funding. Its efforts were not particularly successful, because the representatives from one State wanted the national body to say one thing whilst representatives from another State wanted something different and so on. Was the national body to tell the Government that their proposals were unworkable or congratulate the Government for its foresight? In the end neither message was communicated effectively and the Government used the old and proven method of divide and conquer. It is imperative that we know what we want to say if we are to communicate effectively.

Why do you want to say it?

The second key consideration in getting our message across, is that we must be clear in our minds about the purpose of the message. Why do we want to say it? The reasons can be many and varied. You may wish to communicate in order to educate, to stimulate discussion or to create a particular response.

As carers and as health-care professionals, for example, we want to communicate to educate the public, the community, the medical fraternity and other health professionals about Alzheimer's disease or a related disorder and its effects on the sufferer and the carer. In addition, we may want to communicate at certain times to elicit a particular response – for example in fund-raising. The reasons underlying our desire to communicate determine the way in which we are going to try to get our message across. Therefore it is vital that we remember the answer to this question constantly.

But of course there may be more than one reason. The reasons may vary depending on the target population with which we wish to communicate. Several examples can illustrate this point. Have you ever had the misfortune of finding that a loved one, a spouse, or maybe a parent, who is an Alzheimer's disease sufferer, needs hospitalization for an acute phase of another illness? If you have, you would appreciate the sort of experience which happens too often.

Nurses in acute hospitals are not trained in any detail in illnesses affecting older people such as Alzheimer's disease. The busy nurse, wishing to get on with her routine, is frustrated by the uncooperative manner of the Alzheimer's disease sufferer and endeavours to force the pace. The Alzheimer's disease sufferer, failing to understand the cues, feels frightened and threatened and becomes more uncooperative, even aggressive. The nurse retaliates and compounds what has become a very complex situation, reporting to her superior that Mrs X or Mr Y is totally uncooperative and difficult.

If it has been given at all, the message about Alzheimer's disease or a related disorder has clearly not been understood. The reason for our communication with health-care professionals as in this example is to make them aware of the disease, its effects and appropriate responses.

If however, as a further example, we take an entirely different group of people, e.g. supporters of an organisation, and give them exactly the same message as that which we would give to nurses, we won't communicate. Why? Because we failed to answer the question: "why do I want to say it?". We don't want our supporters over-burdened with the sort of clinical information that we would give to health professionals: we want them to understand and feel the human plight so that they will respond appropriately. We must define the purpose of the message, and it may vary, depending on the audience.

Who do we want to reach?

The third key consideration is the audience or target group. In other words: "with whom do we wish to communicate?" We need to be aware that every organization has many audiences or target groups. We have touched on a couple of these above. But let me illustrate with an example from my own organization, Moorfields Community for Adult Care.

In our formal communication strategies we have highlighted the following target groups:

members of the Board of Management

staff

allied professionals

politicians

bureaucrats

users of our services

residents in our Homes

prospective users and residents

those who give to support our work

those who may give to support our work

and many more target groups. Why is it so important to know who you are aiming at? Because the nature of the target group determines the method of communication to be used. The vehicle for conveying our message may vary depending upon the target group and the purpose. In other words, having determined what we want to say, having defined our purpose and having identified the target audience, we can then decide how to get the message across.

How to get the message across

This brings me to the final key consideration. This question of how to get the message over. Some would call it the methodology, others would call it the medium. Unfortunately, for the inexperienced or the impatient it is all too often the starting point. Someone on staff decides that it would be good to have a new brochure for a particular programme. It sounds great, and before any of the key areas above are considered, the new brochure goes off to the printer. And all too often, the medium used was not the best one for that particular target group!

Some examples may illustrate this point. I will refer again to my own agency. If we decided that we wanted to get a message across to our staff, we would more than likely use an entirely different vehicle for the message than if we were trying to communicate with our supporters. A newsletter, for example, which appropriately addressed issues concerning staff would probably have quite a negative effect on supporters. A symposium, held to canvass issues amongst politicians would be quite ineffective for prospective users and residents. The nature of the target groups must be a key consideration in any communications exercise.

Some basic rules

In summary, we have four key factors in good communication. They may be expressed as the what, the why, the who and the how. What do you want to say? Why do you want to say it? To whom do you wish to say it? How can it best be said? Having looked at these vital fundamentals we need then to address ourselves to some basic ground rules.

Know your subject

First, know your subject. Obviously, if our communication is to be effective we must know what we are talking about. How can we get the message across if we don't fully comprehend the message ourselves? There is nothing more unconvincing than a message giver who clearly does not understand his/her own message.

Sometimes, for example, a speaker is found out at the question time after his paper. He/she may lose all credibility because they are unable to answer any in-depth questions, demonstrating only a superficial knowledge of the subject.

Know your facts

Second, know your facts. Back up your message or argument by presenting facts which are pertinent to the particular situation. For example, how many Alzheimer's Disease sufferers are there in your community? What studies have been done that can back up your figures? (National studies of a broad nature will often suffice.)

Know your audience

Third, know your audience. It would be quite a mistake not to do some homework about the group that you are addressing or aiming to reach. For example, if one wishes to ensure that the nurse in the acute hospital understands the nature of Alzheimer's disease, one needs to know what training programmes have already been put in place. Make yourself aware of hospital policy and be sensitive to the particular ethos of the organization. The way you present your message to such a group of nurses will be very different to that which you would give to an audience of untrained persons who would not understand technical jargon.

Believe in what you have to say

Fourth, believe in what you say. There is nothing worse than an unconvincing speaker or message giver who is equivocal about the subject. How is such a message giver going to convince others? If you are giving a message, give it as if you believe the world depends upon it. A friend recently gave a paper at an important conference. He started off in fine form but lost his momentum and as he finished, he was almost apologetic about his message. He "lost" his audience because he finally ended up being unconvinced about his own message.

Keep it simple

Fifth, keep it simple. Even if we are giving our message to a technically-minded group, it can still be kept simple and we ought to stick to the facts. Sometimes we may have the opportunity of presenting our message on a radio programme. Possibly we may have an opportunity of being interviewed on television. In such situations, the general public will not understand too much about "plaques and tangles". It's sufficient to say that the sufferer has a "degenerative brain failure."

At a recent seminar in Melbourne, an officer of the Corporate Affair's Office, responsible for company legislation, spoke on a recent Act of Parliament affecting retirement villages. He droned on and on, virtually reading from the Act which was very complicated and little understood. Although he was invited to assist peoples' understanding, he was unable to keep it simple and even in question time he responded with further convoluted quotations.

Keep it honest

Sixth, keep it honest. In getting our message across, we must always attempt to state the facts as they are. We shouldn't hide from the truth or try to deceive people. We will earn greater respect and understanding if we keep our communication honest.

Keep it sincere

Seventh, keep it sincere. If we want to get our message across effectively, it must be done sincerely. For example, some of the most effective communication I have ever observed has been when carers simply and honestly state the effect that the disease is having on the life of the sufferer and themselves. Some of my colleagues from Melbourne, Australia can tell you how effective that was when some carers from our Alzheimer's society met with, and spoke to, some politicians recently. The message brought a tear to the eye of more than one and we have witnessed far greater interest in, and support for, the society's work.

Cover all contingencies

Eighth, cover all contingencies. Don't assume people know anything about your subject. Quite often we present a message without covering all the issues, assuming that other people know some of the basic issues because we know the subject from A to Z. This is usually not the case! How often have you been in a group discussion or perhaps a lecture or a conference where a speaker is using jargon that you simply do not understand? It has happened to all of us from time to time. Perhaps many of your audience will know some of the basics, but not all will know.

I can remember at the 1986 meeting of ADI Executive in Paris when I presented the bid on behalf of Australia to host the 1988 meeting at Brisbane. In my preparation for that presentation I tried very hard to ensure that I covered all contingencies and all the selling points, countering any of the arguments that may have been presented against our proposal. We were successful in our bid. Now perhaps it was the excitement of a trip "down under", perhaps it was the thought of visiting the World Expo in Brisbane, perhaps it was the excitement of our bi-centenary celebrations. Or perhaps it was that the message was understood?

Is your message understood?

That leads me to the forgotten element of good communication: feedback. It is imperative that we make every effort to establish if the communication has worked. When you are standing face to face with someone, you can generally gauge if they are absorbing what you are saying. It is much more difficult when communicating with a large group who may be quite remote from you. None-the-less, feedback is your only means of judging whether the communication has worked. If you are asked to lecture on appropriate forms of care for dementia sufferers in acute hospitals and the practice of care subsequently changes, the communication has worked: this is feedback. If you send a letter to your supporters requesting gifts and you receive none, this is also valuable feedback!

I would contend that the feedback we are getting nowadays tells us that we must modify our message from what we may have given some years ago. We may have to become more refined, fine tuning the message as people's understanding of Alzheimer's disease and its problems improves. As their understanding improves, they will be expecting more detail and more precise information.

Conclusion

In a society where there are many competing interests, people will tune out, ignore, or fail to comprehend your message for a variety of reasons. So make it simple, concise and relevant. If you believe in something strongly, stick at it and persevere until you get the message across.

Carers, Professionals and Alzheimer's Disease. D O'Neill ed © 1991 John Libbey & Company Ltd

Chapter 11

DEMENTIA: PRIORITIES FOR CARE, STRATEGIES FOR CHANGE

J Killeen *BSc, DipASS, Director, Scottish Action for Dementia, 33 Castle Street, Edinburgh, EH2 3DN, Scotland*

I welcome an opportunity to share the Scottish experience with a wider audience. Scotland has a population of 5 million and we estimate that it has about 90,000 people with dementia and, of course, a larger number of carers. As in every Western nation, these numbers are going to be increasing until the end of the century and beyond. We feel we have been sitting on a time bomb. We've known over the last 30 years what the demographic changes and trends are going to be and Government reports over the last 30 years have highlighted the needs of older people and, in particular, the needs of people with dementia. I personally have been involved with Scottish Action on Dementia since it was conceived in 1984. My background is that I am a social worker: I specialised in community organisation and development and have worked with a variety of community groups for 20 years. I became involved with dementia through Age Concern where I worked as a training officer for seven years.

Scottish Action on Dementia

What sort of body are we, when did we form and how do we operate? The organization actually grew out of a training conference. It was a conference in which we were sharing coping strategies, in particular how to cope with the most difficult group – the ambulant dementia sufferers. We had 200 people attend out of 400 applicants: it was the very first conference on dementia that had been held in Scotland. There was a lot of sharing of ideas going on, but people were saying to us "It is all very well us learning how to cope better, in fact we are learning a lot and we do know a lot and there are many therapeutic approaches, but we are caring almost alone 24 hours a day, 7 days a week. There aren't the right sort of services and there aren't the right sort of provisions available. The politicians and the managers don't understand what support health-care workers need and what sort of support carers in the community need. So what can be done, what can Age Concern Scotland do?"

Our multidisciplinary conference-planning group decided that it had no right to leave all these questions unanswered, having provided the opportunity for people to air them as they did. We got together and decided to have a forum for action on dementia to which we invited representation from all the Royal Colleges, i.e. of nursing, psychiatry, geriatrics, GPs, and also representatives from voluntary organisations and the whole range of bodies to whom we felt dementia was a very relevant issue. They examined what issues one should be looking at, and we got full support for moving forward with a campaign to improve services for dementia sufferers in Scotland. Alzheimer's Scotland was a founder member.

We represent the whole range of professional bodies, voluntary organisations, some statutory health and social work agencies and a wide range of individuals. We are an independent voluntary organisation and we have the traditional structure of a council, executive committee, full-time director (myself) and a half-time secretary. There are several sub-committees which are looking at the key issues identified in 1984 as being the main ones for attention: training, standards of care, services, rights and legal protection. We also set up sub-groups to tease out issues and clarify objectives, to look at whom we needed to influence and what sort of approaches would be most appropriate.

Interdisciplinary work

A key principle of all our work is that it is interdisciplinary. I think this is something which is extremely important and has given a great deal of weight to what we have had to say. We are a representative body and as such we are listened to by the Scottish Office and by Health and Local Authorities. Our opinion on issues relating to dementia carry a great deal of weight. Our priorities are similar to those of all nations: services to meet individual needs, training and education, standards of care and quality of life, rights and legal protection, financial support for carers and integrated health, welfare and social security policies. All this requires joint planning and joint working at every level. We are trying to communicate with people at every level and it is quite a struggle, but I think this is the way forward. It is interesting to find people working together who wouldn't normally be speaking to each other, such as psychiatrists and geriatricians, social workers and doctors! At the end of our first year a document was produced: *Dementia in Scotland – Priorities for Care – Strategies for Change*.[1].

This was our key policy document which we sent to everybody we wanted to influence and we asked them to respond within a period of four months, to tell us whether they agreed with our analysis of the problems and to tell us what they were going to do about these problems. The responses were collected and published: on the basis of these a symposium was held at which we looked at developing innovative services.[2] At that time, there were no innovative services in Scotland, although there was a lot of good will and a lot of isolated pockets of good practice which had been going on for years. There had been very little progress because dementia had such a low profile.

Identifying needs and actions

Each group has gone through the process of identifying needs and actions. An example of our response to the public perception of the needs of dementia sufferers can be seen by our response to recent changes in the health and social services in Scotland. At the moment the United Kingdom Government is producing consultation papers (white papers) on changes in the National Health Service and changes in Social Welfare Policies and Social Security. All these changes affect people with dementia and we see it as our prime task to look very closely at Government proposals. We are assessing the implications for people with dementia and are working on our public response. We are under a good deal of pressure to get our responses ready in the very short period of time that our Government is giving us to respond. To this end our working groups, which are issues-based, take on the responsibility and are given a mandate by our Executive Committee to work on issues and respond. At the same time we are producing a briefing paper on dementia for wider distribution. We aim to motivate and stimulate our politicians and our member groups by lobbying and working through their networks and through the media so that we are all speaking together with one voice.

Specific issues

Conferences and publications are a useful way of raising the profile of dementia and teasing out issues on a range of problems that are facing professionals and planners. An example is work on legal matters. We have been looking at the law in Scotland and identifying deficiencies in legal provisions for those such as dementia sufferers, unable to make decisions for themselves. What may appear to be a good piece of legislation, such as the United Kingdom Mental Health Act, is actually open to abuse in its interpretation and our group has been able to highlight this. We have produced a guide to dementia and the law:[3] the challenge it puts forward is a very radical alternative to our present system in which, when there is a conflict of interests, things could be sorted out before going to the Courts. Scotland has a system of children's panels, which is a more flexible way of dealing with problems: we would like to see something like that replicated to deal with the problems of people who are not in a position to represent their own interests but who are in the middle of a conflict of interests.

A particular feature of Scottish Action for Dementia is our networking at local level through GLAD: Getting Local Action on Dementia. This is to counterbalance our work at national level: change has to come from below as well as from above. On the policy front over the last few years we have managed to establish dementia as top priority in the Health Service in Scotland through concerted actions and by influencing Government reviews of Services etc. This is illustrated in the government policy document *Scottish Health Authorities Review of Priorities for the Eighties and the Nineties* [4].

Dementia is a number one priority and the document sets out 24 key recommendations for services for dementia sufferers. Scottish Action for Dementia is very aware that this success must not go to our heads. The programme has to be implemented and there is an enormous gap between planning and implementation. We are working very consistently to monitor progress, to look at the way in which the Government is monitoring it, to look what they are monitoring, what sort of standards are we looking for, what policy of service and what sort of measures are being established. These are very difficult and tricky things to work on but nobody else in Scotland is working on them, particularly with regard to the fine tuning of what it is we are asking for and what expectations we want to set for services for sufferers.

Local development

The GLAD campaign is as important strategy for achieving necessary local developments. This is important as there is no universal blueprint for care services, as geography, services and commitments from professional workers vary from area to area. At national level we can not take account of that if we want to have changes and developments in regions. It has to come from people who have access to detailed information locally and can work through their local networks of influence: they can pin-point who it is within their regions they need to influence. In this way forums (such as GLAD) are very important mechanisms for feeding information into the planning process to politicians and for raising public awareness. Carer groups have a crucial role to play. Some of the possible actions are to lobby politicians, develop public education programmes, exchange experiences and ideas and feed consumer views to planners. Scottish Action for Dementia have developed a Starter Pack for GLAD [5] which we launched in advance of Dementia Awareness Week in 1989. Launching publications and promoting concerts are not only fun but also attract media coverage.

Conclusion

Despite our progress, there is still a lot to be achieved. We are not happy with the speed of development or the amount of resources put into services. A lot more work has to be done to raise public awareness of dementia. The new Scottish-based Dementia Services Development Centre promoted by Scottish Action on Dementia will be bringing together information, providing consultation and advice to health and social services and voluntary or state organisations. Based at the University of Stirling it will cater for Scotland initially and will then hopefully provide a service throughout the UK. Eventually it will also contribute to a network of international links with other centres. It will form a sophisticated dementia information exchange and collate information on evaluative research, bringing together briefing packs which would be of very practical use to people who are developing services. The Scottish Office is part-funding this Centre which does not have a big staff team at the moment. It has a director, a field worker, an information officer and a secretary, and really needs a lot more money to be able to carry out a full integrated programme where training can be brought in as well.

We all recognize the need for Alzheimer's Disease International to take dementia on to the political agenda and I hope that everybody will fully support any sort of move in that direction.

References

(1)   Killeen J. Dementia in Scotland: *Priorities for Care, Strategies for Change*. Scottish Action on Dementia, Edinburgh, 1986.

(2)   Hunter D, Norman A, Murphy E, *et al*. Dementia: *Developing Innovative Services in the Community*. Scottish Action on Dementia, Edinburgh, 1987.

(3)   McReadie R, Nichols D, Jacques A *et al*. *Dementia and the Law*. Scottish Action on Dementia, Edinburgh, 1988.

(4)   Scottish Health Service Planning Council. *Scottish Health Authorities Review of Priorities for the Eighties and the Nineties*. HMSO, London, 1988, pp 46-50.

(5)   Davidson E, Crofton E, Killeen J *et al*. *GLAD (Getting Local Action on Dementia) Starter Pack*. Scottish Action on Dementia, Edinburgh, 1989.

For all Scottish Action on Dementia books and a full publication list write to: Scottish Action on Dementia, 33 Castle St, Edinburgh EH2 3DN, Scotland (Telephone: 031-220 4886.

Chapter 12

BUILDING AWARENESS OF ALZHEIMER'S DISEASE AND DEVELOPING SERVICES FOR PATIENTS IN RURAL APPALACHIA: THE KENTUCKY EXPERIENCE

David Troxel[1], *MPH*, **Virginia Bell** [2], *MSW*. [1] *Alzheimer's Association – Lexington/Bluegrass Chapter, 801 S. Limestone #E, Lexington, KY 40508, and* [2] *Sanders-Brown Center on Aging, University of Kentucky, Lexington, KY, 40536-0230, USA*

Introduction

Other papers in this book also discuss approaches to outreach and education about Alzheimer's disease. While the cultures represented are very different, it is amazing how much there is in common: we are all fighting very hard to get the word out about Alzheimer's disease, increase services, help families, and assist persons with Alzheimer's disease. There has been no comprehensive survey of public awareness of dementia internationally. However, in the United States, Alzheimer's disease has become a "hot" disease, one that has attracted much attention. There is still a long way to go, but a few years ago no one knew what Alzheimer's disease was: now there is more and more awareness.

But if the United States is a leader in this area of public education, it is definitely trailing many other countries in the amount of services that are provided. The

National Alzheimer's Association, of which our group in the "bluegrass" area of Kentucky is a chapter, has been very effective in developing support groups throughout the country. There has also been a growth in respite care services, but most of these services tend to be in the private sector and there are very few programmes for people who do not have money. They also tend to be mostly located in urban areas of the United States. The Alzheimer's Association in Kentucky, which serves a large rural area, was determined to reach out to this rural area of Kentucky. This paper describes some of our programme's efforts and offers some very specific suggestions which I hope will transfer to other settings if they are rural.

Rural settings

I think it might be helpful to start off identifying some of the areas of difficulty that we face in America when we are looking at programmes in rural settings. The first one is transportation. While European countries generally have very good public transportation, there are only a few major cities in America that have good rapid transit or public transportation systems. In rural areas many families may not be able to afford a car, particularly in financially depressed areas. There is often no public transportation and older people are particularly victimised because they cannot get to the services that are available. Those older people who do drive, particularly in the mountains in our area, face a hazardous trip if they drive themselves. So transportation is a problem in rural areas.

Lack of medical services is another problem: but it is a problem that has partially eased with the over-supply of physicians in many areas of America. Yet in many rural counties in Kentucky there are still communities without a primary care physician, and there are certainly very few specialists such as neurologists and psychiatrists. A further problem is that general educational levels are low in eastern Kentucky. We have tens of thousands of people in Kentucky who are illiterate, an enduring shame of our society. This situation is of some significance: a brief study that I performed with a colleague looking at some of the standard carer literature on Alzheimer's disease showed that *The 36 Hour Day* requires an 11th grade education to really understand it. This finding gains more significance when we realise that many of the nursing home aides in Kentucky have a fifth to sixth grade reading level. So it is very difficult to take the accepted texts and literature we often see used in educational programmes for Alzheimer's disease, and use them in a rural setting.

The Kentucky way

In 1984 there were just three support groups in the State of Kentucky, a state with 4 million people and a surface area of 40,000 sq miles. It is, by and large, rural except for the cities of Lexington and Louisville. Since then we have made enormous progress, with services progressing from urban to rural areas. Lexington had the first respite programme, the Helping Hand. Today we also have eleven additional Alzheimer's-specific respite care programmes, which is remarkable for a smaller state in the USA.

How did we get to this improved position, particularly in eastern Kentucky? Our Alzheimer's Association began a programme about a year and a half ago which had the following objectives. First, to raise awareness of Alzheimer's disease. Many of our families reported that the doctors and nurses knew nothing about it, and that their neighbours also knew nothing. We felt it was very important to get a message out that to have severe memory loss at any age is not normal and that if you know someone having this problem they must seek medical attention. In effect our message was designed to try to help people who may have treatable dementias. I am sure all of us agree that even if you had to test 100 people with dementia and just found one treatable person, it would be worth the screening of those 100. In addition to raising awareness, other objectives included building support groups and respite programmes. Finally, we also wanted to provide training opportunities for professionals.

How did we achieve these objectives? First of all we actually went to the local people, talked with them about their problems, and did a needs assessment. As a result we hired two local people: we did not bring Lexington City people into the mountains but hired two local residents to be our Regional Co-ordinators. We also established offices in the area and tried to give them a sense of permanence. It has been said that often people or agencies may start a programme in rural communities and never follow through. As a result we were careful to display that we were very concerned about long-term commitment. Finally, Alzheimer's Awareness Days planned with the support of local politicians were held to stimulate interest in the problems of local patients and their families.

Volunteers

Volunteers are an important asset. We tried to involve many people in the rural areas and get volunteers, often not only from family care-givers but also from church groups and professional groups. Despite the fact that many people think that America is very hi-tech, in Kentucky we were about as low-tech as one can be. We literally knocked on people's doors, we stopped at doctors' offices and talked with people. By mobilizing an army of volunteers in a number of county areas going door to door, we managed to get the message to the people. Other approaches included town meetings and utilising local media.

One mistake we made arose out of what seemed to be a big success. On our first awareness blitz we went into a five-county area with about 30,000 people. We had about 75 volunteers carry out the approaches outlined above: media, door to door, a van with "Alzheimer's Awareness Week" and a local phone number painted on it. Incredibly we identified about 180 possible Alzheimer's patients not previously identified. Now to contrast this number Lexington, with a quarter of a million people, only has about 800 people in our Alzheimer's disease support group: so to find 180 potential AD people in a rural five-county area is extraordinary. This seemed to be a success until we began working with these families and realised

81

that there were few medical services nearby, poor transportation services, only two of the five counties had support groups (many people don't like to go to the county next door – in eastern Kentucky, you stay in your own county) and there were no respite programmes in this area. So here we had identified these people and we couldn't necessarily help them. In the end, the situation was not as bad as it might have seemed because we were able to get many to physicians and others travelled to the city for help. We provided all the families with information about caring and tried to help them do a better job as care-givers.

However, it was clear that we weren't really prepared to deal with this big public-health education mission when there were no services in place to help. So we backed up a little bit and during the last year we have been focusing very heavily on creating support groups which we think are the key to everything else. From our experience, families who utilise support groups are more likely to seek help and more likely to go to respite care programmes. In conjunction with the state of Kentucky, five Alzheimer's respite care programmes are now active in eastern Kentucky. The University of Kentucky has started an Outreach Clinic in the heart of one rural area: every two months a neurologist and social work team actually comes to see people – they treat indigent people free of charge. We have also tried to get a contact person in every county even where we don't have a support group – so there is a local person for a family to go to.

The importance of training

Having done this, we realise that we really needed to make a long-term invest-ment in training as well. With help from the Steele–Reese Foundation of New York, we have created something called the Teaching/Learning Centre for Dementia Specific Care, which offers scholarships to ten rural professionals every six months. They come to Lexington for two days of intensive lectures and work hands-on in a day-care programme for people with Alzheimer's disease. Training emphasizes the "do's and don'ts" of caring for persons with dementia. During the next several years we hope to train forty or fifty people very intensively. Not only are we going to train medical professionals but we are going to offer training to clergy, health planners and students. We have also targetted nursing-home aides, where we think there is a major need.

There are some principles for working in rural areas. It is important to have a clear message. Alzheimer's professionals sometime get so tuned into the idea that there is no prevention that they ignore treatable dementias. A most effective message is that memory loss is not a normal part of ageing and to seek help if you are having problems. Other important messages are to advertise the availability and importance of support groups, and encouraging families to use other services. Materials must also be appropriate: reading levels may need to be simplified for a rural area. This is a challenge to all of us to look at our own materials to see if they are appropriate for our population. Appropriate teaching methods are also important: adult learners are different and programmes for care-givers, nursing aides and others should treat them like adults and involve them in the planning of the programme wherever possible. The lecture format is often very inappropriate: role playing can provide a more useful teaching and learning environment.

Attention to the media is also very important. In the USA we are very television-orientated but in rural areas radio is very important. The biggest impact is made when a family member goes public and talks about their problems. One can just feel the walls crumbling down and the "stigma" of Alzheimer's disease dissolving when the Mayor's wife says "my husband has Alzheimer's disease".

Conclusion

My final advice would be to not repeat the mistake we made and plunge into your education programme without first building your services. It is very critical to think upstream in terms of public health: by thinking upstream and looking at the problem at large we can often avoid mistakes. We need to know why there are barriers to services in rural area, to know about transportation and the other features outlined above. It is very important for all of us to move beyond brochures: we need to maintain a sustained effort and to attack from a variety of fronts, not only to increase services but also to increase awareness.

Carers, Professionals and Alzheimer's Disease. D O'Neill ed © 1991 John Libbey & Company Ltd

Chapter 13

QUESTIONS OF LOVE AND CARE – HOW CONTEMPORARY DRAMAS EXPLORE THE NATURE AND EFFECTS OF ALZHEIMER'S DISEASE

Patricia M Troxel *PhD, MA, Dept of English, California Polytechnic State University, San Luis Obispo, CA 93407, USA*

In the final moments of *Do You Remember Love?*, George and Barbara Hollis attend a banquet honouring her as the recipient of the Longfellow Award for outstanding poetry. Barbara, an Alzheimer's patient, is unable to deliver her acceptance speech. Her husband rushes to join her at the podium. With his voice cracking, he reads Barbara's carefully written words, "Don't be afraid to laugh because it is the one thing we have that is ours alone. Our one pure invention. Use it when you think of me. Although I have forgotten many things, I do remember love. Love is our purest gift". While certainly a powerful and poignant conclusion to the drama, this statement offers an important link between a patient's experience of the disease and the artistic expression of that disease. By asserting that humour and compassion are essential to living with Alzheimer's disease, the writer Vicky Patike through her character, Barbara Hollis, reminds us that the artist's style, genre and tone are essential to the effective survival or the "life" of a dramatic enactment of this disease. The work and the patient share a need and a desire to express what may no longer be expressible.

And while most dramas share a classic literary objective, what Horace defined as "to teach and to delight", plays which focus on illness carry a double burden for they must not only artistically express, but they must also impart accurate and

85

specific information about the disease, and transform negative or simplistic audience attitudes and/or responses to that disease. Thus the style and structure of the drama is most often dominated by what is known as Agitprop technique, "agitation and propaganda" rather than traditional entertainment styles that we expect at a good night out. Agitprop theatre stresses the need for direct and immediate action, usually political or social, by the audience. An example of this style can be seen in plays which deal with AIDS, such as Larry Kramer's drama, *The Normal Heart,* which advocates not only major changes in legislation about AIDS but also takes issue with the *New York Times'* reporting of the disease.

Drama and Alzheimer's

Yet for both artists and those who deal with any aspect of disease, it is essential to understand how and why specific literary and performance choices are being made. Why and how does Alzheimer's disease become the centre-point of many recent dramas? And what impact should those dramas have on our awareness of, and response to, this disease?

To explore the why, the how, and the end result, I have selected three recent American dramas; *Do You Remember Love?* an 1985 commercial television drama written by Vicky Patike, *Day-Trips,* a 1988 play by Jo Carson which premièred in 1989 in Los Angeles and *Lucy's Lapses,* a 1987 comic opera commissioned by the Portland Oregon Opera Company with a libretto by Laura Harrington and a score by Christopher Drobny. While all are written by women and feature female protagonists, each offers distinctly different styles and treatments of the subject. Each also suggests the range of dramatic performance venues – from a filmed play to stage-play to opera. We should also note that the composition dates reflect a rise in public consciousness of Alzheimer's disease; AIDS dramas also increase in number as public awareness of AIDS increases.

But my principle interest in these three works is that they display a range of artistic approach to this subject, and as such teach us about the power and impact that Alzheimer's disease has for a modern artist and his/her audience. *Do You Remember Love?* is primarily concerned with imparting information; it is a drama focused on disease. *Day-Trips* deals with a grand-mother, mother and daughter and what the dramatist calls their madnesses; it is a play focused on the individual – the care-giver and the patient. *Lucy's Lapses* is a stylised ironic metaphor for isolation, self determination and loss; it is a comic opera focused on disease as artistic property. Each dramatist enhances our understanding of these foci by making specific choices in drama and performance.

The television drama

Do You Remember Love? offers a story of Barbara Hollis, an eccentric college teacher and poet who begins to experience memory loss, changes in behaviour and personality, and language dysfunction. After she becomes physically violent and on recommendation of a family friend, a psychiatrist, she and her husband,

George, seek diagnosis and treatment at their local medical centre. The battery of tests (all fully and accurately represented) reveal nothing and their neurologist diagnoses Alzheimer's disease. George continues to serve as the sole care- giver despite offers from Barbara's mother, friends and recommendations that he attend a support group. Barbara's case progresses quite rapidly and by the end of the drama, George is forced to acknowledge his own needs, the value of the support group and his family, and his continuing love and support for his wife. Barbara comes to terms with her situation, rejects suicide and in her acceptance speech for the poetry prize acknowledges the fear, the frustration and the joy of her life.

Yet for all the poignancy, compassion and accuracy of the script and the perfor- mances, *Do You Remember Love?* remains simply the story of the disease not the story of the individuals who experience it. In dramatic terms it is a "problem play" – a play of the traditional genre known as the "well-made" play. This type of drama follows a clear, even methodical structure. It usually offers stereotypic characters and shows a move from unhappiness to happiness while reinforcing conventional values. The protagonist always starts from a great height and suffers a great fall. In the case of the play *Do You Remember Love?*, Barbara returns from a pleasant sabbatical to discover she is under consideration for tenure, the height of academic success. As the disease progresses and her health declines, so do Barbara's fortunes and her sense of well-being. The vicissitudes of life characteristic of a protagonist in such a play are dutifully registered in this script. Despite some very powerful performances by Joanne Woodward and Richard Kiley the majority of characters are stereotyped. There is a callous nurse in a nursing home, a jealous colleague, the prodigal son, etc. Since the traditional "happy" ending cannot be offered – there is no cure for Alzheimer's disease – the dramatist constructs an alternative happiness. Barbara wins the greatest poetry award, one given at ten year intervals, and she maintains her understanding of the love and respect in which her family and friends hold her. At the end of the drama we feel as good as we can feel because this play offers us both emotional resolution and intelligent and palatable material about a frightening disease. The artistic drama and style proffer a sense of redemption from the dis-ease which accompanies disease.

The experimental play

In sharp contrast, *Day-Trips* offers us a very experimental dramatic piece. Jo Carson claims that the work is "about dying and madness and duty and the cracks in the world that the dying see that the living don't ... these are stories about my mother, my grand-mother and me. They must somehow stay the real stories they are. I have kept our real names." While asserting the reality of her play, Carson uses a variety of stylised, non-narrative strategies for exploring the situation. She avoids any clear linear sense of beginning, middle and end. Instead she suggests that the cycles, the repetitions that characterise an Alzheimer's patient, are no different from the cycles that seem to occur naturally between a grand-mother and daughter or mother and daughter. She allows each character fantasies which

87

are enacted as if they were real stories. She also weaves the story in and out of time. Despite our awareness of the real time events, we are never certain of any specific time. One exchange of dialogue and action does not lead logically to the next. It is as if Carson helps us to understand how the Alzheimer's patient experiences time by encouraging an audience to see past and present time as simultaneously experienced and equally valued. As she puts it, "experience is cumulative".

Carson does provide a narrator in her autobiographical character of Jo because she is the writer of the piece as well as the participant in it. She narrates because she is the only character with a linear sensibility, because she actually lived as a care-giver and a playwright. She can see the past and present as distinct. Having provided this narrative voice, she often uses it to explain what other characters say, or to provide support or justification for her words or actions. It is Jo as narrator who reminds the audience that "this disease eventually strips off the stuff that makes us human and in the stripping, memories take on a pentimento of the life". In acknowledging pentimento, Jo turns our attention away from a disease taking its course and towards the relationships and experiences of those it touches. This drama explores the individuals not the disease; it is particularly the story of the patient and the care-giver. And as such this drama offers only occasional moments of optimism. The drama returns repeatedly to death, news-papers clippings about suicide, death pacts of care-givers and patients, and Jo's own fantasies about a violent end to the madness of her life with mother and grand-mother. While Alzheimer's disease is the cause of her mother's madness it is also directly and indirectly the cause of Jo's.

The opera

Lucy's Lapses, subtitled "a comic opera in one act", is distinctly different from both *Day-Trips* and *Do You Remember Love?* While the other dramas explore the disease or the individuals who must live with the disease, this piece is interested in the artistic possibilities of the disease. *Lucy's Lapses* is a slightly tangled narrative of Lucy, a 50-year-old mother, her husband Biff, a 50-year-old high school football coach, her daughter Carrie, a beauty contest winner who takes dictation by day and sings in a lounge by night, and their son Danny, an ammunitions expert who is currently in gaol for his explosive activities. We are also aware that she has an off-stage lover, Beau, 19 years old and a high school football player. He becomes the obscure object of Lucy's desire during various recitatives and arias.

Harrington also reveals her set requirements in the instructions which preface her libretto. They include "a large old-fashioned claw-footed bath-tub, a grand piano, an enormous hour-glass filled with mementoes, and bars for Danny's gaol". These set elements typify the slightly exaggerated style of the entire work. They also reflect the dramatist's and composer's concern with Alzheimer's disease as a metaphor for lack of communication and harmony amongst the family and in contemporary society. This is a dramatic world in chaos, one born of an inability to remember the essential connections that make one contented and complete.

That insistence on connection is highlighted by a somewhat ludicrous plot centring around Lucy's desire to put an end to her frustrations, her suffering and her family's embarrassment. Through various encounters with family members, including a major accident in the bath-tub with Beau which Lucy survives but Beau does not, Lucy finally remembers the ultimate connection which her son has been struggling to give her – "electricity and water". Following this revelation she triumphantly dumps the electric lamp into the bath-tub, producing a great explosion and achieving the end she sought from the opening lyrics – her death.

The events seem outlandish and even macabre, and the notion of a comic opera may seem at odds with the subject matter: however, I think it is important to consider what this drama does reveal about Alzheimer's disease. I also don't mean to suggest that the work is devoid of any sensitivity to the disease or the individuals it affects. Midway through the opera Lucy sings a very poignant repetitive melody entitled "Haunted": "The memories haunt me. They come out of the blue. The memories are me. What else can I do?". At the same time, her husband and daughter sing over these repeated lines such phrases as: "You could forget. You could correct. You could erase. Cut and paste". Accompanied by a truly haunting score, this repetitive chorus runs contrapuntal to the insistent descant of the father and daughter and effectively conveys the frustration, anger and defeat experienced by both family members and Alzheimer's patients. While the haunting is clearly intended as a metaphor for an artistic half memory or the memory of a memory, it is no less a real experience. This dramatic piece is composed of vocal music, the traditional symbol for harmony and wholeness, and yet it is linked to a symbol of total disorder and lack of control – Alzheimer's disease. The dramatist and composer make order out of disorder, artistic connection out of frayed ends and most importantly art out of dis-ease. They achieve a kind of *commedia*, if we define *commedia* as happiness and order out of unhappiness and chaos.

Different approaches

To briefly summarise, we have three distinct dramas which focus on Alzheimer's disease and yet each has a special artistic objective often reflected in its method and style of presentation. *Do You Remember Love?* is a traditional drama, presented in a popular medium which essentially seeks to inform its audience about the nature, effects and care possibilities for patients with Alzheimer's. In doing so, it is careful to present diagnosis and treatment. *Day-Trips* is an experimental drama which explores the relationship among female family members including an Alzheimer's patient. It also explores all characters' desires for "release" and despite its experimental style and structure, insists on its place as a real drama about real people. Finally, *Lucy's Lapses,* a comic opera, uses its ironic, macabre and musical style to call attention to the gap between our intellectual understanding and our emotional experience of that disease.

Women, victims and genetics

Before I conclude my analysis of these plays with some comments regarding artistic use and abuse, I should like to point out three important elements these dramas share. All these works are marked by gender, both that of the author and that of the central character/protagonist. In each case, the protagonist, the Alzheimer's patient, is both a mother and a wife, and the author, a woman with experience as a care-giver for an AD patient. As a result there is a feminization of this disease. By this I mean that each work, at some level, forces its audience to address three things. First, there is the subordinate position of the patient, a position frequently linked to a traditional role as the helpless female. Second, there is a victim/martyr stereotyping of the patient and to some extent the care-giver. And third, there is often a genetic anxiety among family members. This may be a fear that is accentuated by a cultural vision of the female as both nature and nurture.

In each case, we are presented with three protagonists and three dramatists who are women. Within the short span of each drama those women become utterly dependent on care-givers as their AD progresses. At no time do we see them function as successful, independent adults. This reinforces a notion of weakness, insufficiency and helplessness which is characteristic of neither the disease nor the feminine in culture. Furthermore this characterisation contributes to a deadly stereotyping of the Alzheimer's patient as a victim or martyr to the disease. One must always distinguish between the notion of tragedy and the tragic if we are to change the attitude that the Alzheimer's patient and his/her family has somehow brought the disease upon themselves. In tragedy, choice and control are essential; a character's desire or decision to go left or right is often what defines tragedy. Tragic is the poignant – a regret or an element of chance. Alzheimer's disease is something that we should associate with that poignancy, that element of chance and not with tragedy or the element of choice. Finally, as Susan Sontag has argued, disease is often presented as a metaphor for an artistic fantasy, not as an illness; it is important to remember that illness is not a metaphor.

Conclusion

There are three important points we need to think about when we are looking at dramas that focus on Alzheimer's disease. First and foremost, we need to see a balance between artistic choices and the presentation of information. We are not simply presenting a disease, we are presenting individuals. Second, we need to avoid a tendency to establish a cause-and-effect relationship between Alzheimer's disease and the patient or the care-giver. In other words, we want to be writing plays about the experience of Alzheimer's disease not about Alzheimer's disease as tragedy. Finally, we need to be very careful that we don't present plays as specifically feminine in choice. We need to see more dramas which present an Alzheimer's patient who is male and has a female care-giver or a patient who is female who has a male care-giver. In all cases we should always be aware that we are seeing ordinary people in extraordinary circumstances: a good Alzheimer's disease drama is one which reminds the audience of the universality, the specificity and the immediacy of the disease.

SECTION 4
Training for Carers

Carers, Professionals and Alzheimer's Disease. D O'Neill ed © 1991 John Libbey & Company Ltd

Chapter 14

TRAINING CARE-GIVERS

C Gendron *PhD*, L Poitras *PhD*, DP Dastoor *MA*, NB Levine *MD*,
*Douglas Hospital Centre, 6875 LaSalle Blvd, Verdun, Qc. H4H 1R3,
Canada*

The immense problem of care giving and its impact on persons assuming this role have become a serious cause for concern for health professionals who work in the field of dementia. Care-takers who, on the one hand, can be considered as therapeutic partners or collaborators in the sense that they care for patients, can also be viewed as potential clients themselves in view of the consequences of their role on their personal life style and emotional life.[1, 2, 3]

The amount of burden or stress which is perceived by care-takers will depend on a number of interacting factors.[4] These include:

(i) the severity of the illness of the care receiver;

(ii) the nature and the quality of the relationship between the care-receiver and the care-taker;

(iii) the family dynamics, when the care-receiver is a family member.

Other factors are:

(iv) the social support network, its availability and its intensity;

(v) socio-demographic variables such as age, sex and ethnic background of the care-giver and care-receiver.

We also need to consider:

(vi) the care-givers' other involvement such as work and their own family problems;

and finally:

(vii) the care-takers' own abilities to deal with stress.

This paper will deal specifically with these abilities to cope with stress.

Coping with stress

These personal abilities play a central role in Lazarus' theory of stress. They are considered as mediators between the stressful event – in our case the care-taking situation – and the way the person will react to the situation. According to the model, the persons' skills (such as communication, interpersonal and social skills), the perception of their role and their strategies to cope with stress in general, will influence the way they will react to their situation. If we extrapolate from this model, it appears that care-takers who lack in such personal resources would be more at risk of reacting with maladaptive behaviour, i.e. psychological distress or physical problems, to any stressful situation. Examples of care-givers at risk are numerous:

(i) those who set **unrealistic demands** upon themselves, who say to themselves "I can do this all on my own, without any help";

(ii) those who have had a **conflicting relationship** with the care-receiver. For example, a patient who has been an alcoholic all his life and who is now cared for by a wife who has a lot of ambivalent feelings (involving guilt and anger) towards her care-giving role, and has difficulty in coping with the situation because of these feelings;

(iii) those who **deny** the severity of the illness and its prognosis and consequently have unrealistic expectations and plans concerning the care-receiver.

Yet another at-risk group are:

(iv) those who have had difficulties in their own past, dealing with problems or stressful situations and have reacted with severe depression or anxiety to the death of a relative, to a divorce or to another personal event.

Our research group at Douglas Hospital did a study of the profiles of a small sample of care-takers. [5] We found that the most skilful copers were those who had superior ability in terms of problem solving. They had an active coping style. They used positive self-statements, and they were rated as internal on the Rotter Locus of Control Scale, which means that they attributed to themselves the control of their situation, rather than leaving it for others to resolve. Based on these observations and on Lazarus' model, our group designed an intervention programme which we call: "SET – Supporter's Endurance Training", specifically for care-takers of Alzheimer patients.[6] This programme focuses on improving the coping skills of care-takers.

Characteristics of the programme

In this intervention, which we devised in 1982, the emphasis is placed on the care-takers' subjective burden, i.e. on the emotional reaction to their situation as well as on their perception of the burden, rather than on the objective burden *per se*. Our intervention was designed to be flexible, adapting to each care-taker's individual needs.

In the first interview with the care-taker, we not only try to identify their needs for respite and support, but also their conception of what the care-taker role is for them as well as their reaction to this responsibility and their perception of the burden. In order to help us in this assessment, we have devised an instrument which we call the Inventory of Hypothetical Problem Situations. This consists in showing the care-taker excerpts of a videotape or photographs of situations which illustrate ten typical problems which are currently experienced by care-takers of Alzheimer patients. Each of the ten vignettes that we show them illustrates a daughter who is taking care of her demented mother. For example, in the first vignette that we show the care-taker, the daughter, is in the process of cleaning-up the sofa on which her mother has just urinated. While looking at this particular vignette, we ask the care-taker three questions. The first question is a projective type of question. We ask them what is the person thinking while she is cleaning this mess? We are trying to see what the care-takers would be thinking through the videotape model. The second question we ask pertains to their coping strategy and coping style in general. We ask them to select one of five statements best describing their own reaction. For example: (a) Would they do nothing in response to such a problem? (b) Would they concentrate on positive thoughts to get through it? (c) Would they be thinking of placing the mother in a nursing home or hospitalizing her, because it is too much of a burden for them? (d) Would they consult others for advice or help? (e) Would they try to find their own original solution to this problem? The third and last question concerns their own problem-solving ability and coping strategy, and we ask them what solution they would have for this particular problem? We do this for the ten problems, each time going through the three different questions.

Assessment

The responses are collated with information from the assessment interview, particularly information on the personal and social history of the care-taker. For instance, finding out what types of problems, such as the death of a child or a divorce, they have had to deal with during their life and how did they react to them? In what ways did the person try to cope with it? What methods did they use? This type of information can be very useful to devise an intervention that is based on the particular needs of each care-taker. With the information gathered we can set-up individual goals for each care-taker and the intervention can be planned accordingly. The intervention focuses mainly on the self-management of the care-taker rather than on the management of the care-receiver. Some programmes use cognitive and behavioural techniques, such as problem-solving and operant conditioning, to improve the care-taking situation. In our programme, we focus mainly on the care-takers themselves and of course, this can have an indirect impact on the care-taking situation.

The approach that we use is very similar to approaches used in industrial settings – the stress management programmes that are offered to managers and to executives in industry, to help them cope with the daily problems.

It is important to mention that this intervention was conceived as only one component of a more comprehensive programme for care-takers and it is seen as a complement to the other types of services. For instance, a complement to education, respite care, support, home care and support groups: it is not seen as a replacement for any of these services. For some care-takers, we found that this intervention may serve as a preliminary step towards the acceptance of further help. For example, a lot of care-takers in our area refuse, at the beginning, to attend support groups, for fear of leaving their relative at home. Some care-takers consider seeking help from others as a failure on their part to be able to cope effectively with their problem. Others will wait until a crisis situation arises, or until they are physically or emotionally totally exhausted, before they seek help. Spouses appear to be the most important target population for this type of intervention since spouses are less inclined to use informal and formal support.[7,8] Wives in particular, seem to have difficulty abandoning exclusive care-giving responsibility and according to Zarit are more susceptible to experience guilt when they choose to do so.[9]

When the care-taker's personal expectations, beliefs and attitudes towards their role are unrealistic and overly demanding, they often will need help to examine, review and take into account their own personal needs and limitations in this situation. New priorities often have to be set in order to help them, not only in relation to their emotional reaction to the situation, but also in order to arrive at a better equilibrium between the patient's needs and their own individual needs. This type of process can require several individual sessions with the care-taker. We usually have eight to ten sessions.

Therapeutic techniques

The therapeutic techniques which we use in our intervention depends on the types of difficulties which are experienced by the care-taker. Among the different cognitive behavioural techniques which are available, four seem particularly useful for care-takers. The first is the relaxation training. Of the several methods available, we use Jacobson's method. The second is assertiveness training.[10] The third is the cognitive approach, where we tend to use Beck's[11] model. Finally, there is the problem-solving training techniques, such as D'Zurilla's[12] approach. We will do briefly an overview of each of these techniques and see how we can apply them to care-takers.

Relaxation training

Relaxation training is a technique that we use to improve the person's capacity to deal with stress by giving them practical means to do so. This part of the training involves more than simple relaxation exercises. Caretakers are also taught to identify and to recognize their personal signs of stress. Do they react with a backache, muscle ache, headache? What is their way of reacting to stress? As well, we try to get them to identify the particular events or situations which seem most stressful for them. For this purpose, we ask the people to keep a diary at home of the most stressful moments of the week, in between the sessions. With the help of this information, we adapt the relaxation technique to the particular problem of the care-taker.

For example, if a care-taker is very anxious when he is feeding his wife, or if he becomes very irritable and anxious at that moment, it may be useful for this person to use a relaxation technique prior to meal time, in order to have a calmer attitude. For another person, it could be useful to use relaxation exercises prior to bed time if this person has difficulty in sleeping and suffers from insomnia from time to time. We ask the care-takers to practice the exercises in between the sessions and then to report back on their experience, so that we can make the necessary adjustment with them.

We find that it is very useful to combine relaxation training with cognitive training. The occurrence of disruptive, negative thoughts or anxiety-provoking thoughts during relaxation can be counter-productive and even greatly diminish beneficial effects of relaxation. So, it becomes very important to address our intervention at these thoughts as well.

Assertiveness training

Assertiveness training is very useful in that, as previously noted, many care-takers have difficulty in asking for help. Some report feeling very uncomfortable asking their family members to help them, saying "Why should I ask them? They should offer me their own help". For example, parents will often avoid asking their children for help, for fear of disturbing them, saying that they are already involved with their family, their work and their own obligations, so they should not be involved in the burden. The problem may be different in that a more equitable sharing of caring tasks is necessary when many people are involved in care-giving, not only in the care-giving itself, but in helping the care-giver also.

The first step in the assertiveness training is to assess the care-takers interpersonal and social skills, so that we can have a good impression of what the problem is. In order to do this, we often use role playing. For example, a care-taker might tell us that it is difficult for her to ask her sister to help in the care of their mother. We would ask her to pretend that the therapist is the sister and to speak to the therapist as she would to her sister. We often observe that the care-taker is not sufficiently clear in her requests. For example saying: "Well, maybe one day you can come and see mother and help me", instead of saying: "Well you know I would really appreciate it if you would come once a week to help me with mother". So, the way the person is addressing the sister has a very important effect on the result of the request. In some cases, we also do family interventions for this type of situation in order to gain a better understanding of the family dynamics. It is sometimes very helpful in sorting out the exact nature of the care-taker's problem, and also provides guidance in the sharing of tasks and responsibilities.

A second step in the assertive training intervention involves finding out the motives of the care-taker for not asking for help. Do they feel guilty? Do they fear refusal? Do they want to avoid indebtedness to someone who would answer their call for help? All these kinds of reasons need to be discussed during the sessions. For the training itself, we use role playing, discussion and occasionally, self-help books, for care-takers who enjoy reading. The assertive training technique itself involves explaining, modelling and demonstrating to the care-taker what an assertive behaviour is. So the therapist needs to be quite active in all these techniques. Many sessions may be necessary and progress can be slow. The care-taker has to be trained and there is a lot of practice and trial-and-error, and therapists need to give a lot of feedback so that the person will learn the desired behaviour. It is also very useful and desirable to use the person's problems as examples for role playing instead of hypothetical situations because, then the person can really transfer whatever is learned in a training session into their home environment much more easily than if hypothetical situations are used.

It can be very useful to combine the assertive training with problem-solving training. For example, if a care-taker is asking for more leisure time or for more participation from another member of their family, the person needs to be not only assertive, but also to be a good negotiator in order to negotiate the time with this person. This type of behaviour may require problem-solving training in order to help them in their decision-making process. The combination of the two techniques – assertiveness and problem-solving – can also be useful in cases of spouses who have difficulty in assuming their new decisional and assertive role. This is particularly true for the spouse who relied on her husband to take decisions all their life, and after all this time it is difficult to assume this new role without any help or guidance.

Cognitive techniques

Cognitive techniques are a very important part of the training because according to Lazarus' model, a lot of the adaptation or adjustment to stress is influenced by our cognitive processes, i.e. those processes by which we appraise a situation, and evaluate our personal capacities to deal with it successfully.[13] For the care-taker, this may mean the person will be very much influenced by what the role of care-taker means to him. Does he feel he has the capacities to do it and also does he feel he can do it effectively? So, this section of the training programme concentrates on the person's attitudes, their beliefs and expectations concerning their role. It concentrates on their internal dialogue and, more specifically, on the negative thoughts that they may have, especially in stressful situations.

An important step is to help the care-taker learn to recognize their personal style of internal dialogue. Do they tend to predict the worst catastrophes or to dramatize whenever a problem arises? With the use of positive self-talk and other cognitive techniques, the care-taker can learn to view his/her problems in a different light. Through such training, it is hoped that the care-taker will have a more positive outlook in response to problems, highlighting their own capacities to deal with difficulties. "I can do this: there is no point feeling sorry for myself: maybe tomorrow will be different" are good examples of positive self-statements. Role playing is used to illustrate the internal dialogue during the session. Again, we ask the person to practice at home, as a lot of practice is involved in all these techniques.

Problem-solving training

The last technique is problem-solving training. This kind of technique can be used when the person tends to panic, to become angry in reaction to a problem or to ignore the problem. Problem-solving abilities can be assessed during the first session. Questionnaires can be used, of which there is a whole variety in the literature. The training itself involves more than just helping the care-taker to find appropriate solutions to their problems. We try to initiate the person into the different steps of the problem-solving and decision-making process. The format is not theoretical: we ask the person to bring their personal problems and we try to encourage them to resolve these personal problems.

At the same time, these problems become models for the learning of the process of problem-solving. The care-taker is taught to clarify whatever problem arises, to attempt to identify the problem before labelling it, and to obtain additional information to further understand it. For example, if at some point the patient becomes incontinent of urine, it may be important for the care-taker to ask questions such as: "When did the problem start? Is it only at night? Does it happen once a day? Is it only when he is in his bed?", etc..., in order to envisage the different possible solutions. These may be to consult a physician to see if it is a urine infection or begin a toilet training schedule, etc... . Depending on the accurate identification of the problem, the solutions can be very different, and it gives the care-taker a better idea of the different solutions possible if the precise nature of the problem is clear. As a last step, the care-taker tries one of the solutions and evaluates its effectiveness.

It is important to keep in mind with all of these techniques that the successful acquisition of any of them will depend on multiple rehearsals of these techniques. Much will also depend, of course, on the care-taker's motivation and desire to improve these skills. Some care-takers will protest at first that this is useless, and that they will never learn this, and why should they learn? Or else, they complain that they are too old to learn, etc... . This reluctance has to be dealt with during the first session in order for them to accept this kind of training.

Conclusion

We evaluated our programme in 1986, using a single-case design methodology, and we found positive results and positive changes among carers who received the training on a measure of assertiveness, a measure of anxiety, perceived tolerance time (the length of time they would think they could cope with these difficulties), and also on their coping style.[14] The results suggested that skills training with care-takers was an approach that was worth further development. We are still in the process of doing research on this particular package. We are developing a group intervention, as the group format has the advantage of being more economical than the individual session format.

In conclusion, there is a need for large-scale outcome studies that would evaluate the relative effectiveness of different components of a comprehensive programme designed for care-takers. For instance, the effects of educational approaches, counselling strategies, stress-management interventions, family based behavioural techniques, support groups and relief services on the care-taker's coping abilities need to be evaluated. From a clinical point of view, it would also be helpful to obtain the profiles of care-takers who respond best to each type of intervention.

References

(1) Fadden G, Bebbington P, Kuipers L. The burden of care: the impact of functional psychiatric illness on the patient's family. *Br J Psychiatry* 1987, **150**, 285-292.

(2) Gilleard CJ. Problems posed for supporting relatives of geriatric and psychogeriatric day patients. *ACTA Psychiatr Scand* 1984, **70**, 198-208.

(3) Levine NB, Gendron CE, Dastoor DP, et al. Existential issues in the management of the demented elderly patient. *Am J Psychother* 1984, **38**, 215-223.

(4) Ory MG, Williams TF, Emr M, et al. *Families, Informal Supports and Alzheimer's Disease: Current Research and Future Agendas*. Dept. of Health and Human Services Task Force on Alzheimer's Disease, U.S., 1984.

(5) Levine NB, Dastoor DP, Gendron CE. Coping with dementia: a pilot study. *J Am Geriatr Soc.* 1983, **31**, 12-18.

(5) Levine NB, Gendron CE, Dastoor DP, et al. Supporter endurance training: a manual for trainers. *Clin Gerontologist* 1983, **2**, 15-23.

(7) Gilhooly MLM. Senile dementia: factors associated with care-giver's preference for institutional care. *Br J Med Psychol* 1986, **59**, 165-171.

(8) Barush AS. Problems and coping strategies of elderly spouse care-givers. *Gerontologist* 1988, **28**, *677-685*.

(9) Zarit SH, Todd PA, Zarit JM. Subjective burden of husbands and wives as care-givers: a longitudinal study. *Gerontologist* 1986, **26**, 260-266.

(10) Lange A, Jakubowski P. *Responsible Assertive Behaviour*. Champaign II: Research Press, 1976.

(11) Beck AT, Rush AJ, Shaw BF, Emery G. *Cognitive Therapy of Depression.*. New York: Guilford Press, 1979.

(12) D'Zurilla TJ. Problem-solving therapy. In: Dobson KS, ed, *Handbook of Cognitive-Behavioural Therapies*. New York: Guilford Press, 1988.

(13) Lazarus RS, DeLongis A. Psychological stress and coping in aging. *Am Psychologist* 1984, **38**, 245-254.

(14) Gendron CE, Poitras LR, Engels ML, et al. Skills training with supporters of the demented. *J Am Geriatr Soc* 1986; **34**, 875-880.

Carers, Professionals and Alzheimer's Disease. D O'Neill ed © 1991 John Libbey & Company Ltd

Chapter 15

LESS INSTITUTIONALIZATION AND LOWER STRESS AFTER A DEMENTIA CARERS PROGRAMME

H Brodaty *MD, FRACP, FRANZCP,* **M Gresham** *BAppSci (OT),*
Department of Academic Psychogeriatrics, Prince Henry Hospital, Little Bay, New South Wales 2036, Australia

Introduction

The unremitting burden of dementia falls mainly on the shoulders of families. As carers become demoralized, isolated, psychologically distressed and socially impaired, they become less able to support affected relatives at home. Interventions designed to alleviate the carers' burden and improve their coping skills may improve their quality of life and that of affected persons as well as delaying patients' placement in institutional care. We report a prospective controlled-intervention study of an intensive ten-day residential training programme for carers. The aim of the study was to assess the effects of training families in how to care for patients, usually spouses, suffering from dementia. We describe the details and effects this training course, the Dementia Carers' Programme, and compare the effects of the programme with two control groups – a Memory Retraining Group and a Waiting-List control group.

Dementia Carers' Programme

In the Dementia Carers' Programme, groups of four patients and carers were admitted together for ten days of intensive training. Organizing training and support for carers has many facets. We used several approaches. Group supportive psychotherapy sought to relieve carer psychological distress by allowing carers to ventilate feelings and to attend to grief, anticipatory mourning, carer burn-out and guilt. Medical staff provided carers with information about medical aspects of dementia such as diagnosis, prognosis and medication. Nurses talked to carers about various nursing skills, e.g. the approach to someone who is incontinent. A welfare officer outlined welfare services and the use of domiciliary services. We discussed legal and financial aspects of dementia – wills, emergencies, durable power of attorney. Other training included information about exercise from a physiotherapist; diet from a dietitian and the use of practical aids and safety and organization in the home from an occupational therapist. As there was so much information to absorb, carers received printed material as well.

One priority was to attempt to relieve marital stress as poor marital relationships can exacerbate the strain of spouses: 96 per cent of carers in this programme were spouses. We did this by discussing strategies in management of difficult behaviours, by helping the spouse to ventilate feelings of frustration and by holding an extended family session. In order to mobilize family support, we asked that as many of the people as possible who were concerned with the patient come in for this session. Up to 20 people would come into the room and talk about how this whole network could work together to help look after the affected relative in a very practical way. It was very interesting to note the dynamics that emerged. Some families came together in a very positive way. In other families feuds started or dormant conflicts erupted; these could be difficult to handle.

Isolation, assertiveness and coping skills

Another difficulty reported by carers is their isolation, which we attempted to combat by introducing carers to the Alzheimer's Disease and Related Disorders Society, by forming carers into potential small self-help groups of four, and by discussing possible ways that carers could nurture and maintain contacts. We specifically tried to make carers feel comfortable about taking time away from their sick spouse or relative. We found that assertiveness training for carers and help in the adoption of new roles was particularly helpful, especially for women, many of whom had never been the public face of the family. In many cases they were not used to talking to bureaucracy, handling finances or taking on the new roles that arise when one becomes a carer and takes over the other partner's roles. The next part of our approach was to train carers in coping skills such as communication and use of activities. However, it was not sufficient to teach carers about such strategies: it was also important that they practise them. As both carers and patients were living in, this was done during the course. For example, having been taught the basics of communication with a dementia patient, carers could video-tape and then analyse their communication with patients. It was thus not merely theoretical, but very practical with a lot of feed- back.

Patients and control groups

Meanwhile the patients were involved in their part of the programme: environmental reality orientation, memory retraining, reminiscence therapy and general ward activities. The two control groups were the Memory Retraining Programme, where the patients were admitted on their own and underwent the patient programme outlined above; and the group who had been on the waiting list for the Dementia Carers' Programme for six months.

Results

There were a hundred pairs in the programme, only four of whom were not included in the analysis because of insufficient data. Seventy-three per cent of the patients had Alzheimer's disease. There dementia was mild, as evidenced by their average score of 1.1 on the Clinical Dementia Rating scale and their mean Mini Mental State Examination score of 17 out of 30. Carers were slightly younger, and a surprisingly high proportion (52 per cent) were male. They were predominantly middle class. About 35 per cent were already members of the Alzheimer's Disease and Related Disorders Society prior to entering the study. All participants entering the programmes completed them.

All patients deteriorated over the twelve months of follow-up. No matter what we did, or to which programme they were allocated, patients declined in a linear fashion on all measures used – the Mini Mental State Examination, the two Blessed scales, the Clinical Dementia Rating scale, the Activities of Daily Living and the Problem Behaviour check list of Gilleard *et al.* If we were unable to influence the patients' cognitive and behavioural decline, could we make any impression on the psychological morbidity of the carers? Our main hypothesis was that we could decrease their psychological strain by our residential training programme. We measured this with the General Health Questionnaire (GHQ), on which a high score suggests psychological morbidity, and a low score psychological well-being. There was a steady decline in GHQ scores over a twelve-month period for carers in the Dementia Carers' Programme. So when carers received training, psychological well-being improved. In contrast, GHQ scores rose over the twelve months among carers in the Memory Training Programme, i.e. the carers without formal training suffered an increase in psychological morbidity. These differences were statistically significant ($p < 0.01$). Curiously, the psychological health of the carers who waited six months to receive training remained static.

Less institutionalization

The second stage of the study was a census carried out on the patients about thirty months after the programme had finished. Five patients had died at home and twelve in institutions, but there were no significant difference in the number of deaths between groups. However, there was a very significant difference in the number of people staying at home compared to those admitted to nursing homes or similar institutions. Sixty-five per cent of those in the Dementia Carers' Programme were still at home thirty months after entry into the trial. In the Memory Retraining Group, where carers had received no training, 25 per cent were still at home, an almost three-fold difference. The Waiting-List group had an intermediate result, with 40 per cent of patients still at home. Although these are approximate figures the difference between carers receiving training and the carers not receiving training was highly significant.

Conclusion

This Dementia Carers' Programme has the capacity to lower the rate of institutionalization, while decreasing carer psychological strain. Carer psychological strain has been shown to decrease after institutionalization of the patient, but we found that we could decrease the carer's psychological strain and demoralization while keeping the patient at home. We also found that consumption of health services such as medical care, medication, respite care, day centres and hospitalization were either not increased or even less for both patients and carers from the Dementia Carers' Programme over twelve months of follow-up. We have subsequently reported this intervention was cost effective. Thus a multi-disciplinary, intensive training course for carers leads to less institutionalization of patients, less strain on carers and possibly less use of health services.

References

Brodaty H, Gresham M. Effects of a training programme to reduce stress in carers of patients with dementia. *British Medical Journal* 1989, **299**, 1375-1379.

Brodaty H, Peters K. International Psychogeriatrics, 1991 (in press).

Carers, Professionals and Alzheimer's Disease. D O'Neill ed © 1991 John Libbey & Company Ltd

Chapter 16

EDUCATING ALZHEIMER'S DISEASE ASSOCIATION HELPERS TO SHARE THE CARE

E Kingsley, *School of Nursing, Curtin University, Bentley, Western Australia*, PM O'Connor, *Home Respite Service, Alzheimer's Disease and Related Disorders Association of Western Australia, Subiaco, Western Australia*

Confidence is a vital prerequisite for successful caring. Confidence is engendered when workers know that they have the skills and support necessary to perform their work. Training and support are central to the efficient delivery of service to Alzheimer's Disease and Related Disorders Association (ADARDA) clients and their carers. Without an adequate introduction to the service and an orientation to the disease and without the necessary skills and ongoing support in their work, ADARDA helpers will not be able to give optimum service or receive optimum benefit from their work.

Education, support and administration are three major components of an agency's role in dealing with staff and volunteers. For new ADARDA helpers, the educative function is paramount as few recruits have previous training or experience in the area. Once helpers have become competent and confident in their role the agency's supportive role takes prominence. Working continuously with people with Alzheimer's disease can be stressful and helpers need consistent training and support to overcome any problems which might arise from the nature of the work. Overriding these two functions is the agency's administrative role which is to ensure that the delivery of care is of the highest quality and that the caring experience is a positive one for both clients and agency helpers.

107

Foundations of education programmes

In determining the type and nature of education and training that is required to ensure high quality service delivery, a first step is to consider the concepts of education and to determine the level, scope and content that is most appropriate for each type of helper and to the nature of work that they perform. All programmes must be:

(i) relevant to each helper, their existing knowledge and skills;

(ii) adequate for the tasks they will be called upon to perform;

(iii) appropriate to their level of client and/or carer contact;

(iv) delivered in such a way that the helper feels confident and supported as they fulfil their caring role.

This paper describe the training of three categories of helpers who work directly and indirectly with ADARDA clients and care-givers in Perth. They are the home respite carers, the ADARDA telephone advisory volunteers and the community-based home-service volunteers.

Obviously the home respite care-giver who works full-time with clients will have a different education and training compared to the volunteer who works in the office and answers telephone queries about Alzheimer's disease or the community home support volunteer. To a varying degree all will need some knowledge of Alzheimer's disease and how to relate with clients and/or their carers. They will also need to develop skills which are appropriate to the level and type of contact that they have with the clients. They learn the caring skills which are essential: for giving direct care for the client: for supporting the care-giver and to ensure their own well being. Four general concepts are central to the training of all ADARDA helpers: confidence, communication, caring and good old-fashioned common sense! These concepts are reflected in each of the training programmes.

Home respite carers

Home respite carers are paid helpers who work with Alzheimer's disease clients and their care-givers. They are employed through Commonwealth and State Government funding. Most work is performed in the client's home but respite workers also take clients on social outings and to appointments with the doctor, etc. They offer personal care and diversional activities for the client and practical informational and affective support for the care-giver. Their objective is to help provide for the physical, emotional and social needs of both clients and care-givers and to act as a link between the family and official health and welfare services.

Home respite carers undergo a full-time two week training programme prior to commencing duty. They then have weekly training and support sessions with other carers and with their coordinator. Their initial training programme includes skill sessions on Alzheimer's disease and information on current trends in research and care. It also has a heavy emphasis on the practical, behavioural and affective aspects of dealing with clients and carers and also in meeting their own needs.

Respite carers are educated on the normal process of ageing, on Alzheimer's disease, and on behavioural problems associated with the disease. They are trained in the skills of personal, practical, behavioural and diversional care. Effective communication skills are paramount and they are trained in the use of touch, movement, massage and music. They visit residential and support agencies where they observe "hands-on" care of patients. The legal and ethical aspects of their work are explored.

They are alerted to the reactions that care-givers experience when a loved one has Alzheimer's disease and to the burdens they experience in their role. They visit many community services and are taught how to act as a link between the care-giver and the formal health and welfare systems. They are also taught their role in meeting the carer's social, emotional and spiritual needs.

The obvious ethical, behavioural and administrative functions that the respite carer needs to know in order to perform their work are stressed. They become confident in their role: they are taught how and when to be assertive, to effectively manage their time and to limit their involvement to a manageable level. For their own well being, they are taught stress management, autogenic relaxation, aware-ness of their own needs and utilization of all available resources to meet those needs.

Our home respite carers have registered lower than expected levels of stress in their work. We feel that the content of the training, the weekly support sessions and the availability of 24-hour contact with the coordinator were contributing factors. The respite carers stated that the training they received had been at the appropriate level and scope for their work at the end of the course and again after three months in the field. They expressed a desire for further knowledge and skills to help them to develop their caring role.

ADARDA telephone advisory volunteers

These volunteers work on a part-time basis in the office of the ADARDA. They manage the office, prepare the society newsletter, answer queries from carers and the public and maintain a library of books and videos for public use. Their public relations role is to assist the public with information and to speak on AD at a wide range of organizational meetings and training programmes. If carers require more in-depth information than the volunteer is able to give, or if the volunteer assesses that one-to-one help with counselling is required, the caller is referred to the adult coordinator who is located nearby.

Their training programme consists of eight weekly sessions. These are followed by two sessions of supervised practice in the office where the worker is supported by a more experienced volunteer. When all training has been successfully com-pleted the volunteer joins the regular office roster. These volunteers often work together and they receive support from their contact with each other and with

109

their coordinator. Their major role is in listening, in being empathetic and in referring the care-giver to the relevant service or agency. The content of their training course reflects these functions.

Most telephone volunteers have had a family member who has Alzheimer's disease and they have some knowledge of the disease and the caring role. Information on Alzheimer's disease and its symptoms, methods of care, the stresses of caring and on coping with behavioural problems is given to reinforce their existing knowledge and to fill in any gaps in this knowledge. The history and objectives of ADARDA are also discussed.

Volunteers are taught the rudiments of interviewing with an emphasis on empathy, listening and effective telephone communications. Ethical principles and standards of volunteering are discussed. It is strongly emphasized that although volunteers may give advice, carers must be encouraged to make their own decisions. They are introduced to many community resources and are instructed on referral procedures. Office techniques, the recording and documentation of activities and the legal and ethical aspects of their work are also taught.

Home support volunteers

These helpers work with agencies that care for a variety of aged clients in the community. There is no one volunteer agency that provides services exclusively for patients with Alzheimer's disease: however, any agency that provides a service for the aged will have a high percentage of their clients with some level of dementia. ADARDA is contemplating the establishment of its own volunteer services and the training needs of these volunteers will be different again from those of general community service volunteers.

A week-end residential training programme is held on a regular basis for community volunteers who come from a variety of agencies. This mix of agencies gives volunteers some understanding of the role and function of other agencies. The social contact between volunteers is the beginning of a number of friendships and social networks. The training programme covers the topic of volunteerism, dealing with specific categories of clients and with the importance of self-care for volunteers. There are sessions on volunteerism looking at motivation, expectations and satisfactions and dissatisfactions of volunteers with their activities. We also discuss the ethical, attitudinal and behavioural standards of volunteers who work with the aged in their own homes. Then we look at the attributes and the needs of specific client groups: normal ageing compared with pathological ageing, mobility, safety and dealing with grief and loss in old age. Apart from dealing with the needs of the general aged population, we emphasize the needs of the ethnic clients, of those with dementia and particularly the needs of family carers. In all our courses there is a special emphasis on the need for volunteers to care for their own health and development. The programme includes stress management and relaxation for volunteers. Ongoing support is the responsibility of each individual agency: most of them hold regular support and training courses.

Evaluating the programmes

Evaluations of the volunteer programmes have been positive: pre- and post-course evaluations with the Palmore Test on Knowledge of Ageing show that not only does the level of knowledge concerning the aged improve but there is also a significant improvement in the attitudes of volunteers towards the elderly. These results have been more positive for the residential than for daytime courses.

The three specific programmes have been evaluated by attendees and by those conducting the programmes. The courses are continually revised to meet the changing needs of helpers and clients. The evaluations suggest that the programmes are adequate in style, depth and content to meet the needs of various helpers in their specific roles and functions.

Virtually all the paid employees recognize their need for education and training. Some volunteers, such as gardeners or handymen, do not feel that they need training, stating that: "it is all a matter of common sense". However, after attending a course, all of our volunteers have recognized that there are always new and additional aspects of working with the aged that they can learn.

Community service work is often performed in isolation and helpers have limited contact with others in the course of their activities. Some feel alone in their work and the support of the coordinator and regular contact with other helpers is to their overall satisfaction. All helpers appreciate support and acknowledgement of their work. Regular training and support meetings are a relatively new idea in some areas and the response from both volunteers and paid workers has been very positive. They state that they feel adequately trained to do their work, they feel supported and come to feel that they are an integral and important part of the helping group. They also enjoy the education, training and social components of the meetings.

Conclusion

Although the three specific programmes may be successful, there is no room for complacency. Family carers are probably the most important ADARDA helpers: they are full-time workers, giving practical and affective help and are the ultimate volunteers. To meet their needs, it is vital they also have access to training and support. Support groups do exist and various training and information sessions are held: these activities are positive but are currently conducted by whoever has the time and the interest on an ad hoc basis. To meet these needs of family carers is the next area for future development. Carer education and training must be coordinated and expanded to give optimal support to the carers of people with Alzheimer's disease.

Carers, Professionals and Alzheimer's Disease. D O'Neill ed © 1991 John Libbey & Company Ltd

Chapter 17

TRAINING STAFF TO CARE FOR PATIENTS WITH ALZHEIMER'S DISEASE

C Weber, *Corinne Dolan Alzheimer Center at Heather Hill, 12340 Bass Lake Road, Chardon, Ohio 44024, USA*

The course described in this paper was originally planned for unit staff (primarily nursing assistants) of a nursing home in-patient unit for dementia patients. It has been modified to be used with both professionals and home-care staff as well.

Basic approaches

The first goal of the sessions is to create a group atmosphere to help shape the attitude of staff towards their work. We all know that working with demented persons is difficult – but it can be creative and fun, and this is the spirit that we try to create in the class sessions.

There are three basic approaches to staff training. The first is aimed at nursing assistants and focuses concretely on techniques such as facilitation of activities of daily living, communication and approaches to problematic behaviours. A second approach, which is usually reserved for professional staff, focuses more closely on Alzheimer's disease and the dementing processes, and is presented in a more academic format. The third approach combines both approaches. We believe that staff responses to patient behaviours and situations will be both sensitive and effective if they combine an intellectual understanding of the disease process (including development of a conceptual model of brain function) with technical skills, creativity and empathy.

Eight of the ten one-hour sessions include a didactic component but much of the time is spent in participative and experiential way. We try to mix media to enhance the learning process. Each session begins with a discussion of the homework from the previous session. That provides review as well as a transition to the new session.

Course content

The first lesson is on normal ageing. The second is on normal brain function. The third lesson is on the dementing illnesses with a focus on Alzheimer's disease. The fourth lesson is on memory. The fifth reviews previous lessons and utilizes a confusion-simulation game. The sixth lesson is on communication and communication techniques and looks at environmental influences.

The seventh lesson is on behaviour with an emphasis on its connection to communication. This lesson, as well as many of the others, relies heavily on the willingness of the instructor to act out various parts. We find that the further the instructor is willing to go in this respect, the more the student will engage. It is particularly useful in demonstrating what staff often do wrong and why (from the patient's perspective) it doesn't work. Students can also criticize the instructor's performance initially, rather than each other's performance. This is much less threatening.

An example which illustrates potential reactions aroused by restraints on wandering is for the instructor to ask one of the patients to leave the room. The instructor then shouts: "Help, she is escaping!" and dashes after the student, grabs her from behind, and tries to drag her back into the room. We then talk about her feelings and reactions. At times a student struggles or becomes combative. The logic of this behaviour in a "normal" person is discussed in relation to our perception of it in a demented person.

The eighth lesson is on techniques for approaching problematic behaviours. In other courses this topic is broached much sooner: we feel that the advantage of presenting it after the previous seven lessons is that by this time the students do not perceive many behaviours as problematic. Even though some behaviour may be related to the disease process, students understand that many of these behaviours are actually the result of staff behaviour. They learn a number of techniques for changing their own behaviour in order to reduce behaviour problems or problematic behaviour in patients. The ninth lesson is on the family and focuses on developing empathy and understanding. The last lesson combines a summary, graduation and evaluation. I believe that graduation is important in developing staff self-esteem.

Useful teaching techniques

It may be useful to describe in more detail some key techniques that we found helpful. For example, the aim of the second lesson on normal brain function is for students to develop a conceptual model of brain function in which specific types of memory, ability and function are processed in discrete areas. The students try to understand that behaviour and performance depend on the integrity and integration of these areas. After a short lecture we look at brain maps, discuss brain areas such as Broca's area, and talk about the types of dysfunction which may occur in a person who has had damage in one of those areas. The instructor begins with a stimulus like a knock on a door. He then tries to list as many real or imagined areas in the brain that might interact in order to result in a response of answering the door. This might be phrased in the following way by the instructor: the ears hear the sound and send a message to the sensory alarm centre; the sensory alarm centre goes to the general alert centre and reports that something is going on; the general alert centre asks the sensory centre what the problem is; the sound sensory centre asks the sound memory centre to identify the sound; the sound memory centre says it is a "knock", not a door bell or the telephone bell; the thinking centre associates knocks with doors and asks the planning centre to do something; the planning centre asks the social control centre what is the appropriate response to a knock on the door, and so on.

We work creatively through as many possible areas of the brain and their functions and connections. I do not worry about the students learning technical names or locations of brain areas because it is the concept we are developing and not an exercise in terminology. The students then do the same type of exercise in small groups.

Finally we play a game that is a little bit like the child's game of telephone, where people represent various areas of the brain responding to the stimulus. The advantage of this approach is that they not only develop a conceptual framework for understanding the dysfunctions related to dementia, but they also have a good basis for breaking down tasks into minute steps or segments when we work on activities-of-daily-living (ADL) skills.

Role play

Our goal in the next lesson is for the students to understand various aspects of dementia such as memory loss and agnosia and for students to relate to these aspects as symptoms which care-givers can treat. In this lesson and in most of the following lessons, we build on a role play in which one student is given the role of a patient and is also given some aspect of dementia like visual agnosia or receptive aphasia to act out. The others do not know what the handicap is and they try to find out by interacting as carers with "the patient". In doing this they have to learn the various aspects of dementia, as does the patient/student who is acting out that role. As the course progresses, so does the role play: it becomes more complex and multiple handicaps are assigned to "patients". These are often combined with competing patient-staff agendas. An example would be a hungry patient and a staff member with instructions to give the patient a bath. The others try to guess what is going on. Feelings of the patient are discussed as well as the effectiveness of staff technique.

The student/patient must be instructed to be him-or herself. There was one course where the students mimicked some of the patients on the unit with varying disabilities instead of feeling the disability from within. The lesson is not internalised in the same way if they do that. The instructor must push them back into their own personality and role in order to experience the exercise from their own point of view. This helps the students to develop empathy and understanding for the patient's experience.

Staff are thus encouraged to look very closely at a patient's behaviour in order to try to guess what aspect of dementia is portrayed. This develops a questioning attitude among staff as to whether specific behaviour is a dementia-related problem, or whether it relates to the staff's reaction to it. Staff also get the opportunity for feed-back from the "patient", about their approaches and techniques which is not normally available. They get suggestions from the rest of the group about how they might have acted differently, giving them a chance to explore some of the techniques for handling problems that they will use with patients. Other students often get so involved that they jump in and want to help out or intervene in the interaction – a group dynamic that we are trying to develop with our staff.

Acknowledgements

The course described in this paper arose from a grant by the Robert Wood Johnson Foundation to develop our Alzheimer's Centre. We owe much to Dr. Joseph Foley for his support and expertise.

Carers, Professionals and Alzheimer's Disease. D O'Neill ed © 1991 John Libbey & Company Ltd

Chapter 18

COMMUNICATION IN CARE

M Greenwood *MB BS FRCPsych, Consultant Psychiatrist, Middlesex Hospital, Mortimer St, London W1N 8AA, United Kingdom*

We continuously hear that there should be training for carers, but who is going to provide this training? Wherever you come from and whatever your politics, I am sure you must agree that the amount of money available for health care is limited. So how do we make the best use of the resources that we do have? Is money well spent on training? The majority of people looking after those with dementing illness whether in hospital, in residential homes, in the private or voluntary sector or indeed in their own homes, have had no special training either in problems of ageing or in the problems of dementia. In addition, they have a poor self image. If they are paid, it is poorly and their worth is not recognised by society. I thought that one way of improving this low self image would be to offer some training. I admit my motives were not wholly altruistic. As a Consultant Psychiatrist with responsibility for developing a comprehensive service for the elderly in one part of Central London, I thought it would help me as well as the carers if I could assist those working with elderly people to cope better with their dementing illness. Indeed, by increasing the carer's knowledge and skills I hoped some of the demands on my services would decrease.

Setting up a training course

I had no special expertise in setting up training courses of this type. So I consulted with colleagues from different backgrounds – from the health service, from the local authority, the social services department, the housing department, some voluntary agencies and relatives – and we held a seminar called Co-operation or Collapse. The aim was to identify our problems and improve our mutual working relationships. It was no great surprise that the outcome of this meeting underlined the lack of even basic training for carers. By this I mean all carers – relatives, paid, unpaid, semi-professional, whatever. However, training costs money. Recognising this, the British government has made funds available to local authorities specifically to train their residential care workers. Many large establishments like the National Health Service offer some training to their own

117

employees but small organizations may not be able to run their own schemes. There is little cross fertilization of ideas between people working in the same area but from different backgrounds. Our meeting highlighted the need for training for workers from all backgrounds – health authorities, social services, those from the voluntary sector, those from the private sector and relatives.

But how could we fund such a scheme? We have been lucky enough to obtain support from a charity. With the help of the Joseph Levy Charitable Foundation, I was able to appoint an education and training officer and we have been running courses for the past eighteen months on the mental and physical well-being of elderly people.

How did we do it? I looked around for existing informal teaching programmes and I discovered that the Professor of Geriatric Medicine at another teaching hospital in London was teaching the basics of geriatric medicine to care assistants from the private sector, also using charitable monies. With his programme as a basis, we devised one with a much stronger emphasis on the psychiatry of old age and the problems associated with dementing illnesses. We decided to make the programme appropriate to as wide a range of carers, both formal and informal, as possible, for we recognized the value of sharing of similar experiences in different settings. Our handout stated that carers from any background would be welcome and that previous psychiatric or medical training was not necessary. Speakers were selected who had undergraduate teaching experience and we collected a sufficient number so that they are not called upon too frequently.

Atmosphere and catering

A special effort was made to ensure that the atmosphere was warm, welcoming and non-threatening. We recognised that the course would attract people who were unused to talking in public: therefore it was important that the total group should not be too large with small enough discussion groups for everyone to talk comfortably. For the majority of people who attended, this was the first course they had ever been on. The number who could attend was restricted to thirty, allowing for a potential 10 per cent drop-out. The catering has been taken over by various ex-carers who wish to give their time freely to support this venture. It has been possible to provide tea, coffee and lunch two days for less than £3.00 per head. People are encouraged to introduce themselves on the first day to break the ice. The main group is also sub-divided for friendly discussion and to encourage rather shy individuals to voice their views. We emphasise the importance of making the carer feel cared for and appreciated if he/she is to give of his/her best.

The running of the course depends enormously on a good co-ordinator. It is impossible to set up such a venture without having an organiser dedicated to this role. We were lucky enough to recruit an educationalist from a nursing back-ground. Despite her own administrative skills and the use of modern technology, she required additional secretarial time. The venue for the meeting is also important. It must not be too threatening either in size or in position. We chose the vacated Day Hospital Building at the entrance to the grounds where my longstay unit is sited. This is also useful as viewing of this National Health Service longstay facility for the care of those with severe dementia is an optional element on the course.

Practicality

The emphasis on the course has been on practical help. Active participation is encouraged. A good example of small but significant difficulties often put in the way of communication of elderly people is well demonstrated by this particular exercise: a small group of participants is placed in a straight line and asked to give feed-back on an activity they previously had been involved in. On one occasion, they sat in silence. A few mutterings were heard and then one young man who was seated at the end of the row who had not spoken at all earlier in the morning burst out in great fury "How could we possibly discuss a topic seated like this in a straight line?" The point was extremely well taken.

At the request of participants, we now provide handouts to supplement the different sessions. Many of the carers do not possess appropriate text books and feel rather uneasy at the thought of reading one. We have some basic equipment and we make use of the enormous range of teaching materials, including audio-visual aids, readily available. Production of our own teaching materials would be very costly in terms of time and money.

I pointed out earlier that no one body accepts the responsibility for this type of cross-boundary education and therefore there is no formal allocation of money. In our case the charity pays the salary for the training officer and her secretarial help but we must aim to make the course self-financing. We pay a nominal sum for the use of the empty hospital building, and charge £30.00 for two days but this is heavily subsidized. This is far below the economic rate but even this heavily subsidized figure is too much for many small organizations to fund their workers and on one occasion, a special jumble sale was apparently organized to pay for a worker to come. With charitable monies from other sources, we have purchased equipment including a photocopier and a computer which are invaluable.

Advertising

How have we advertised our course? Initially we informed the various agencies with whom we had contact, and the local, private and voluntary institutions as well as the statutory ones but it does seem that in many cases, the original invitation was lost on the desk of some rather high-placed administrator and never actually came to the attention of the basic practitioners. Most people do not retain information: if it is sent out too early, reminders then have to be sent. At the suggestion of someone who attended the course, we now take out an advertisement in a fairly simple magazine read by many managers of homes. We have not used the main nursing or social work press where a small advertisement costs at least £50.00. We are also immensely grateful to the Alzheimer's Disease Society

119

of England who give us free publicity in their newsletter. Personal invitations and response to the advertisements continue to produce more than adequate numbers to fill our places.

We decided on a two-day course as being a compromise which people and organizations would find acceptable. Half-day release over a longer period is more difficult to organize in terms of off-duty especially taking into account travelling time. More than two days away from work interferes grossly with the carer's own work.

Evaluation

How useful has our course been? We have now been running the course on a two-monthly basis since April, 1988. We have also run one second-level course and the response has been such that we shall be repeating this later on in the year. We have given an evaluation form to each attender and from the subjective reports, the course has been well received. How it has altered the practical abilities of the carers has not been possible to work out but unsolicited feed-back from some managers has reported that workers do feel much more confident and competent. We commissioned an independent evaluation by the Age Concern Institute of Gerontology at Kings College, London and that has shown that we are indeed fulfilling a big need. I personally find it most heartening to see the pleasure that the majority of people experience during the two days of the course accompanying the increase in their self-confidence, the knowledge that they do indeed possess certain skills and the recognition that they are appreciated.

The Department of Employment Training Agency in England now is trying to standardize a national vocational qualification for carers. This is in anticipation of the dearth of school leavers and younger people willing to go into various caring professions. This consists of different levels of academic and practical competency. They hope to provide an umbrella frame work which will allow some standardization of existing courses and we hope that with minor modification, our course will be able to qualify.

Conclusion

Although our initiative is but a drop in the ocean, yet I hope that I have demonstrated that with conviction, co-operation and support from a charity, you can set up a worthwhile training scheme for carers.

SECTION 5
Improving the Environment

Carers, Professionals and Alzheimer's Disease. D O'Neill ed © 1991 John Libbey & Company Ltd

Chapter 19

THE DESIGNED ENVIRONMENT AND THE ALZHEIMER PATIENT

JL Shroyer *PhD, Chairperson, Department of Merchandising, Environmental Design and Consumer Economics, Texas Tech University, Lubbock, Texas*

This paper arises out of a collaborative project on Alzheimer's disease initiated by Dr JT Hutton, who brought together a group of individuals from various research backgrounds at Texas Tech University and Texas Tech University Health Sciences Centre to look at the different areas which affect the individual with Alzheimer's disease. As a result of several research grants we have had the resources to conduct interior-design related experiments in the living environments of individuals diagnosed with Alzheimer's disease. We have worked closely with several nursing homes in the West Texas area to identify specific environmental design factors which can positively or negatively affect the well-being of these special individuals.

The designed environment

The designed environment is a major factor in our everyday life. For the non-demented individual, the physical environment includes our homes, work places, community service facilities, and recreation facilities such as libraries, churches, parks, etc. However, for the person who suffers with dementia of the Alzheimer's type, these environments become a source for increased confusion and ultimately frustration. This frustration may often result in socially unacceptable behaviours such as screaming, hitting etc.

Despite the large number of individuals with Alzheimer's disease and other dementing illnesses, recent studies have not specifically addressed the environmental design requirements of Alzheimer's disease victims. Although recent US government hearings and reports suggest that social and organizational characteristics of institutions could postpone the time when a patient with AD becomes bedridden and requires skilled nursing care, there appears to be minimal recog-

123

nition of the possible impact of designed environments, both home and institutional, on the functioning and well-being of these individuals

Although conjecture exists among behavioural and medical scientists as to a clear cause-and-effect relationship between the housing environment and behaviour and medical health, certain assumptions, based on animal research, human observation, behaviour mapping and user perception, seem to be generally accepted. Although many of the conclusions are based on observations in mental facilities, the findings are applicable to some degree to other environments. Analogies can also be drawn from studies of the effects of the home environment

INTERIOR DESIGN CONCEPTS		
	INTERIOR DESIGN FEATURES	**OBJECTIVES**
A	CLUSTER FURNITURE ARRANGEMENT	ENCOURAGE SOCIAL INTERACTION PROMOTE SENSE OF SECURITY
B	CIRCULATION PATHS FREE OF LOW OBJECTS	PROMOTE SENSE OF SECURITY & COMPETENCE
C	8' PARTITION TO BLOCK VIEW INTO LARGER SPACE	PROMOTE SENSE OF SECURITY REDUCE SPATIO-TEMPORAL CONFUSION
D	RESOURCES (DINING & BATHROOM) ARE CLEARLY ACCESSIBLE & AT A DISTANCE CONSISTENT WITH COMPETENCE	REDUCE DISORIENTATION REDUCE CONFUSION
E	CHAIRS & SOFAS WITH ARMS & HIGH STRETCHERS BETWEEN FRONT LEGS; STURDY, NON-COLLAPSIBLE DESIGN FURNITURE WITH ROUNDED CORNERS & EDGES AND UNCOMPLICATED DESIGN	PROMOTE SENSE OF SECURITY PROMOTE PERSONAL SAFETY & WELL-BEING REDUCE CONFUSION
F	PORTABLE TABLE LAMPS FOR HOME-LIKE ATMOSPHERE AND EFFECTIVE, GLARE-FREE ILLUMINATION	ENHANCE SENSE OF SECURITY & WELL-BEING CONTRIBUTE TO SAFETY
G	FULL-LENGTH DRAPERIES FOR TRADITIONAL APPEARANCE AND DAYLIGHT & HEAT CONTROL	PROMOTE SENSE OF SECURITY & WELL-BEING IMPROVE COMFORT CONDITIONS
H	TALL PLANTS FOR AESTHETIC INTEREST AND DIFFUSION OF DAYLIGHT	CONTRIBUTE TO PERSONAL COMFORT REDUCE MONOTONY
I	SCREEN TO REINFORCE CLUSTER ARRANGE-MENT AND REDUCE GLARE	ENHANCE PERSONAL COMFORT AND SENSE OF SECURITY
J	SUPERVISORY ACTIVITY CONVENIENTLY LOCATED	CONTRIBUTE TO PERSONAL SAFETY

	OTHER
	  MINIMIZATION OF DOORWAYS
	  ELIMINATION OF CHANGES IN FLOOR
	    SURFACE
		REDUCE CONFUSION & FRUSTRATION

	AVOIDANCE OF SHARP COLOUR CONTRASTS
	    CONFUSING PATTERNS, FINE DETAIL
	  WARM COLOUR SCHEME
		COMPENSATE FOR AGE-RELATED VISION CHANGES

on the cognitive development of children. These investigations have assessed factors such as the organization of the physical and temporal environments and the opportunities for variety in daily stimulation. These research studies may have important implications for the design of prosthetic environments for patients with Alzheimer's disease who may be experiencing a variety of physical problems. For example, impairment of orientation and judgement would suggest that there should be a highly structured or formal framework underlying the use of life spaces.

Researchers have consistently identified several environmental variables that

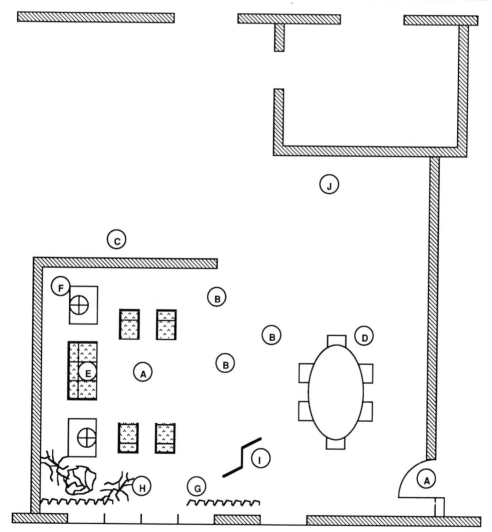

Fig.1 Interior design considerations, and their rationale, for a care facility for patients with Alzheimer's disease.

are consistently deficient, including illumination, colour, furnishings and layout, textiles, architectural features and climate control.[4] Any one of these elements, if problematic or inappropriately applied, can further complicate the life of the individual with dementia. Not only may certain environmental features be a threat to safety, but they may also produce anxiety which can amplify cognitive deficits.[5] Cohen noted that certain behavioural approaches (e.g. using environmental cues) can have some advantages over drugs in the treatment of cognitive impairments common in dementia of the Alzheimer type. She has identified the need to review the patient's environment, to define potential threats to safety or sources of emotional stress, and search for adaption. Additional studies have emphasized that encouragement of independence, self-sufficiency and social interaction is critical to prolonging functions.[7] Concomitant changes in the social environment may also be required to increase the chances that the patient can remain in the home environment and the community. Appropriate adaptations can benefit both the patient with dementia and the carers.

Recommendations

We undertook a programme of empirical multi-method research on the characteristic behaviours of Alzheimer patients, conducted in collaboration with a neurologist, a psychologist, and a lighting specialist Our findings suggested both limiting and facilitating factors that may help mitigate levels of confusion and disorientation.[8] These factors include background elements, spatial arrangement and design of furniture components. We suggest the following recommendations (see Fig. 1).

(i)   Avoid using large open multi-purpose spaces; utilize activity-specific spaces.

(ii)   Provide clear circulation pathways.

(iii)   Plan adequate and safe space for wandering/pacing.

(iv)   Emphasize forms and shapes of particular importance (e.g. doorways).

(v)   Enhance safety by specifying furniture components with rounded or chamfered termination points and edges.

(vi)   Avoid curved and angled lines on walls which can affect physical balance.

(vii)   Specify textures which aid in grip and balance (e.g. non-skid floor surfaces).

(vii)   Increase the quantity of light.

(ix)   Design lighting layouts to reduce glare and brightness contrast.

(x)   Avoid light patterns which reflect images on to walls and floors.

(xi)   Select a colour palette for interior space in conjunction with colour temperature and a colour rendering index of light sources.

(xii)   Reduce unnecessary use of confusing sounds in the environment.

(xiii) Specify sound absorptive materials in institutional settings.

Vision limitations are not uncommon in Alzheimer's patients.[9] These limitations suggest the need for large design patterns or solid colours in upholstery and textiles for visibility, interest and appeal. The use of larger patterns and hues with higher reflectance values for the furniture upholstery allows the Alzheimer victim to see objects more clearly and thus reduces the probability that he or she will bump or fall over furniture components

Conclusion

There is still much misinformation and a lack of understanding about the environmental needs of individuals with Alzheimer's disease. Recognizing that an imperfect fit exists between the living environment and its user is an important step in the design process. Even more important, however, are the approaches applied to design solutions. We need to ask the question – does the environment promote understanding or fear? Appropriate environmental design components and elements may enhance the health, welfare and functional ability of the dementia victim.

References

(1) Alzheimer's disease: Joint Hearing before the Sub-committee on Health and Long-Term Care of the Select Committee on Aging and the Subcommittee on Health and Environment of the Committee on Energy and Commerce, House of Representatives, 98th Congress, first session. Washington DC, US Government Printing Office, 1984.

(2) Alzheimer's disease: Report of the Secretary's Task Force on Alzheimer's Disease. Washington DC, US Government Printing Office, 1984, DHHS publication no (ADM) 84-1323, 1984.

(3) Elardo R, Bradley RH. The home observation for measurement of environment (HOME) scale. *Development Review* 1981, **1**, 113-145.

(4) Liebowitz B, Lawton MP, Waldman A. Evaluation: designing for confused elderly people. *AIA Journal* 1979, **2**, 59-61.

(5) Weldon S, Yesavage JA. Behavioural improvement with relaxation training in senile dementia. *Clinical Gerontology* 1982, **1**(1), 45-49.

(6) Cohen GD. The mental health professional and the Alzheimer patient. *Hosp Community Psychiatry* 1984, **35**(2), 115-116, 122.

(7) Reifler BV, Wu S. Managing families of the demented elderly. *J Fam Pract* 1982, **14**(6), 1051-1056.

(8) Schroyer JL, Hutton JT, Anderson GM. The Alzheimer patient: interior design considerations. In Hutton JT (ed), *Alzheimer's Disease and Related Dementing Disorders*. Texas Tech Alzheimer's Center, Texas, 1987.

(9) Hutton JT. Eye movement and eye fixation testing in dementing disorders. In O'Neill D (ed), *Carers, Professionals and Alzheimer's Disease*. London, John Libbey, 1991,

Further reading

AIA Foundation. *Design For Aging*. Washington DC, The AIA Press, 1985.

Calkins MP. *Design For Dementia*. Owings Mills MD, National Health Publishing, 1988.

Carers, Professionals and Alzheimer's Disease. D O'Neill ed © 1991 John Libbey & Company Ltd

Chapter 20

A SPECIAL DAY CENTRE FOR THE CONFUSED ELDERLY IN MELBOURNE, AUSTRALIA – THE FIRST FIVE YEARS

JA Tulloch, *Mount Royal Hospital, Victoria, Australia*

The Gatehouse Day Centre was initiated following a survey of confused, elderly people in two municipalities in Melbourne, Australia in 1982. The survey was conducted by a group of health-care professionals involved with care of the elderly. The suburbs are predominantly middle-class and are well supplied with geriatric day hospitals, day-centres and psychiatric day-hospitals. However, it was found that dementia sufferers who were incontinent, disturbed or prone to wander were unable to be accommodated in any of these settings. It was decided to provide a day-care service specifically for this type of dementia sufferer which would provide some relief to their carers. In June 1983 a public meeting was held and a committee representing local health-care workers, local councils, psychiatric and geriatric services covering the area, and carers of demented people was elected to organise this type of service. The target group were sufferers with moderate to severe dementia who were living at home with carers and who were unsuitable for available forms of day-care. Behaviour disturbances and incontinence were not exclusion criteria.

The aims of the service were (i) to provide a therapeutic community atmosphere for the attenders; (ii) to provide respite care for the carers; and (iii) to manage behaviour disturbances using environmental and handling techniques rather than sedating drugs where possible. The local psychiatric hospital kindly provided a rent-free house in its extensive grounds. The house is about half a mile from the hospital proper, separated by sports grounds and fields and is at the end of a quiet road, making it ideal for the purpose. The house has two living rooms, a dining-room and a kitchen large enough to accommodate a large kitchen table. The bedrooms of the house are upstairs and are not used by the day-centre. The stairs are blocked off by a gate to prevent access. The garden is large and was quite overgrown. Modifications to the house include 5-foot perimeter railings, dead locks on the front door and upgrading of the downstairs bathroom to include a toilet with hand rails and a shower recess. After renovations the house was considered suitable for use by up to 10 participants per day.

After applications for government funding were refused, funding for the first year of operation was obtained from voluntary donations and charitable trusts. Eventually enough money was raised to commence operations and the service was widely advertised to local general practitioners, local hospitals, elder-care workers as well as through local media outlets.

The day-centre accepted its first patients in June 1984. The day-centre operates on two days per week (Tuesday and Friday) from 9.30 a.m. to 3.00 p.m. The staff employed initially were: (i) the coordinator, who was a state-registered nurse (SRN) who was employed for 20 hours a week; (ii) an assistant (untrained) for 13 hours a week: and (iii) a cleaner for two hours a week. We did not specify that the coordinator should be an SRN: we were looking for the right type of person, but with some form of professional training. The coordinator works one other session apart from the Tuesday and the Friday to allow time for home assessment of new referrals, preparation for the programme and shopping for provisions for the catering. The assistant works from 9.00 a.m. to 3.30 p.m. on Tuesdays and Fridays. As funding became more secure further staff were employed: a further assistant for 8 hours a week and the cleaner also worked as an assistant from 12.30 to 2.30p.m. on Tuesdays and Fridays. The extra staff employed allows for 4 staff members at the busiest time (12.30 – 2.00 p.m.) and allows for splitting of the groups to fulfil more individual needs of the attenders.

Assessment for attendance

All new referrals are assessed at home by the coordinator prior to their first attendance at the day-centre. This allows the coordinator to assess their functional capacity in their own home environment and to make an assessment of family relationships. Where necessary referral is arranged to local geriatric or psychogeriatric services. However, most clients have been seen by one of these agencies prior to referral to the day centre. After assessment at home, plans are made for the first attendance, usually in the company of a spouse or a carer. At this stage all participants will have a personal file made up, consisting of a photo album with photographs of significant people in their lives, and of significant events for reminiscence purposes. If the carer is unable to provide transport, transport is provided by the day-centre, using taxis or a small community bus owned by one of the municipalities that the service covers.

Programme

The timetable for the day is fairly consistent on most days but tries to accommodate individual participants' abilities and skills. The philosophy of care is to encourage independence by working together with the staff and participants to run the house. For example, rather than staff pouring tea and coffee with milk and sugar as they know each participant likes, the participants are encouraged to pour their own tea and coffee and to add their own milk and sugar as they wish. Incontinence is managed where possible with regular toiletting although changes of clothes and showering may be necessary. Regular medication is controlled and given by staff during the day.

As the participants arrive at the door they are met by staff and hang hats and coats on a stand that sits just inside the front door. This demonstrates to participants that they are coming to stay for a while. Following this all staff and participants have tea together. Then follows a period of discussion and reality orientation. All staff and participants introduce themselves and this leads on to a general discussion of the weather, temperature and season. With the renowned changeability of the weather in Melbourne this provides a ready source of discussion! Then attempts are made to discuss current news events or life events affecting any of the staff or participants, e.g. birthdays or anniversaries. This often provides an opportunity for reminiscing about similar events in the past.

After this discussion time all staff and participants move into the kitchen of the house to help prepare lunch. The hallmark of this is the preparation of the Gatehouse soup! This is a mixed vegetable soup and all participants take part in cutting the required raw vegetables into small pieces to make them suitable for soup. Despite the use of sharp knives and graters this activity has not resulted in any significant injuries in 5 years of operation. After this preparation has been completed the ingredients are combined in a big pot and left to simmer while participants conduct another activity.

This next activity may be gardening if the weather is fine or inside activities such as listening to music or reminiscing using participants' personal files. The men especially enjoy digging the garden, slashing long grass or watering. A small vegetable garden is kept with limited success. Prints and posters on the walls inside are used as aids to reminiscing: old and familiar tapes and records are also used. During this time some of the participants help to set the dining room for lunch. At about midday all participants and staff sit down for lunch, starting with the soup that they prepared earlier. Clearing the table and washing up then become a community activity – the participants seem to enjoy being useful members of the team.

After lunch those participants who do not need a rest go with all except one staff member for a walk in the extensive grounds of the hospital. As mentioned before, the Gatehouse is about half a mile across fields and sports grounds from the nearest building: there is plenty of scope for walking in the country and observing nature. One of the living rooms of the house is fitted with two sleeping divans allowing those participants who need a rest after lunch to have one.

131

After returning from the walk there is just time for another cup of tea before transport starts arriving for home. When relatives come to collect their family member there is usually an opportunity for friendly discussion of what they have done that day and any problems that they may be encountering. The coordinator becomes an extra support for the carers through these discussions. Once all the participants have left, the staff clear up and collapse exhausted from six-and-a-half hours of non-stop activity.

Statistics

The average attendance at the day-centre in the year 1988-1989 has been 8 per day. At present 12 people are attending; 8 for 1 day per week and 4 for 2 days per week. A total of 23 people have attended; of these 12 are still attending, 6 have moved to residential care, 3 are no longer attending and 2 have died. Periods of attendance in the past have extended up to 3 years, but 6–12 months is the average.

The initial funding for the day-centre was solely by charitable donation. With the perceived success of the service, government funding became available after the first year of operation. At present, funding for up to 80 per cent of costs is provided by the Australian Commonwealth Government's Home and Community Care Programme. This is a funding programme aimed at various support mechanisms to help maintain aged and disabled people in their own homes rather than in expensive residential care. The extra 20 per cent of costs is provided by donations, fund-raising and cost-savings where possible. The actual cost of attendance at the day-centre is approximately A$50. Participants contribute A$5 for each attendance, although no participant is excluded if they are unable to afford this.

Costs of the service are kept as low as possible by working staff without tea and lunch breaks and by employing extra staff just for the busiest times of the day. Whether these work practices can be continued if the industrial climate becomes more militant is uncertain, but all staff employed at the day-centre so far have been loving, dedicated people who have been willing to work under these conditions.

Evaluation

Formal evaluation of the impact of the dementia service on sufferers and carers has been limited. We have applied several times to the government for funds to allow this to be done, but have not been successful with our applications. However, carers have demonstrated great support for this service by the extra voluntary work that they have done to help it. The only formal project of evaluation was presented at the 4th Alzheimer's Disease International conference in Brisbane. This study assessed carer stress before and after attendance at various day centres, including the Gatehouse Day Centre. The total results showed no significant reduction in stress levels with attendance at day-centres. However, since the day-centres studied varied considerably, it is difficult to draw conclusions about the effectiveness of any one particular service. Thus the question whether participation in this type of day-care reduces stress in carers or improves levels of functioning in participants remains unanswered. The even larger question as far as governments are concerned, as to whether day-care allows a longer period of home-care as opposed to institutional care also remains unanswered. The committee of management of the Gatehouse Day Centre regards support of the community carer as a high priority, regardless of costs.

Since its inception in 1984 the Gatehouse day-centre has provided a model for many other day centres which have since opened in the state of Victoria, Australia. We were very fortunate to have employed as our first co-ordinator a state-registered nurse who was full of ideas as to how demented patients could be managed. Over the years she has been able to test her ideas in practice, and has developed a programme which seems to meet the needs of clients and carers very successfully. After guiding this programme for the first four years, she has now gone on to become a teacher for staff responsible for running activities programmes for demented people in institutions. In this position she is able to spread her enlightened management techniques to an even larger audience.

This type of day-care programme depends for its existence on dedicated staff members who are able to work without rest-breaks for extended periods of time. Volunteers do have a role to play, but need to be instructed and well-trained. For instance, we had an elderly man who visited once a fortnight to play the flute for the participants, which they seemed to enjoy. However, a volunteer who does not fully understand the importance of encouraging independence rather than dependence in this group can do more harm than good by providing well-meaning assistance to the participants.

Although funds are available for extra days of opening, we have been reluctant to do this for two reasons: firstly, we have done surveys of carers, and have found that one or two days of care seems to be as much as they or the participants can cope with, and secondly, we are very aware of the probabilities of staff burnout, with dropping of standards, if staff are required to do this type of work on a full-time basis. The service operated 52 weeks per year, however, since a break in the programme is considered to be disadvantageous to both carers and participants.

In the last five years the Gatehouse day-centre seems to have filled a gap that existed in the services for the demented elderly at home. We believe that day-care centres should be small, local and personal to avoid undue travel time and to allow better carer support. The concept of having a programme geared to familiar tasks such as running a house or garden seems to be appropriate for this group of people.

Carers, Professionals and Alzheimer's Disease. D O'Neill ed © 1991 John Libbey & Company Ltd

Chapter 21

ENVIRONMENTS FOR PEOPLE WITH DEMENTIA NEW ISSUES, NEW SOLUTIONS

U Cohen, G Weisman, *School of Architecture and Urban Planning, University of Wisconsin-Milwaukee, P.O. Box 413, Milwaukee, Wisconsin 53201, USA*

Alzheimer's disease and related disorders have a major influence upon the provision of housing and health care for the elderly. Over two and a half million Americans suffer from dementia that is sufficiently severe to require continuous care, and more than half of all nursing home beds are occupied by people with dementia. Despite this clear need, research-based guidance for the planning and design of environments for people with dementia remains exceedingly limited.

Holding on to home: Designing environments for people with dementia (Cohen & Weisman, 1991) represents the synthesis of three related research projects focused on environments for people with dementia and the possibilities available in the design of environments for this population. Aimed at design, social service, and health care professionals, *Holding on to Home* addresses the process of preparation, planning, programming, design and construction, and use and post-occupancy evaluation of current environments for people with dementia. Four fundamental goals have guided the authors' efforts to design therapeutic environments for people with dementia:

(i) to provide an understanding and appreciation of the therapeutic potential of the physical environment in the care of people with dementia;

(ii) to build, to the greatest extent possible, upon both clinical experience and empirical research in the formulation of principles for planning and design; and

(iii) to develop generalizable principles for planning and design that are responsive to basic environmental needs of people with dementia and their care-givers and to therapeutic and organizational goals.

(iv) to illustrate the architectural application of these principles across a broad range of facilities, including private residences, day-care centres, group homes, and long-term care facilities.

Linking Alzheimer's disease and environmental design

Alzheimer's disease and environmental design seem, at the outset, to be two very disparate topics: the relationship they bear to one another may be quite unclear initially. This article can provide only a brief answer to such an important question. A basic understanding of the relationship between architecture and Alzheimer's disease depends upon three fundamental premises.

Firstly, it is essential to recognize that the role of the architectural environment need and should not be limited to the mere provision of physical shelter. Thoughtfully designed architectural environments represent potentially valuable, albeit typically under-utilized, therapeutic resources in the care of people with dementia. Indeed it has been argued that many of the behaviours attributed to Alzheimer's disease are, in part, a consequence of counter-therapeutic settings. There is empirical and theoretical support to suggest that even modest modification of traditional room and unit layouts, along with complementary modifications in the organizational environment, can slow or in some cases even reverse the declines expected over time in the behaviour of people with dementia.

Secondly, it must be recognized that the physical settings occupied by people with dementia do not exist in isolation; rather, they are integral parts of a larger, complex system and must operate in concert with the social and organizational dimensions of this larger system. Thus, *physical environments* for people with dementia must be considered in the context of social, behavioural and organizational variables.

Finally, there is great value in recognizing the residential qualities of environments for people with dementia. Many such facilities, while well-intentioned, do not, as a consequence of their medical or institutional characteristics, serve the best interests of people with dementia. All therapeutic settings should retain the positive attributes of home to the greatest extent possible.

Principles for planning and design

The design of environments for people with dementia must take into account their special and specific needs, the distinct goals of their care-givers (family members and staff care providers) and the organizational environment. The design principles developed by the authors address critical issues (e.g. wandering behaviour) and provide directions for solutions (e.g. meaningful wandering path) responsive to the needs of residents and care-givers. Appropriate solutions will vary with the nature of the population to be served and the specific environment under investigation. The design principles contained in *Holding on to Home* offer suggestions that cover the entire design process, from general planning principles (e.g. suggestions for tapping local resources), to general attributes of the environment

136

(e.g. recommendations for a noninstitutional image), to building organization (e.g. recommendations for small groups of residents), to specific activity areas (e.g. domestic kitchens). The following list describes some of the selected design principles from *Holding on to Home*.

(i) Eliminating environmental barriers. Physical and cognitive impairments associated with dementia often make movement through and use of the environment difficult. It is critically important to eliminate these barriers to negotiability in environments for people with dementia. In addition to traditional solutions such as ramps and handrails, environmental interventions may include clear and consistent information and easy-to-operate handles and controls.

(ii) Things from the past. Familiar artefacts, activities and environments can provide valuable associations with the past for people with dementia, and can stimulate opportunities for social interaction and meaningful activity. Rather than being limited to a simple "rummage box", the *total* environment may potentially be used to trigger reminiscence.

(iii) Sensory stimulation without stress. Levels of sensory and social stimulation in environments for people with dementia should not differ dramatically from those encountered in domestic environments. Both sensory deprivation and overstimulation are conditions to be avoided. The physical and the organizational environment can both be designed to regulate stimulation, providing interest and challenge without becoming overwhelming. Opportunities should be provided for increasing or reducing levels of stimulation to respond to changing needs and tolerance levels over the course of a day.

(iv) Opportunities for meaningful wandering. Wandering is a relatively common behaviour among people with dementia. Too often in the past it has been viewed as a problem, and resulted in the use of chemical or physical restraints. A far more positive approach is to view wandering as an opportunity for meaningful activity. Both physical and organizational environments should be supportive of such activity, providing appropriate settings with secure and well-defined paths.

(v) Public to private realms. People with dementia should be able to select from among a variety of spaces falling at distinct points along a continuum of public to private realms. Such a continuum, created through both architectural and administrative means, facilitates resident control of sensory and social stimulation, and may reduce perceived intrusion of individual personal space.

Design application

The following plan is one of several illustrative designs described in *Holding on to Home*. The plan (Fig. 1, overleaf) illustrates the application of many design principles in the context of a respite and day care centre.

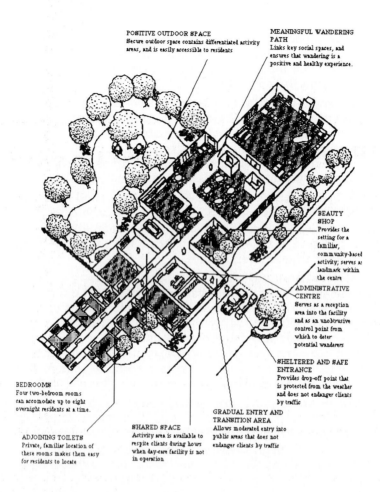

POSITIVE OUTDOOR SPACE
Secure outdoor space contains differentiated activity areas, and is easily accessible to residents

MEANINGFUL WANDERING PATH
Links key social spaces, and ensures that wandering is a positive and healthy experience.

BEAUTY SHOP
Provides the setting for a familiar, community-based activity; serves as landmark within the centre

ADMINISTRATIVE CENTRE
Serves as a reception area into the facility and as an unobtrusive control point from which to deter potential wanderers

SHELTERED AND SAFE ENTRANCE
Provides drop-off point that is protected from the weather and does not endanger clients by traffic

GRADUAL ENTRY AND TRANSITION AREA
Allows moderated entry into public areas that does not endanger clients by traffic

SHARED SPACE
Activity area is available to respite clients during hours when day-care facility is not in operation

BEDROOMS
Four two-bedroom rooms can accomodate up to eight overnight residents at a time.

ADJOINING TOILETS
Private, familiar location of these rooms makes them easy for residents to locate

Fig. 1. Day-care and respite centre: design considerations.

Bibliography

Cohen U, & Weisman GD. *Holding on to Home: Designing environments for people with dementia.* Baltimore MD, The John Hopkins Press, 1991.

Cohen U, Weisman G, Ray K, Steiner V, Rand J, & Toyne R. *Environments for people with dementia: Design guide.* Washington, DC: Health Facilities Research Program, AIA/ACSA Council on Architectural Research, 1988.

Carers, Professionals and Alzheimer's Disease. D O'Neill ed © 1991 John Libbey & Company Ltd

Chapter 22

PURPOSE-BUILT UNITS FOR THE CARE OF THE CONFUSED AND DISTURBED ELDERLY. DEVELOPMENT AND EVALUATION

R Fleming *BTech, Dip Clin Psy,* **J Bowles** *RN, Department of Health, New South Wales (South Eastern Region), PO Box 300, Goulburn, New South Wales 2580, Australia*

In 1986 the government of New South Wales gave the go-ahead for the construction of the first purpose-built unit for the care of the Confused and Disturbed Elderly (CADE) to be built in New South Wales. This unit was opened in June 1987 and was intended to be the first of a network of such units. These were to provide care for dementing patients who were no longer being admitted to the psychiatric hospitals as a result of legislative changes. Since then the policy of developing the CADE unit network has continued with 8 more units planned for construction within the next 12 months and a further 21 during the course of the implementation of the 5-year plan for mental health services. While these units as a whole will provide services for the elderly with dementia, care of the elderly chronically mentally ill with non-dementing illness will take place in similar but specially-dedicated units.

The design of the units has been based on the experience of caring for the mobile, confused elderly in the wards of the traditional psychiatric hospitals. This gave ample information on features to be avoided. More constructive advice and information was available from other units that had moved towards providing care in more domestic settings. Among these the Lodge programme, run by the

Uniting Church and guided by Brian Moss, was very influential. The particular contribution of the design of the CADE units lies in the recognition of the need to provide an environment that feels like home to the residents but which is prosthetic in nature.[1]

Design principles

The eight principles on which the design of the units have been based can be summarised:

(i) Smallness. Groups of eight patients have been found to be the optimum size for the care of the mobile, confused and disturbed elderly.

(ii) Domesticity. The environment should be as homelike as possible, recognizing that the residents will be living there. All of the facilities found in an ordinary house need to be provided, including a kitchen, laundry, bathroom, etc. As many of the demands of ordinary domestic life should be passed on to the residents as they can cope with, e.g. food preparation, cleaning, washing etc.

(iii) Closeness to the community. The chances that the residents will continue to be part of their social network after admission should be maximized by providing for their care in small units in their own community rather than in large centralized units that put a geographical and social distance between them and their family.

(iv) Reduced extraneous stimulation. The dementing person experiences difficulties in coping with a large amount of stimulation. The unit must be designed to reduce the impact of stimulation that is unnecessary for the well-being of the resident: for example, entry and exit doors used for deliveries and staff movements should not be visible to the residents; doors to treatment rooms, cleaners cupboards and storerooms should merge with the background. Similarly, power points and controls that should only be used by staff should not be visually prominent. This approach both reduces stimulation and avoids tempting the residents into situations that could cause them difficulties.

(v) Highlighting of important stimuli. Stimuli that are important to the residents should be highlighted. Toilet doors should be distinctive and aids to recognition should be provided on bedroom doors and some light switches.

(vi) Simple environment with total visual access. Confusion may be reduced by caring for the confused person in a simple environment. The simplest environment is one in which the resident can see everywhere that she wants to go to from wherever she is. This principle practically eliminates the inclusion of corridors in the design: if combined with a strategically-placed staff room, this approach results in the staff being able to see the residents almost all of the time.

(vii) Provision for "planned" wandering. Wandering is a feature of the behaviour of the dementing person, rather than fighting against it, it was decided to design the unit so that it could take place safely. A pathway, defined by the layout of furniture, the provision of two doors to the garden and paths around raised flower beds were provided. The need for this feature in practice has been much less than was originally expected.

(viii) Familiar decor. It is well known that the dementing person recalls the distant past more easily than the recent past. It follows then that their experience of recent furniture designs and decors must be less congruent with their present mental state than their experience of decors that they enjoyed in their younger days. To ensure that their experience of their surroundings is in keeping with their mental state the decor of the units resembles those found in homes in the 1940's and 50's.

These principles were used to design Peppertree Lodge, the first CADE unit. It is a sixteen bed facility, divided into two sub-units of eight.

The Peppertree Lodge experience

Twenty people were admitted to Peppertree Lodge in the first 15 months of its operation. Fourteen came from a psychiatric hospital, 3 from the hospital supporting the local geriatric assessment team and 3 from the local district hospital. They had a mean age of 76 with a range of 62 to 88. Twelve were men, 8 were women. Those who came from the psychiatric hospital had had a mean length of hospital stay of 3.9 years (1 month to 21 years).

The diagnoses on admission were: senile dementia [8], Alzheimer's disease [5], chronic brain syndrome [1], dementia of uncertain aetiology [1], dementia associated with alcohol abuse [4], cerebral haemorrhage [1]. All residents were active and mobile on admission: nine were described as aggressive. They all had significant problems with self-help skills, orientation for person, place and time. The problems posed by their wandering and/or 'interfering' behaviours made them unsuitable for care in traditional nursing homes. Ten were incontinent of urine and 6 of faeces.

All of the residents of Peppertree Lodge are regularly assessed on the Psychogeriatric Rating Scale (PRS).[2] This is a measure of disability in the key areas of physical problems, self-help, confusion, behaviour, sociability, psychiatric symptomatology and staff dependency. The inter-rater reliability of the PRS when used by trained raters ranges from 0.9 for the behaviour sub-scale to 0.98 for self-help and sociability. The validity of the confusion sub-scale has been assessed using the Mini-Mental State Examination:[3] the PRS correlated at a value of -0.84 with the Mini-Mental State Examination.

Progress

All available residents were assessed (i) prior to admission, (ii) within the first month, (iii) between the second and fourth months, (iv) with their case reviews within the seventh to twelfth months, and (v) finally reviewed between the thirteenth and fifteenth month. Ten residents were present at all measuring points. Figure 1 summarizes the changes that took place in the 10 residents assessed at all measuring points. A reduction in scores indicates a reduction in disability and points at which the scores are significantly different ($p < 0.25$, one tailed) from the pre-admission score are circled.

All of these residents remained in Peppertree Lodge during the course of the study

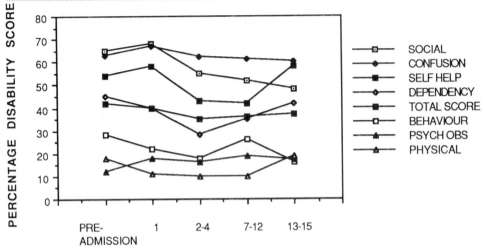

Fig.1. Changes in PRS scores over the first 15 months in the ten patients with the longest residence.

but one of them was transferred to a nursing home almost immediately after his last assessment. Of the twenty residents admitted during the first 15 months, 3 went on to nursing homes after becoming physically frail, one died of a heart attack and another from a cerebral embolism.

Information is also available on the changes that took place in seven of the long term residents during their stay in the psychiatric hospital prior to admission to the CADE unit. They had been assessed with the PRS over a fifteen month period spanning 1985 and 86 (Fig. 2).

This data indicates a steady deterioration in all areas except confusion. The deterioration in the physical score is statistically significant ($p < 0.05$, two tailed). When the 1985 scores are compared with the scores of the same people at the end of the fifteen month period in Peppertree Lodge the means of five of the seven sub-scales and the total score show an improvement. This suggests that the fifteen month stay in Peppertree Lodge reversed the deterioration in the areas of self help, behaviour, sociability and nursing dependency bringing the residents back to a level of functioning that they had not enjoyed for more than three years. Physical condition and psychiatric symptomatology did not improve.

Conclusion

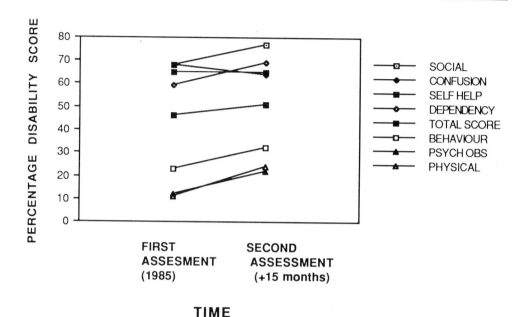

TIME

Fig.2. Changes in PRS scores over 15 months in a psychiatric hospital.

The principles of design that informed the development of the CADE unit appear to have been established as being useful. The unit has facilitated staff in the provision of high-quality care to mobile, confused and disturbed elderly people. The staff report a high level of satisfaction with their environment and it is encouraging that staff turnover is low.[4] The CADE approach is now being adapted by a team of people, including psychiatric hospital staff, for the provision of replacement wards for long-term patients in psychiatric hospitals. Detailed plans are available for units for patients requiring a simple, secure environment with higher supervision needs: plans are also available for units catering for those who, while requiring hospital standard care, can enjoy more privacy than the standard CADE unit provides. The units are being designed as 16-bed modules that can be put together in various combinations to meet the requirements of different patient populations.

References

(1) Fleming RW, Bowles JR. Units for the confused and disturbed elderly: develop-ment, design, programming and evaluation. *Australian J Ageing* 1987, **6**(4), 25-28.

(2) Fleming RW. The Psychogeriatric Rating Scale: a practical tool for assessment, monitoring and programme development. *Australian J. Ageing* 1990, **9,** 62-65.

(3) Folstein MF, Folstein SE. "Mini-Mental State" a practical method for grading the cognitive impairment of patients for the clinician. *Journal of Psychiatric Research* 1975, *12, 189--98.*

(4) Fleming RW, Bowles JR, Mellor S. Peppertree Lodge, some observations on the first fifteen months of the first CADE unit. *Australian J Ageing* 1989, **8**(4), 29-32.

SECTION 6
Carers' Initiatives

Carers, Professionals and Alzheimer's Disease. D O'Neill ed © 1991 John Libbey & Company Ltd

Chapter 23

RESPITE CARE OF DEMENTIA PATIENTS AND THEIR FAMILIES

WJ Wiley, *President, Alzheimer's Disease and Related Disorders Association, Honolulu, Hawaii, USA*

When Alzheimer's disease strikes a family member, both patient and care-giver suffer. The needs of the patient are so great that the care-giver experiences physical fatigue as well as psychological stress. If the health of the care-giver declines, the patient may not be adequately cared for.

Coping with multiple loss

The purpose of our group respite demonstration project has been to provide relief for care-givers and at the same time care for the patient in a positive way. In the Honolulu groups we provide assistance for families whom we know are suffering many losses. Spouses lose what they hoped would be the "golden years" of their shared retirement. They lose the companionship of a beloved spouse whose personality is slowly disappearing. They lose the benefit of the skills their partner used to provide such as financial, driving, homemaking.

The patients' losses are also great. Beginning with the loss of memory of the recent past and forgetting the skills of living, they lose the ability to read, to figure, and to analyse. They lose their awareness of time, space, direction, and identity. Their bodies may no longer tell them when they are too hot or too cold, whether they are hungry or full.

Judgements, inhibitions, recognition, know-how disappear. Recollection of events, language, and relationships progressively dwindle. Every new loss is a restriction on the freedom of both patient and care-giver. The respite group effort is designed to provide stimulation activities not usually possible in home care. We help patients maintain the skills they still have for as long as possible. By reinforcing the habitual social activities that patients have known, we foster participation and fun, interaction and closeness, sensory stimulation, exercise and relaxation. Movement to music and singing are enjoyed by nearly all patients.

147

Those who no longer remember their own names nevertheless remember the words and tunes to the old songs they sang as young people.

Goals

Our goals for participants are social interaction, maintenance of skills, self-esteem, and enjoyment with a minimum of physical restriction. Our goals for care-givers are time off and rest, support and counselling, a chance to view their patient more objectively, the attainment of humane patient management skills, and pursuit of their own activities.

When we recruit staff and volunteers (many of whom are previous care-givers), we look for qualities such as a sense of humour, flexibility, compassion, patience, creativity, and most of all the willingness to enter into the "reality of the patients". To accept the "new reality" of patients with symptoms of dementia, we must be willing to allow them to return to the past, to return to child-like abilities and activities, to sympathize with their agitation and fears (even paranoia), to acknowledge, *not deny*, their experience of hallucinations and delusions, and to accept the inevitable narrowing scope of their existence.

Those who give respite care must be willing to allow unconventional behaviour (unless it endangers the health or safety of the patient). We are conditioned to do things in a certain way; to follow customs of dress, behaviour, and language. Our patients will lose their knowledge of, and their ability to comply with, conventions. Scolding, preaching, nagging, punishing, pleading will not have meaning for the patient most of the time. He or she may not understand a concept, or even the words we speak. When an ability is gone, it probably cannot be retrained. Real care requires a lot of loving and allowing patients to be what they are.

Group Respite Demonstration Project

A 1987 survey of day-care in Hawaii showed that about 400 individuals were participating in adult day-care programmes. Monthly costs varied from $335 for social day-care to $1000 for day-hospital care. Despite the high costs, all programmes were operating at capacity or had waiting lists. About 25 per cent of all participants had some form of dementia. Several demographic trends in Hawaii suggest the need for more day-care programmes. We have the nation's longest life expectancy, a relatively low number of nursing home beds per 1000 elders, a high cost of living, and a large proportion of women in the work force. The most conservative projection estimates that day-care programmes need to serve as many as 900 clients by 1990 and 1000 clients by the year 2000. This paper reports on a volunteer Group Respite programme in Honolulu operated by the Honolulu chapter of the Alzheimer's Disease and Related Disorders Association (ADRDA). It is the only Honolulu day-care programme that restricts admission to adults with dementia. It costs participants $2 per 4-hour session and was begun in 1986 in response to a demand for low-cost, dementia-specific day programming by the Association's membership.

We will first provide a description of the programme followed by a report on a study of patients and volunteers, and finally a discussion of the implications for similar programmes. The author wishes to acknowledge Phyllis Hormann-Schaefer, family support coordinator, the Alzheimer's Association - Honolulu Chapter, for her assistance in the design and implementation of the Group Respite Programme, and Kathryn Braun, executive director, Honolulu Chapter, for her analysis of the survey data.

Programme

The Honolulu Group Respite programme uses volunteers who provide one-to-one attention to the clients under the supervision of a paid respite coordinator and a part-time assistant. In September 1986, the programme provided four hours of supervised activities and social opportunities on one day a week at a church. In 1987, a second day was added at the church and another 4-hour programme was started at a nearby senior centre. A fourth 4-hour programme is being started at a community centre. Each programme provides supervised activities and social opportunities for five to ten clients in a safe stimulating environment. The care-givers can use this time to attend to personal business, knowing that their patients are in good hands.

All volunteers attend an initial 4-hour training session on Alzheimer's disease and other dementias, communicating with dementia patients, managing difficult behaviours, and minimizing catastrophic reactions. Role playing is an important tool used to convey information and demonstrate patient management techniques. Policies and procedures for respite volunteers and information about the Honolulu Alzheimer's Association are also presented. Additional in-service training sessions are held at regular intervals and all Group Respite volunteers are expected to attend.

Each patient's family must complete a registration form and sign a waiver of liability. Care-givers may use our programme exclusively or in combination with other forms of respite. For example, of the 26 participants currently in the programme, 10 use the group respite only; 8 use group respite and in-home respite; 1 uses group respite and day-care; 2 use group respite, in-home respite, and day-care; and 5 live in care homes.

Goal and routines

The programme's goal is to provide adults with dementia with the opportunity to socialize and participate in activities to their maximum potential. In all activities, the process of participation is more important than the products that may emerge from the activity. Thus, all patients participate in all projects, without pressure to keep up with any preset standards. Participants seem to blossom in this programme; visitors have commented that the patients look so normal in this setting that they cannot distinguish the patients from the volunteers.

149

Table 1. Characteristics of Group Respite Patients (N=44)

		frequency	mean
GENDER:			
	Male	6 (36%)	
	Female	28 (64%)	
Lived with:			
	Spouse	18 (40%)	
	Children	15 (33%)	
	Other relative	3 (7%)	
	Paid care-giver	9 (20%)	
Dementia dx:			
	Alzheimer's	42 (95%)	
	Brain tumour	1	
	Parkinson's	1	
Medications:			
	Medical	21 (47%)	
	Psycho-active	15 (33%)	
Aware of memory loss		4 (9%)	
Problems with:			
	Eating	9 (20%)	
	Toiletting	9 (20%)	
	Sleeping	17 (39%)	
	Wandering	18 (40%)	
	Aggression	15 (35%)	
	Anxiety	3 (7%)	
Enjoyed exercise		32 (73%)	
Length of participation (months)			5.07
Reason for discharge			
	not discharged	20 (45%)	
	kept home		
	placed	7 (16%)	
	died	7 (16%)	
	distance	4 (9%)	
	felt "out-of-place"	3 (7%)	
		3 (7%)	

Sessions follow a routine. Families bring participants to the group programme between 9 and 9:30 am. Patients join the Morning Circle to socialize with each other and volunteers. Each participant and volunteer wears a brightly coloured name tag. Patients' tags are distinguished by a red heart on the front and emergency information on the back (name and phone number of the Group Respite programme and of the family care-giver, social security number, date of birth, and hospital preference). After all participants have arrived the group plays active ball games and does exercises to music until 10 am. Participants and volunteers then move to small groups (2 patients and 2 volunteers per table) for a refreshment break. At this time conversation flows easily, although the content may seem unintelligible and the comprehension level of each individual patient varies.

After the break the group may do one or a combination of things including arts, crafts, puzzles and other quiet table activities, visiting pre-school children in another part of the church, or going for a walk. Sometimes the restless participants go walking while the calm ones participate in table activities. Crafts and other fine motor activities are reduced to one-step tasks and completed in an assembly-line fashion. Participants are assigned tasks within their functional ability. Some may be content to participate as observers. When a client shows no interest in the activity, options are provided. In this way, flexibility and spontaneity are incorporated into the basic structure of the day.

At 11:30 am the group reconvenes for a half-hour of singing, dancing, and story telling followed by lunch which the families send with their patients. Volunteers assist participants who need to be reminded to eat or need to be spoon-fed. Patients are involved in helping the staff or helping other participants whenever possible, which promotes feelings of self-worth. Families collect their patients between 12:30 and 1 pm.

Funding

Donated space and volunteers keep costs low; the budget for the first 2 years was $32,000. The projected budget for the third year is $40,000, allowing us to employ a full-time coordinator, expand services from 3 days a week to 5 days a week, and complete a "how-to" guide for churches and civic organizations that wish to establish similar Group Respite programmes. This translates to about $3.50 an hour per client. To date, the programme has been funded as a demonstration through individual, foundation, and government grants (including $5,000 from the National Respite Care Demonstration Program of ADRDA).

Program liability insurance costs about $1,000 a year per site, which has caused us to think of ways to spin-off the programmes rather than take full responsibility for their operations. By the end of the demonstration period, we hope the programmes will be adopted by the churches and centres where they are currently located and that they raise fees to cover the cost of hiring a regular programme supervisor at each site. The Honolulu ADRDA will continue to provide training for volunteers and to act as a consultant to the groups.

Patient and volunteer characteristics

As a relatively new programme in Honolulu which depends on volunteers, the Alzheimer's Association was interested in determining the kinds of patients and volunteers who were successful in the programme. Thus, information from patient and volunteer registration forms was correlated with several measures of success. The sample included the 44 patients and 16 volunteers who had participated in the programme between December 1986 and March 1987.

Table 1 displays the characteristics of the 44 patients. The average age of patients was 76.5 years and two-thirds were women. Forty per cent were living with spouses, one-third with children, 7 per cent with other relatives, and 20 per cent with professional, paid care-givers. Most had a diagnosis of Alzheimer's disease: one participant's dementia was caused by a brain tumour and another had dementia of Parkinson's disease. In addition to a dementia-related diagnosis, one-third of the patients had heart disease and less than 10 per cent had one or two other conditions such as diabetes, pulmonary conditions, vision or hearing impairments, arthritis, urinary tract problems, or psychiatric disorders. Although a number of patients were not taking any prescription medications, almost half were taking drugs for medical problems and one-third were taking mood-altering drugs and/or sleeping pills.

Almost all of the patients were not aware of their memory disorders, but were still able to feed and toilet themselves and make their needs known. Most were reported to enjoy regular exercise (primarily walking). The majority (79 per cent) experienced short-term memory loss, a third were easily distracted, most were disoriented to time and place but not person, 35 per cent were aggressive, 40 per cent were problem wanderers, and 7 per cent were anxious.

Length of participation

The average length of participation was 5 months. Of the 44 patients in the sample, 20 were still attending the programme at the time of data analysis. Of the 24 who were no longer attending, 7 had become too difficult to care for at respite and were kept at home, 7 had been in nursing or care homes, 4 had died, 3 had stopped attending because of distance, and 3 stopped attending because they felt out of place at the programme.

Longer length of participation was not associated with any of the patient characteristics. However, significant associations were identified between patient characteristics and each of the reasons for leaving the programme. Patients who were kept home because they were too difficult to manage were likely to be male, to be unaware of their memory impairment, and to have aggressive behaviour, problems sleeping through the night, and problem wandering behaviour (i.e. refusing to return to the programme or being disruptive or unsafe). Patients who were placed in nursing homes had problems similar to this group, except that they were less likely to have lived with their spouses. Those who stopped attending because they took a turn for the worse and subsequently died were taking more medications than other patients, were likely to be male and to have problems with eating and toiletting. Patients who stopped coming because they felt "out-of-place" were likely to be aware of their memory impairments and were likely to be living with spouses.

Compared to patients who had stopped attending, patients who were still in the programme at the time of data analysis were likely to be female and less likely to have problems with eating, aggressive and unsafe wandering, and sleeping through the night. Taken together, these findings suggest that there is a class of dementia patients who do best in Group Respite – those who are no longer aware of their memory problem but who can still toilet and feed themselves, who sleep through the night, and are not problem wanderers.

Table 2. Characteristics of Group Respite Volunteers (N=16)

		frequency	mean
Age (years)			55
Gender:			
	Male	3 (20%)	
	Female	13 (80%)	
Education:			
	High school	6 (37%)	
	Some college	3 (19%)	
	Finished college	7 (44%)	
Past care-giving experience:			
	None	3 (19%)	
	Cared for elderly family member	7 (44%)	
	Professional	6 (37%)	
Motivation:			
	To help others	11 (68%)	
	Career interest	2 (13%)	
	Looks enjoyable	3 (19%)	
Length of participation (months)			10.06
Still involved with programme		13 (81%)	
Success rating (from 1=not successful to 5=very successful)			3.69

Volunteer characteristics

Table 2 displays the characteristics of the 16 volunteers associated with the programme. Most (80 per cent) were women, two-thirds of whom had attended college; their average age was 55. Three had no prior experience caring for older adults, 7 had cared for an older family member, and 6 had professional care-giving experience. In answer to the question, "why do you want to be a respite volunteer", 11 (68 per cent) reported that they wanted to help others and/or to do something worthwhile, 2 reported that they wanted experience in social services in order to help make a career choice, and 3 reported that they thought they would enjoy working with older people.

The average length of stay for volunteers was 10 months. At the time these data were analysed, 3 volunteers had dropped out. The drop-outs were younger and had little previous care-giving experience compared to those who stayed. Reasons for leaving included travel distance, poor personal health, and transfer to other volunteer opportunities.

Volunteers were rated on their successfulness on a 5-point scale by the programme staff. High-scorers were more likely to have cared previously for an elderly family member and to have reported that they joined to help others and do something worthwhile. These findings are not surprising: we would expect successful volunteerism to be related more to altruistic motives and past experience than to demographic variables.

Implications for other programmes

To those who are thinking of starting a volunteer group respite programme, we offer the following suggestions:

(1) We feel that this low-cost, group respite programme can be easily replicated. One needs to identify people who have time to volunteer, who want to help others, and have had past care-giving experience. Men are an asset to the programme but women are easier to recruit. We suggest these volunteers be drawn from the local Alzheimer's Association membership or perhaps from the membership of a religious or civic organization. For example, two church groups have asked us to help them start group respite programmes. They already have pools of volunteers with a mission to help others. They also have insurance that covers church activities. We recommend they hire a co-ordinator who can be paid from fees collected from the participants.

(2) We feel that this programme offers a viable respite option to families of dementia patients. Its low cost is appreciated by the families, who may use this service alone or in combination with other respite programmes. We recommend, however, that group respite programmes as we have described restrict admission to dementia patients who have minimal need for professional attention and personal care. Accepting patients who need a lot of assistance with toiletting, walking, and feeding may cause burn-out in volunteers and may present a danger to patients and volunteers. While it is very hard to turn away families who need

relief, a programme dependent on donated space and labour must not over-estimate the amount of personal care it can provide. Of course, we recommend that the coordinator be knowledgeable about other programmes to which families can be referred. At the same time, we have found that participants who are still aware of their memory loss feel out-of-place in a programme designed to manage dementia patients. These adults may be better suited for day-care programmes which serve alert as well as demented adults.

Conclusion

The Group Respite programme as demonstrated in Hawaii is one resource in a continuum of services available in the community for dementia patients and their families. It also provides an opportunity for civic and religious groups to contribute to their immediate communities by replicating this low-cost programme as a major project. The demand for respite services always seems greater than the supply, especially for dementia patients. The Honolulu Group Respite programme represents one useful model in meeting the increased need for services.

Chapter 24

THE THREE-DIRECTIONAL BENEFIT OF IN-HOME RESPITE

PM O'Connor, *Co-ordinator Home Respite Service, Alzheimer's Disease and Related Disorders Association of Western Australia, Subiaco, Western Australia,* **EJ Kingsley,** *School of Nursing, Curtin University, Bentley, Western Australia*

Introduction

Members of the Alzheimer's Disease and Related Disorders Association (ADARDA) in Perth, Western Australia, had registered the need for in-home respite for family care-givers since the inception of that organization in 1982. This mirrored the previous experience of the Western Australian Veterans' Affairs Department who had set up a Dementia Sitters' Programme in 1984; and reports from the United Kingdom and United States. In a survey of 1715 families, 64 per cent of care-givers rated home respite as their first priority of needs to be met.[1] Caregivers identified reliable, competent respite care as the single, most important service needed to prevent premature, long-term placement.[2, 3]

Goals of home respite

The primary goals, therefore, of the ADARDA (WA) Home Respite Service are:

(i) to care for the person with dementia in safety and security, and
(ii) to provide support and respite to the primary care-giver.

This is achieved by the provision of a trained home respite carer on a regular basis once a week for up to six hours. In April 1988, ADARDA (WA) attracted funding of $133,200 from the Home and Community Care Programme, a joint State and Federal Government initiative designed to bolster community support for the frail aged and disabled. The service was open to any person with a medical diagnosis of irreversible dementia. Although it was aimed at providing respite for ageing spouses, self respite was also acceptable, and people living alone in the community could be served.

Since the service started in August 1988, over 230 enquiries have been processed. The co-ordinator has made 140 personal visits of assessment of which 120 have received services, 11 on an occasional basis, and 109 on a regular basis. Evening, weekend and overnight stays in times of crisis are now available due to increased funding. Most referrals have come from social workers, care-givers and Silver Chain district nurses. Because of the hidden costs of caring for a person with dementia, and the age of the target group, no fee is charged, although donations are encouraged.

Priority is not assigned according to need but on first come, first served basis.[4] As Gaynor observes, "respite care given when the care-giver's health fails is not true respite".[5] Thus, respite ideally should start from the earliest time possible. The service can only serve a small number of clients. However it has expanded faster than reports of other services,[6,7] and it is vital that a high quality service and input are maintained.

Four of the six carers were recruited from the Veterans Home Service Programme which had lost its funding. They had undergone a Dementia Sitters training programme and had four years experience. Others were selected from advertisement, and range from single women in their late twenties to married women in their fifties, and one male carer. These paid carers have proved reliable, consistent and motivated, and loyal to the service. Training was provided initially by a two weeks programme covering the needs of the person with ADARDS, the care-giver, and the home respite carer. The qualities of caring, commitment, commonsense, communication and observation were emphasized.

Methodology

Three major approaches were used in this descriptive study to assess and evaluate the Home Respite Service.

(i) Care-giver satisfaction with the Home Respite Service.

(ii) Perceived benefits and satisfactions of the Home Respite Carers. Data was collected via questionnaires from 30 care-givers and 12 Home Respite Carers; informal interview and focus-group discussions with both family care-givers and home respite carers.

(iii) Client disability rating related to the "estimate of risk" of entry into long-term care. 120 entering clients were assessed according to a Functional Independence Rating scale and assigned an estimate of risk of admission to hostel or nursing home care. Anecdotal and qualitative evidence was collected from care-givers and compared to the level of risk to estimate the success to the service in deferring client admission to long-term care. As clients enter long-term care data will be collected on clients who have received respite services and compared to those who did not.

Only two eligible applicants for service were refused services.

Results

The three beneficiaries of the ADARDA Home Respite Service were the person with ADARDS, the primary care-giver and the home respite carer.

Benefits to the client

The benefits to the client were both direct, by attending to a person's physical, social and emotional needs; and indirect, by supporting the care-giver's health. Evidence relating to these benefits was collected by reports from home respite carers and a questionnaire circulated to care-givers.

Respite carers reported that their clients recognized and warmly greeted them from one week to the next, despite severe short-term memory loss. Clients co-operated and joined in simple games or household tasks. They were able to carry out simple instructions and attempt puzzles. Shared activities such as singing, dancing and in one case tennis, brought moments of obvious enjoyment. Clients showed pleasure in simple outings such as feeding ducks and going for a walk.

All care-givers indicated that they felt that the client benefited from the ADARDA Home Respite Service. Care-givers also felt that the client was comfortable with the home respite carer. They were confident that the client was well looked after – i.e. the level and scope of the Home Respite Service was both sufficient and satisfactory. They found the carers to be caring, patient, reliable and dependable, well trained and competent.

These factors influenced the care-givers satisfaction, on behalf of the client, in the level, scope, quality and amount of care that the client received. Because the care-givers felt satisfied in these areas they were happy and confident in leaving the person with ADARDS in the Home Respite Service's care.

Benefits to the care-giver

These fell into three categories:

(i) those which relieve stress

(ii) those which help the practical aspects of caring

(iii) those which help the affective aspects of caring.

Fifty per cent of care-givers stated that respite helped a great deal in reducing the strain of caring for the person with ADARDS, whilst 38 per cent felt it helped a lot. 4 per cent felt it only helped somewhat and 8 per cent a little. It is noted that the care-givers who rated the lower levels of satisfaction were not regular users of the service but had only used the service once or on an intermittent basis. Care-givers commented that the service "reduced the strain of constant care" and that the "situation would have been intolerable without this service". Another said that she "would crumble physically and mentally" without the service.

Practical aspects were helped by information about ADARDS and learning how

159

to cope with behavioural difficulties. Male care-givers appreciated the extra time and trouble respite carers took to ensure good grooming, dressing and appearance. The respite carers are preparing a book of simple recipes for men who take over the role of cooking as well as a directory of services which will come into the home such as hairdressers, podiatrists, etc.

Care-givers particularly appreciated help with the emotional burden of caring so amply illustrated in the following comments:

> *In my case sexual matters have been and still are a big problem at times. I handle it the only way I can. Then I feel guilty, and unfortunately that is when I want out. He puts me into Coventry which is terrible. He won't eat or drink which now I don't worry about (he will when ready), and my doctor can't help me – I've asked. L's stroke is of a crying and depressing nature. He is completely changed and I have to learn to get to know him all over again. Incontinence – I just change sheets and wash with no comment. He now hates me to be out of his sight which is also extremely wearing. Otherwise we get along fine.*

Respite relieves the care-giver of caring responsibilities for a space of time and according to one care-giver, "gives you time for yourself", "gives freedom" to renew friendships, attend a symphony concert, visit the library, continue writing a book, attend art classes, or even in a 80 year-old spouse's case, to play tennis. Family members may join together to enjoy an outing, hitherto impossible. Care-givers found the sharing of care important, expressed by the following comments – "The situation would be intolerable without your support" and "it makes you feel you aren't alone". Having someone to listen with objective empathy gives permission to talk of problems, complain. Five minutes "letting off steam" can defuse a potential crisis. The acknowledgement of the burden by the care-giver can lessen guilt of wanting to get out – it gives permission to get away from it all, even if for a short period.

Benefits to respite carers

The following benefits were expressed by the home respite carers in order of rating. (i) General satisfaction of being a home respite carer for people with Alzheimer's or a related disorder. (ii) Besides this, they felt there was an emotional benefit in the friendships developing from the care-givers and their families and with other respite carers. (iii) They liked the sense of belonging to the Home Respite Service, which for some carers was a "way to avoid loneliness" and for another "very rewarding to be accepted like family – most important in a new homeland". (iv) There was an affective benefit in the giving and receiving of love and kindness. Satisfaction in performing their role successfully has resulted in a growth of self-esteem and self-concept for women who have been out of the workforce for some time.

In regard to stress experienced at work, home respite carers felt some frustration in not being able to help enough, in not having enough time, some tiredness and sadness in the situation. Overall, however, they were not stressed – "So far, I'm free of any stress caused by client or by the system, or have been able to deal with it successfully."

Summary

From the above discussion, it appears that care-givers were satisfied with the level and quality of care of their relatives with Alzheimer's disease. This may be due, in part, to the fact that the service is available when they need it, and is provided free of charge.

Caregivers reported reduction of the level of their stress, partly through the physical help, but also through the brief periods of "freedom", and the sharing of the burden with someone who understands through the same experience. Care-giver support keeps patients at home for longer periods, and until they need extensive care.[8]

Home respite carers felt that they were adequately trained in scope and level for their work. They have unexpectedly low levels of stress and actually enjoy their work, and feel that they have a positive role to play. This surprising lack of stress may result from weekly group sessions, relaxation or stress management training.

Flexibility has been a large ingredient of success of the scheme, both in the provision of services and the adaptability of the carers. The home respite carers are not tied to an award, are multi-skilled and flexible. Evening and weekends are offered as alternatives and appreciated. One couple chose to have one evening out together instead of daytime respite. This significantly lessened their stress and maintained their relationship.

Despite all efforts made to provide respite as soon as possible, the sort of obstacles found by other programmes still exist.[6, 7] Reluctance of care-givers to accept help demands timing and patience. The problem of disseminating knowledge of the service has been addressed by numerous talks to community organisations, hospital and community nurses. The general practitioner of each person receiving services has been notified. The use of leisure time has to be actively encouraged particularly with elderly spouses.

Care-givers have great need of stress management training, coping strategies and relaxation skills. These care-givers have reported better sleeping, and more positive attitudes towards caring.

Future directions

The use of a more holistic, less medically oriented approach may see the development of more innovative and imaginative ways of communicating and interacting with these confused people. Respite care needs to be flexible and prepared to meet the changing needs of care-givers. Use of evening, weekend and longer terms of respite should be expanded. Working families need consideration if they are to share the burden of caring. The same sort of choices that have been developed in the child-care field should be considered.

Support for care-givers should be instigated from the beginning, when spouse or parent is diagnosed, if burn-out is to be avoided. Individual counselling, relaxation training, stress management and coping strategies should be the norm rather than the exception. ADARDA can provide much in the way of information about ADARDS and community resources and special support. Besides the vital care-givers' support groups, special groups focusing on unresolved emotions, social groups for male carers and special groups for children are waiting to be developed. The home respite carers' needs are best served by ongoing evaluation of the service, the development of training and maintenance of extensive support to prevent burn-out and stress.

A successful home respite service is only part of a range of services which need to be more fully developed in order to provide much more choice to families faced with the daunting task of caring for a person with ADARDS. A more concerted, co-ordinated approach is necessary if an impact is to be made.

References

(1) U.S. Office of Technology Assessment. *Losing A Million Minds – Confronting the Tragedy of Alzheimer's Disease and Other Dementias.* Washington DC, US Government Printing Office 1987, pp 31, 152-154, 248.

(2) Heagerty MA, Dunn LM, Watson MA. Helping care-givers care. *Aging* 1988, **358**, 7-8.

(3) Upshur CC. An evaluation of Home-Based Respite Care. *Mental Retardation* 1982, **20**(2), 58-62.

(4) Argyle N, Jestice S, Brook CPB. Psychogeriatric patients: their supporters' problems (1985). *Age and Ageing.* 1985, **14**, 355-360.

(5) Gaynor Sandra. When the care-giver becomes the patient. *Geriatric Nursing* 1989, May/June, 120-123.

(6) Middleton L. Training respite workers for Alzheimers' families. *Aging* 1987, **356**, 24-26.

(7) Dunn LM. Respite: preventing burnout. *Advice* 1989, **2**(6), 2-4.

(8) Smallegan M. There was nothing else to do. Needs for care before nursing home admission. *The Gerontologist* 1985, **25**(4), 364-369.

Carers, Professionals and Alzheimer's Disease. D O'Neill ed © 1991 John Libbey & Company Ltd

Chapter 25

DEVELOPING THE FIRST SPECIALIZED ALZHEIMER'S DISEASE FACILITY IN THE UNITED STATES

S Gilster *BS*, A McCracken *PhD, Alois Alzheimer Center, University of Cincinnati, Ohio, USA*

The Alois Alzheimer Centre, dedicated to the care and study of Alzheimer's disease and other dementias, opened on 1st May, 1987, and was the first specialized comprehensive facility of its kind in the United States. The centre is an 82 bed, long-term care facility. All the beds in this facility have been licensed for "skilled-care" so that we might accommodate people throughout the course of the disease process. This means that they would not have to be transferred to another skilled-care facility. The population served in the centre is a population who must have a primary diagnosis of Alzheimer's disease or dementia. We have developed a specific diagnostic work-up to identify those individuals with reversible dementia who are then referred to appropriate services.

Design considerations

In the United States, debate continues on the most appropriate structural design for specialized units and facilities. Until recently, dementia units were housed in sections of existing long-term care facilities that were sectioned off or segregated for a special population. In addition, in the United States there are a few free-standing facilities that are totally dedicated to caring for persons with Alzheimer's disease and dementia. As such a facility, we have had a great deal of experience looking at physical environment and the impact upon individuals with dementia. In the United States, one specific design for dementia utilizes the concept of individual bedrooms surrounding a central core. This central area contains all of the dining and activity space for the individuals residing on the unit. Although the population residing in units and facilities with this design are readily observed by staff, there have been difficulties verbalized in utilising this physical design as well. To date, there is not enough research to demonstrate the most effective physical plant for individuals with Alzheimer's disease. In fact, many who demonstrate successful special-care programmes in traditional facility structures argue that programming and not structure is the key to a successful programme. We feel that both play a vital role, and look forward to the publication of research from the specially-designed units and facilities that will demonstrate the effectiveness of physical structure and specialized programmes.

Our centre is a renovated structure, an elementary school building abandoned due to a declining enrollment. This building was selected as it houses a number of beneficial physical components that serve to improve upon the care for individuals with dementia. The building and setting were chosen for a number of reasons. Firstly, the location: as it sits on seven acres of land and is sited in a residential community. It is very quiet and peaceful, a conducive emotional atmosphere particularly for individuals with cognitive impairment.

Although easily accessible by major thoroughfares, it is not sited on a major highway. Therefore, it is safer for the population which we serve, particularly those who like to wander outside. The passage ways are very wide, allowing for wheelchairs and easy passage for the people who wander within the facility. This is useful, as our philosophy about wandering is to allow the clients to wander at will throughout the facility. Another advantage of the facility is the size of the rooms. The rooms are very large – as they were converted school rooms – and are about 200 to 400 square feet (19–37 square metres). They can accommodate a number of pieces of furniture and items from home that personalize the environment for the resident. The rooms are used therapeutically as well. If an individual is anxious or upset or seems to be fearful, they are taken back to their rooms where staff talk to them about pictures that are on the wall or items of furniture in their rooms that are very meaningful for them, in order to calm them. This has been very effective in reducing anxiety and decreases our need to resort to chemical and physical restraints in this population.

Security

A physically and emotionally secure environment is important. The Alois Alzheimer Centre developed an alarm system in conjunction with an independent contractor which tied in all six exit doors within the facility, and some gates to courtyards, into a centralized system. This system is in the main area of the building, inside the nurses station. An alarm goes off when an individual goes out a door, and a visual alarm goes off to indicate which door the patient has opened. When he/she walks out of the door, they walk into an enclosed courtyard with a locked and alarmed gate. This security system permits a great deal of freedom and choice of movement for our residents, not only within the facility, but outside as well. Although structural design to provide a home-like, secure and pleasant environment is important, our experience has been that staff selection, staff training and the development of individualized programmes are critical.

We know that staff need to be flexible, relaxed, compassionate and willing to "go that extra mile". No two days and no two individuals are alike and often we have to go beyond the role of our typical responsibilities to meet the individual needs of the people that we serve. We encourage staff involvement and believe that all staff, and especially the carers, are the vital links in a successful programme. Training staff to care for individuals with dementia is carried out when they are first appointed and continues as in-service training.

Activities and behavioural management

Another programme that is very important and which plays a major role in the centre is our activity programme. Alzheimer's disease patients are a population who can not effectively manage their leisure time: too much idle time leaves them restless and anxious. We gear our activities to be meaningful, enjoyable and to allow for individual accomplishments and successes. Our motto for the centre in the area of activities is "Never say never". These activities are carried out not only within the facility but also outside of it. Patient groups have visited a fire museum, art museums, the zoo, the symphony orchestra, ballets and apple-picking among other activities. They get a tremendous amount of enjoyment from this. When we can not go out we bring it in! This happened on a delightful snowy day when everyone seemed to want get outside and get their hands in it. Unfortunately it was a little too cold to do that so we laid out some plastic sheets, brought in buckets of snow and built some snowmen. There is nothing that we will not try!

Behavioural management without the use of excessive medication and restraint has not been as much of a problem as we had expected in the centre. We experience less aggressive behaviour and catastrophic reactions than expected from reports in the literature. This may relate to the level of staff training and the emotional environment that exists within the facility. We believe that an environment where individuals feel safe, secure, and accepted for who they are at that moment reduces the behavioural problems that are often encountered in this disease.

A dementia specific day care and in-facility respite programme was also developed and offers help to families to maintain individuals at home for as long as possible. Both have been very beneficial, not only for the families, but also for the people participating in the programmes. They have maintained a level of functioning while developing relationships and friendships with people within the programme and the facility.

Disease progression

Critical events such as functional and cognitive losses will occur in time and families grieve with every loss. Families need support at times like this, and support is provided through a number of programmes. We try to deal with families in realistic and positive terms. Instead of disabilities we talk about capabilities. Emphasis is placed on new ways to communicate with their family members and to share their lives with them. They are not going to be able to share thoughts and emotions in the same form over time, so we keep families involved through meetings, activities and gatherings so that they can share and enjoy being with one another without the pressure of constant verbal communication.

In time, however, the disease progresses and families are left to make decisions regarding life support and care. To complicate an already complicated issue, the centre has individuals from all over the United States: therefore, families are spread throughout the country. Many families are not in agreement with the level of care techniques and life-supporting measures which should be provided. Potential problems may arise with families where we need to balance their wishes against the potential liability for the facility should one of the family members not agree with the course of action. This is a major problem in the United States in many bioethical areas. The centre finally established a policy to help us in individual situations where there is a conflict, in consultation with numerous groups including clergymen, the Alzheimer's Association, families, legislators and lawyers. Families are asked to establish guardianship of the person through the courts as a result of this policy. This caters for the incompetent person for whom decisions have to be made: if the family decide a guardian, then the centre is kept out of the dilemma.

Staff programmes

The centre has developed a few other programmes to motivate and stimulate our own staff and to enhance their knowledge of caring for individuals with Alzheimer's disease and dementia. First, we have conducted numerous seminars and have developed a panel of expert speakers that has helped to decrease the myths and fallacies that surround this disease. As a resource centre, we have taught people from all over the country and Japan who are interested in starting programmes or who were involved with programmes themselves. Through our affiliation with the University of Cincinnati as a teaching nursing home, we provide a site for students for hands-on training. No amount of theoretical study about Alzheimer's disease substitutes for the experience of working with patients and carers to understand the impact on individuals and on families. Research at the Alois Alzheimer Centre focuses on care strategies rather than on medical therapies.

Conclusion

There is a great deal that can be done to improve the quality of life for individuals with dementia and for their families. In special care areas where there is a commitment to this specific population, we know that we can make this difference work for patients and their families.

SECTION 7
Therapy

Carers, Professionals and Alzheimer's Disease. D O'Neill ed © 1991 John Libbey & Company Ltd

Chapter 26

NON-DRUG THERAPY IN DEMENTING ILLNESS

S Hart *MSc, PhD, Department of Psychology, Severalls Hospital, Boxted Road, Colchester, Essex CO4 5HG, England*

The title of this paper covers a very broad brief. I do not propose to provide a detailed examination of this vast field: instead I will refer to particular non-drug or psychological approaches and use these to illustrate the points I wish to make. I believe it is important for me to discuss some of the methodological and conceptual issues surrounding interventions attempted to date, and those to be attempted in the future. This paper will pose a number of questions, but will not provide answers to all of these, because in many cases those answers must await the efforts of future researchers and carers.

Non-drug therapy in an organic condition

The first question to be confronted must be whether non-drug approaches have any place in the treatment or management of patients afflicted by dementia, since most dementia-associated conditions are biologically based and involve neuronal degeneration and neurochemical changes. This question can be answered in the affirmative on the basis of empirical observations and on theoretical grounds. It is worth stressing that drug and non-drug approaches to management and treatment of dementia are not dichotomous alternatives, nor should these be mutually exclusive. Ultimately both produce their effects via the same mechanisms. Drug treatments designed to produce symptomatic relief act directly on neurons to alter the activity of neurotransmitter systems and as a consequence modify cognition, emotion and/or behaviour. Psychological approaches seek to effect change in cognition, emotion and behaviour, but alterations in these must involve modulation of neurotransmitter dynamics in the same neural substrates. Ultimately, therefore, psychological interventions act in a similar manner to pharmacological agents, albeit more indirectly and over a different time scale.

Hence a combined approach to treatment, and a broad sense of perspective, is likely to be most helpful to the victims of dementia.

What psychological interventions have been attempted and have they worked?

Table 1. Examples of non-drug approaches to the treatment and management of dementia

Alterations of the physical environment
Reality orientation and validation therapy
Reminiscence therapy and life review
Behaviour modification
Cognitive therapy
Distraction and diversion tactics
Art therapy
Exercise

Many non-drug intervention strategies have been applied (Table 1). Attempts have been made to alter the physical environment of patients with dementia, some with the aim of increasing social interaction and engagement and others with the goal of circumventing the need for cognitive abilities that have been lost. For example, furniture has been re-arranged to facilitate social interaction. Pathways have been provided to allow those so disposed to wander while remaining safe from harm and minimizing the disruptive effects of their wandering upon other patients' or carers' activities. Labels and signs have been provided on doors and walls and particular routes marked out on floors to enhance orientation. External memory aids such as notebooks and calendars have been made available. Use of such aids will be particularly relevant to individuals in the early stages of a degenerative process and may allow them to maintain their role in society for rather longer than would otherwise be possible. For many this should enhance psychological well being.

Reality Orientation

However, evaluating the effectiveness of non-drug (and indeed drug) intervention strategies has proved a major problem. This can be illustrated with respect to Reality Orientation (RO) which is the most popular, most talked about, and most intensively researched psychological approach to the treatment of individuals with dementia. RO is based upon the assumption that certain kinds of basic orienting information are essential if a person with dementia is to function at a reasonable level.

Twenty-four hour RO involves carers using the opportunity provided by every interaction to present individuals with dementia with information about time, place, their own identity and that of others around them, as well as to comment upon what is going on at the time of the interaction. More frequently RO has been applied on a sessional basis in what might seem to be a rather artificial context. Sessional RO involves intensive work, usually with a small group of individuals, for short periods of time. Although generally advocated as a supplement to 24-hour RO, it has become an intervention in its own right and the evaluative studies that have been carried out have not produced clear evidence of obvious advantages for 24-hour RO. This somewhat surprising finding may have occurred, as Hanley has suggested, because 24-hour RO has not really been applied properly[1]. It is quite difficult to sustain the positive attitudes, attention and effort that are needed to keep this up all day long. Woods and Britton expressed the situation succinctly when they noted that "Twenty-four-hour RO has not been tried and found wanting, indeed it may never have been fully tried!".[2]

This has implications for the training of care-givers. Various writers have highlighted the importance of the reactions of staff. In attempting to account for discrepancies between the positive anecdotal reports of those involved in RO programmes and the disappointing results indicated by the supposedly more objective outcome measures of controlled studies, they have asserted that the principal effects of RO are to enhance the morale and enthusiasm of staff. This is not an insignificant achievement in itself. Indeed the recipients of care will almost inevitably benefit indirectly as a consequence of improved care-giver morale.

Reminiscence therapy

Another form of therapeutic intervention that is fairly widely practised is so-called reminiscence therapy. From a theoretical point of view this springs from Butler's idea of the necessity of a life review as death approaches.[3] In reviewing past achievements and failures individuals ideally arrive at a state of reconciliation and integration in readiness for impending death. By and large, however, what takes place in reminiscence groups is focused upon nostalgia with story-telling and relaying of information rather than promotion of a critical and more personal reappraisal of the past and of the roles individuals have played in this.

Thornton and Brotchie reviewed published studies addressing various aspects of reminiscence and concluded that there was little evidence of an age-specific increase in reminiscence activity, that the function of reminiscence was unclear and that the role of reminiscence as a therapeutic activity was in doubt.[4] On the positive side they affirmed that reminiscence groups were generally enjoyed by both care staff and patients. One notable benefit deriving from such activity was that care staff came to have a much greater knowledge about and understanding of the individual histories of those in their care. This must, of course, make some contribution towards preserving the individuality, dignity and worth of those who, having been afflicted by dementia, come to be placed in institutional care. Furthermore, any activity that can bring pleasure and enjoyment to the victims of dementia is to be welcomed in its own right, quite apart from whether it improves cognitive functioning or behaviour. In other words, whether one sees reminiscence therapy as a failure or as a useful activity depends to a very large extent upon what one holds to be the goals of therapy and how one chooses to define achievement thereof.

What we have seen little of to date is the true application of Butler's notion of the

171

Life Review which must, of necessity, be individually directed, rather than occurring as a group activity. This has been applied increasingly to patients with functional illnesses such as depression, but seldom to those with dementia. Individuals with dementia will require much greater effort from care-staff as they will have difficulty in sustaining the necessary cognitive effort required to direct their thinking processes and pursue a coherent line of thought. Nevertheless my own experiences, mostly with patients with pre-senile dementia of the Alzheimer type, has made me wary of the notion that people with dementia necessarily lack insight, even though they may be unable to articulate their thoughts and feelings in a form that we would readily recognize as "insightful". Therefore it is important that we do not *automatically* forego any attempt to facilitate a process of life review in patients with dementia.

Behaviour modification

Behaviour modification, based upon the principles of learning theory and using applied behavioural analysis to identify those environmental contingencies which might promote and/or maintain specific behaviours, remains "an unfulfilled potential" in relation to the treatment and management of problem behaviours associated with dementia.[2] It has been applied very successfully in the field of mental handicap or learning difficulties and has dramatically improved the quality of life for many. However, behaviour modification has often been portrayed by its critics as a dehumanizing technology which exerts repressive control and as such is incompatible with a philosophy of "normalization" or "social role valorization", that is "the use of culturally valued means in order to enable people to live culturally valued lives".[5] Increasingly this philosophy is also being invoked in relation to the care of elderly people with dementia. I would argue that the supposed incompatibility between normalization and behaviour modification is more apparent than real and arises from previous misapplications of behaviour modification approaches. The emphasis within behaviour modification has very much turned away from the use of negative reinforcement and aversive strategies to the use of only positive reinforcement, a position which is completely consistent with humanistic approaches to care.

Sensitively applied, behaviour modification offers tremendous potential for managing some of the behavioural excesses, such as shouting, screaming and aggressive behaviour, which can be manifested by the victims of dementia.[6, 7, 8, 9] It may be of use in relation to their behavioural deficits also, such as lack of eating or inappropriate eating behaviour, failure to dress, etc.

Neuropsychological deficits and behaviour

The behavioural excesses and deficiencies of the victims of dementia undoubtedly have their roots in the disturbances of neuronal functioning produced by Alzheimer's disease and other dementia-producing conditions. Indeed I would emphasize the potential contribution of often unrecognized neuropsychological deficits to a number of such problems, for example apraxia in relation to feeding and dressing problems and agnosic problems in relation to socially unacceptable eating behaviour.[10] However, the expression of behaviour is always an interaction between biological and environmental factors. Hence it is important to determine neurological factors as well as environmental contingencies that might be contributing to promotion and/or maintenance of behavioural deficits and excesses in any given individual.

It is also important to realize that the relative weightings of biological and environmental factors will differ from one individual to another in relation to any particular behaviour. Within a given patient their respective contributions will differ as the disease progresses. Hence the need for assessment procedures and management interventions which are focused upon individuals first and foremost and which make a wholistic appraisal of the clinical picture.

Studies of efficacy of non-drug approaches

Despite many positive reports of beneficial effects, the empirical data amassed to date on the efficacy of non-drug approaches to the treatment and management of individuals with dementia has been less than adequate. Methodological shortcomings abound and may seriously compromise the validity and therefore the utility of the data that have been collected. These problems are best documented for investigations of RO.[11] A problem that is frequently encountered is lack of adequate controls. It is insufficient to simply have a no-treatment control condition, as one cannot distinguish between specific beneficial effects brought about by the treatment as opposed to non-specific effects of increased attention being directed towards subjects during its delivery. Any alteration in routine, almost irrespective of what it is, may produce some change in subjects' behaviour and possibly some degree of improvement.

Another problem is that the subject population under investigation is all too often inadequately described. Furthermore, groups have very frequently been heterogeneous, not only in terms of including patients whose dementia syndromes derive from different aetiologies, but also with respect to the severity of subjects' impairments. Much remains to be done also in terms of evaluating the efficacy of therapeutic interventions in non-institutional settings, e.g. in the individual's own home.

When we consider the specific aims set out and dependent measures employed in various studies, it becomes apparent that it is all too easy to lose sight of what must be the overriding goal of all non-drug (and indeed of pharmacological) interventions, namely to enhance the overall psychological well-being of those whom we seek to treat. This means not only enhancing their level of cognitive functioning, but also and no less importantly, their sense of autonomy, individuality dignity and self-esteem. In other words we are dealing with life satisfaction, quality of life and quality of care. These are admittedly elusive concepts that are difficult to define in terms that allow for collection of empirical data that can be

173

presented to the general managers and politicians who hold the purse strings, and who rightly demand accountability and demonstrable value for money.

Community or institution?

One of the major driving forces behind the move towards care in the community has been the belief that the highest quality of life can be achieved by maintaining people in their own homes, close to their origins, to their families and friends, and to places that are familiar to them. However laudatory the principle of care in the community, its practical implementation has often fallen far short of this ideal. Families may well be glad to retain elderly people at home with them, but they have the right to expect that their efforts will be recognized and that support will be readily available. Caring is a costly business in emotional, physical and financial terms.[12, 13] The well-being of the victims of dementia is intimately linked to the well-being of those who care for them.

In recognition of the morbidity associated with caring, importance is rightly being attached to determining how best to provide care for the carers. There is much interest in psychological approaches to reducing the burden of care by providing carers with better techniques to manage the problems posed by dementia and to enhance their own sense of control and capacity to cope with the stress of the "36-hour day". This includes instruction in basic techniques of behavioural management, explanations of aberrant behaviour in terms of underlying neuro-psychological deficits and guidance regarding how to circumvent these, cognitive interventions to help carers reconstrue the behaviour of their dependents and their own responses to the tasks of caring so as to maintain their self-esteem and reduce stress.[14] It is also vital that carers be helped to maximize the relief they can obtain from intermittent respite care, and this includes assuaging the guilt that many experience when they seek something for themselves. Efforts are being made to provide carers with information in a language and format that is meaningful to them and which they perceive is relevant to their own problems.

However, the time may come when it is in the interests of all concerned, the person afflicted by dementia, his/her carer(s), family and the community at large, to have that person removed from the home environment and placed in an alternative setting. Ideally this would be close to relatives and friends who could continue to participate in the process of caring, though less intensively. Such establishments would ideally be run, not on institutional lines, but rather with an emphasis on individuality, taking account of the needs of each resident and exploiting any residual assets or strengths that might be available in order to meet these needs. Individuals would continue to be cared for in the community and, more importantly, as members of the community.

Considerations of care in the community have all too often focused upon the word *in* but much more important than where care is provided is the manner in which it is delivered. It is all too possible for a small "domestic" setting to become as much an institution as any large hospital, nursing home or residential facility if it is run along "institutional" lines. Conversely, hospitals, nursing homes and residential facilities can be run so as to provide the highest standards of care in physical and psychological terms. I would suggest that it would be a sad reflection on our society if we were to construe recipients of care in hospitals, nursing homes etc. as having left the community.

The task of caring is a monumental one. It is a monumental task not only in terms of the magnitude of the physical and emotional investment required, but also in a more abstract but none-the-less profound sense. I refer here to the monument that will remain when the demented individual has finally succumbed to death. By this I mean that the way in which that person is remembered will depend to a large extent upon how the task of caring has been executed and the costs associated with it.

Training

Finally I would like to address three important issues, namely training, bereavement and early diagnosis. We cannot overemphasize the importance of training to achievement of the goal of high-quality care for those afflicted by dementia. I would suggest that initial and in service top-up training events should be compulsory for all care staff, irrespective of their position in management and/or professional hierarchies. Training involves much more than transferring skills to those who are in direct contact with patients – important as this is! Training affords an opportunity to critically examine both care practices and, more importantly, the philosophy of care which guides the way in which these practices are implemented.

It is the philosophy of care that guarantees preservation of the individuality, dignity and worth of the person being cared for. It is all too easy to intellectualize about a problem while ceasing to experience its devastating impact, or our own potential roles in dehumanizing individuals. When faced with the inevitable day-to-day demands of providing care, theory and practice can all too easily become dissociated from one another. The effectiveness of training has to be evaluated, not just in terms of short-term measures such as knowledge gained and attitudes expressed. Ultimately the effectiveness of training will have to be measured in terms of enduring changes in the day-to-day behaviour of care staff and improvements in the quality of life of those in their care.

Bereavement

When the topic of bereavement is raised it is usually in relation to the needs of carers, their anticipatory grief and sometimes guilt at their lack of grief when the person they have cared for dies. It is right that we should consider and attempt to cater for such needs. However, I would like to suggest to you that we also need to consider the needs of dementing individuals themselves, in relation to the loss of their own abilities and roles, and in relation to their loss of companions. It is all too readily assumed that those with dementia are protected from these losses by their lack of insight. However, there are reports of patients with severe dementia manifesting marked behavioural alterations following the death of fellow patients in institutional settings.[15,16] We must recognize these needs and respond creatively by adapting the techniques of bereavement counselling and therapy that are usually applied.

Early dementia

My last point concerns the challenge of early cases. We have heard much about increasing public awareness of Alzheimer's disease. A spin-off of heightened public awareness will be that increasingly in the future we shall be faced with the task of caring for the psychological needs of people at a much earlier point in the progression of their disease, at a time when their cognitive deficits are not yet sufficiently global to warrant a diagnosis of dementia. How are we to counsel such individuals, to provide them with a realistic appraisal of their future without inspiring panic or despair, to provide them with the information necessary to allow them to set their affairs in order, to prepare their families for the impending changes so that they too can adapt and cope with the burden of caring?

Conclusion

Much has already been achieved by way of non-drug interventions to enhance the well-being of those afflicted by dementia – and of their carers – but there can be no grounds for complacency. Much remains to be done.

References

(1) Hanley IG. Theoretical and practical considerations in reality orientation therapy with the elderly. In, Hanley IG, Hodge J (eds) *Psychological Approaches to the Care of the Elderly*. London, Croome Helm, 1984.

(2) Woods RT, Britton PG. *Clinical Psychology with the Elderly*. London, Croome Helm, 1985.

(3) Butler RN. The life review: an interpretation of reminiscence in the aged. *Psychiatry* 1963, **26,** 65-76.

(4) Thornton S, Brotchie J. Reminiscence: a critical review of the empirical literature. *British Journal of Clinical Psychology* 1987, **26,** 93-111.

(5) Wolfensberger W. The definition of normalization: update, problems, disagreements and misunderstandings. In, Flynn RJ, Nitsch KS, (eds), *Normalization, Social Integration and Community Services*. Baltimore, University Park Press, 1980.

(6) Stokes G. *Shouting and Screaming*. London, Winslow Press, 1986.

(7) Stokes G. *Wandering*. London, Winslow Press, 1986.

(8) Stokes G. *Incontinence and Inappropriate Urinating*. London, Winslow Press, 1987.

(9) Stokes, G. *Aggression*. London, Winslow Press, 1987.

(10) Holden U. *Neuropsychology and Ageing*. London, Croome Helm, 1988.

(11) Holden UP, Woods RT. *Reality Orientation: Psychological Approaches to the "Confused" Elderly.* Edinburgh, Churchill Livingstone, 1987.

(12) Hart S. Psychology and the health of elderly people. In, Bennett P, Weinman J, Spurgeon P, (eds), *Current Developments in Health Psychology.* London, Harwood Scientific Publishers, 1990.

(13) Creedon M. Economic consequences of Alzheimer's disease. In *Carers, Professionals and Alzheimer's Disease.* London, John Libbey, 1991.

(14) Bayles KA, Kaszniak AW. *Communication and Cognition in Normal Aging and Dementia.* London: Taylor & Francis, 1987.

(15) Haycox JA. Bereavement and severe dementia. *Lancet* 1987, ii, 405-406.

(16) Summerfield D, Smellie N. Bereavement and severe dementia. *Lancet* 1987, i, 1097.

Carers, Professionals and Alzheimer's Disease. D O'Neill ed © 1991 John Libbey & Company Ltd

Chapter 27

ENHANCING LIFE FOR INDIVIDUALS IN A SPECIALIZED ALZHEIMER'S FACILITY THROUGH CREATIVE BEHAVIOURAL MANAGEMENT

D Torgersen *BSN*, **S Gilster** *BS*, **A McCracken** *PhD, Alois Alzheimer Center, 70 Damon Rd, Cincinnati, Ohio 45218, USA*

Enhancing life for those with Alzheimer's disease is a major goal for all carers. Individuality must be a mainspring of care plans for those with dementia: each person is unique, with unique approaches required to meet their needs. An individual plan of care has to be created for each patient if we are to meet these needs. A second important factor in dementia care is that there is more to life than memory: there are also will, desires and preferences. Individuals can express these qualities even in the later stages of the disease. A third challenge is to ensure the appropriateness of our interventions. Inappropriate actions may escalate behavioural issues whereas appropriate actions may help to diffuse them. Without appropriate interventions the patient's helplessness and dependency increases: his/her impairment and emotional distress will also increase. In this paper I would like to outline our approach to some common problems in caring for patients with Alzheimer's disease.

Training

The development of teaching strategies and interventions poses a challenge for those who care for and about individuals with Alzheimer's disease. Training of personnel is critical in contributing to the quality of life of our patients: all personnel should be included in the training programme, from the receptionist at the desk who answers the phone to the typists in the business office. Training of staff should be a continuous process. Our programme covers a range of topics from the disease process to behaviour modification interventions. Other approaches to training programmes are presented in this book. A basic tenet of our training is that: "When you have met one Alzheimer patient, you have met one Alzheimer patient". Because of each patient's individuality and uniqueness, we work on a daily basis to bring their quality of life up to the level which we ourselves would want as individuals.

A special effort is made to celebrate the parts of the person that remain intact, regardless of the severity of the disease process. The families provide us with family histories: using these we are able to deal with antisocial behaviours and the anger and frustration that result from this disease. Successes are praised because these individuals often fear that their families are going to abandon them.

The behaviours of demented individuals vary with the stage of the disease process. For example some patients experience a lot of anxiety when admitted to our facility as a result of the change of environment. They are less able to make sense of their experiences and of their new environment. We do not rush our residents and rarely use our intercom system except in emergencies as it can be very distracting for them. A lot of time is spent reassuring patients, with a lot of touch and hugging and special care. Our family carers have been the experts and continue to be the experts for us. As we have learnt so much from them, we want to promote that family security even after they are placed in the facility: so our families are very involved.

Wandering and delusions

Wandering is a typical issue: it is a part of the disease process. For some it may represent the fear of being lost, for others it may be based on previous life styles. One gentleman who begins to wander every afternoon about three o'clock was a school bus driver: he obviously felt that it was time to go and get the children. What we learn from their previous life styles and past helps us realize what triggers this behaviour. Some patients run away from stressful situations and some use wandering for physical stimulation. Examples of these might be former joggers and runners. Our approach is to provide a safe, secure area for them where they can wander if they choose to do so. Safety is a prime consideration and obstructing furniture should be avoided in hallways to prevent injury. It is worth trying to find out what triggers the wandering behaviours. Sometimes it is a question of hunger or a need to go to the toilet. In other cases, something in the environment may trigger the wandering impulse: for example, a suitcase left behind in the room may trigger an impulse to leave. It is worth removing suitcases and coats and any object – even boots – that might trigger the desire to leave. Another therapeutic approach to wandering is redirection of energy and participation in activities that enable release from the frustrations and over-stimulation that sometimes occur. Our parachute game is very simple but allows the patients to get rid of some of that energy.

Delusions and hallucinations present a different problem. The delusions can often give a clue to a valued activity that the individuals were involved with before they became cognitively impaired. We have a lady who is a nurse who had spent most of her career in paediatric nursing who would often try to find children to take care of. By giving her a couple of dolls that look like babies to take care of, she is not only less delusional but has also remained continent for a year. At night she gets up and as she checks the baby, she remembers to toilet herself and it has been a real success for her. To help with hallucinations we do what we can to correct those feelings of fearfulness in the environment by acknowledgement of these feelings and by reassurance.

Sundowning and catastrophic reactions

"Sundowning" has attracted a good deal of attention in caring circles recently. It is often due to fatigue or inability to cope with the confusing environment at the end of the day. Patients lack the sensory appreciation of changes in the environment to give them vital orientation as night falls; toiletting may also act as a trigger for sundowning reactions. We have been able to improve the symptoms of sundowning by changing the lighting in the facility as night comes on. Activities may help to distract attention: simple activities such as music and failure-free activities in the evening and late afternoon are useful in providing appropriate stimulus. Sometimes just a change in environment is sufficient: enjoying a snack in our outside area is another diversional activity for our sundowners. These measures help us to change our method of approaching the individuals who are affected by sundowning.

Catastrophic reactions represent the most severe form of behavioural disturbance and can pose a major problem for patients and staff. We do not see as many catastrophic reactions as we had anticipated in our facility, and this may be due to staff training. Some catastrophic reactions may be related to the environment but they may also herald an acute illness in the same way that increased confusion or agitation may precede a urinary tract infection. A calm approach works well with catastrophic reactions. Sometimes patients need to be removed from their situation and we use their own rooms for this purpose. This is particularly effective because they are allowed to bring their own furniture and photograph albums to their rooms. These factors make the room a good place to take people to avoid catastrophic reactions. Alternatively an outside area may be used: the change of environment will often help to alleviate such a reaction.

Conclusion

Individuals with Alzheimer's disease need to feel a sense of place. They need to find something they can do right. They want to know they can still give happiness and they need pleasurable times created for them. Our unit tries to give them a sense of place, and to find things that they can do right. They still need to know they can develop stimulating relationships. We must forge a bridge that will maintain a path to each person's uniqueness. Individuals will respond appropriately if treated as human beings and enabled to play an active role in their own care for as long as possible.

Carers, Professionals and Alzheimer's Disease. D O'Neill ed © 1991 John Libbey & Company Ltd

Chapter 28

THE HELPING HAND DEMENTIA-SPECIFIC RESPITE MODEL

V Bell *MSW,* D Troxel *MPH,* N Cox *MSW, Sanders-Brown Center on Aging, University of Kentucky, Lexington, KY 40536, USA*

The Helping Hand is a day centre and in-home programme, sponsored by the Lexington/Bluegrass Chapter of the Alzheimer's Association with close ties to the Alzheimer's Disease Research Center at the University of Kentucky. It is a social model, providing safe, creative companionship for persons diagnosed with a non-treatable memory problem who are living at home but who are unable to stay alone. The day centre is open from Monday to Friday from 8.00 a.m. to 5.00 p.m., and the in-home service is by arrangement between family and staff. The programme fees are $10.00 for a half day, and $20 for a full day. The programme is staffed primarily with volunteers.

Origins

When we started we were all alone. Only a handful of day-care programmes existed in the country for persons with non-treatable memory problems. The search for a model on which to base our programme took staff through the United States and to Great Britain. While we liked many programmes which treated the Alzheimer's patient as a valuable human being, we rebelled against some centres where persons with memory loss were kept in an environment that, while safe, did not stimulate the individual or strive to bring out the best in the person.

Surprisingly, this concept that programmes should consider the needs of the individual with Alzheimer's disease was radical at the time. Most day-care centres existed primarily to provide the family care-giver with a break, or respite, from the onerous task of care-giving. We believed that the Helping Hand could provide the desperately needed respite and a rich environment for the programme participant with a memory disorder.

We rejected the term "inappropriate behaviour" to describe behaviours which resulted from legitimate feelings of anxiety, frustration and even anger. What could we offer that could possibly help to change those feelings to more secure, safe and valued ones? If we could find the answer to this question, we felt that the patient's behaviour would improve. We feel that our greatest accomplishment has been to build self-esteem in memory-disabled persons and as a result to prevent most of the "hard to manage" behaviour. From the beginning, we viewed each participant as a unique individual – an adult, not a child, with feelings, life-long traditions and methods of coping in daily life. We are aware that most participants have at least a lingering sense of their life story until very late in the disease process.

Assessment

A good assessment of the patient's functional level is most important. To expect too little from a person is as frustrating as expecting too much. What can the person do? What are his limits? Having an excellent way of communicating and relating is of little use if it is not matched to the patient's communication ability. Ongoing assessment is also important, as a person's functional level may change with time. We have given much attention to matching a person's functional level to all aspects of our programme.

A life-story for each participant is essential. It is important to identify which names of persons, places or things that the person may still recognize if recalled by a companion. Place of birth, parents, family, early childhood, pets, school days, spouse, children, career, favourite colours, songs and hobbies are examples of the kinds of information that can be used throughout the day to give the participant a feeling of being a part of the group and still in the flow of life. The life-story and the functional level of a person can guide the selection of meaningful activities and time together. A bridge player with mild memory loss may still enjoy playing a game with an understanding partner. A severely demented person who once enjoyed a game of cards may now enjoy "playing with" the cards. Look for surprises in the following areas for activities and programming: music, poetry and old sayings, dancing, old skills and memories, and games involving hand-eye coordination!

Language is such an everyday kind of activity that we tend to take it for granted. Every time that we carry on a conversation, we do a staggering amount of information processing. Memory loss makes this process more and more complicated. Therefore conversations need to be simple, slow, sincere and with as much non-verbal input as possible. A further helpful development is the growing appreciation of the power of non-verbal communication with Alzheimer's disease. To use an old cliché, actions speak louder than words, and what a person sees, hears, tastes, smells and feels should convey the message that all is well and that every person is valuable. Communicating effectively, verbally and non-verbally, can build self-esteem and improve behaviour.

Volunteers

"He requires care that is thoughtfully planned and executed, his social relationships are complex, difficult and often unpredictable – just as might be said about any of us – and his immediate needs range from those related to bare survival to remnants of mature and sophisticated development represented, for example, by the enjoyment of music.[1]" Who can give the individual attention that an Alzheimer's person needs to function at his highest level? In the Helping Hand, some 75 volunteers give sensitive, loving one-to-one care. These volunteers are carefully chosen, and attend a 16-hour study session on topics such as normal ageing, Alzheimer's disease and related disorders. family coping with dementia, and communicating and relating to the memory-disabled person. In addition to a half-day each week with their Alzheimer's friend, the volunteers may become good friends with the family care-giver, serve as a teacher to visiting students working in the programme or serve on planning committees.

Initially many believed that the volunteer model could not work. Items which caused particular concern were whether the volunteers could cope with a task that even family members find daunting, and whether volunteers could be dependable. These worries have been resolved. The five volunteers who had been with the programme in 1984 are still with us. They have been dependable, and so have the seventy others in the programme. They bring with them the interest and expertise of a variety of ages. These volunteers have helped to reverse stereotypes of persons with Alzheimer's disease.

Conclusion

Since its inception, the Helping Hand has been a laboratory of learning. As Nancy Mace has written: "We know that life can be bearable and sometimes filled with laughter, love and joy despite the devastation of dementing illness.". We have shared this experience in the Helping Hand programme. We hope that the hundreds of observers who have come to our programme from nursing homes, hospitals and other settings have left with a challenge to rethink their approach to the care of persons with dementia.

Reference

(1) Howell, M. Caretakers' views on responsibilities for the care of the demented elderly. *J Amer Geriatr Soc* 1984, **32**, 657-660.

Carers, Professionals and Alzheimer's Disease. D O'Neill ed © 1991 John Libbey & Company Ltd

Chapter 29

AT RISK COMMITTEE

Vicki Rose, *Social Worker, Norwich Social Services, Norwich, Norfolk, England*

My role as a social worker in a multi-disciplinary geriatric team is to ensure that the clients remain in the community in the care of their relatives or friends for as long as possible. In practical terms, regular and frequent planning, coordination and follow-up are required. This means that we focus only upon individual clients by name, their circumstances and their needs, and organize a definite plan of action. The development of community-based services tailored to address the needs of Alzheimer's patients and their carers requires that these services should be coordinated, effective, relevant and caring. Ideally this drive for effectiveness should be based on a client-centred perspective. The philosophy of our service is based on the principle that a person with dementia should be able to live at home for as long as possible with the support of community-based services, rather than in an institutional setting that can often reduce individuality in areas such as choice, privacy, independence and dignity. The aim of the At Risk Committee is to improve the quality of life of Alzheimer's sufferers and their carers, enabling them to remain in the community and avoiding premature or inappropriate admission to institutional care.

Inappropriate admission to institutional care

Three reasons for inappropriate admission to institutional care have been identified:

(i) a person's lack of knowledge of existing community services resources;

(ii) a person's inability to mobilize local resources to meet their individual needs;

(iii) local resources that lack the degree of co-ordination needed to meet the gaps in client's needs, as these agencies may act autonomously in assessment and provision of service.

The formation of the At Risk Committee addressed these issues. Autonomous community based services now have a formal structure that allow for full consultation between the various services. These meetings contribute to decreasing the problems associated with a fragmentation of community-based services. Through client cases being discussed in a forum with participation by the agencies providing services to the client's home, gaps or changes in existing care plans to meet the individual's need can be identified earlier, and a plan of action can be decided upon and implemented by the relevant agency. These client-centred meetings attempt to reduce crisis responses to a client's change in circumstances. A coordinated approach of this type to assessment and structured implementation of services to clients who are often consumers of multiple community-based services would assist in decreasing unnecessary or early admission to institutional care. By pooling each agency's specific knowledge and ideas, particularly with regard to gaps in services to individuals, a more comprehensive overview of local resources can be achieved, involving both main stream and voluntary services.

Informal communication

Prior to the establishment of the At Risk Committee, there was no formal structure or network mechanism for communication between community-based agencies who had the potential to service the Alzheimer client and their carers. Informal communication channels existed that allowed for a very limited flow of information. This informal mode of communication is certainly an important aspect of any service provided it is part of an effective service. However, it does not address the need for a coordinated approach involving all services that have the potential to be involved with a particular client group. With the existing client group, multiple use of community service is the rule. Consequently, when multiple service usually occurs, it relies solely upon informal networking and communications channels. It is not the most effective or efficient way to deliver a service in assisting unmet needs. An example might be a case where the home care service attends and the district nurse visits, but no one has addressed the need of whether they need meals on wheels. A formal mechanism is therefore required to facilitate communal meetings between community service providers where discussion centred on clients own unmet and changed needs can occur.

The absence of such a mechanism necessitated the establishment of a formal committee that was composed of service providers. The committee was started in July, 1986 by the Geriatric Assessment Team in Lismore, Northern South Wales. An explanatory letter was sent to the service agencies in the Lismore area outlining the need for a formal structure to facilitate coordinated services. The agencies, recognizing the benefits in the form of this committee, responded positively. Attendance at the meetings has reflected strong commitment. Each agency has to provide an effective service. The establishment of the committee has been successful due to each agency's commitment to (i) regular attendance at meetings, (ii) participation in multi-disciplinary discussions and service planning and (iii) ability to focus primarily on the needs of the client. One is not there to talk about the latest policy of government, one is there to talk about the client's needs.

Formal communication

Any group of complementary organizations which share clientèle but do not have a formal system of co-ordination will find it difficult to perform well. In the welfare area this is especially so as, due to the less tangible and changeable nature of the market, the consumers are the primary beneficiaries of a coordinated service approach. Secondary beneficiaries are the persons directly involved or responsible for this sort of delivery. The benefits gained from a coordinated service approach can be demonstrated with the structured forum for communication. Review is important, otherwise the care providers cannot specifically address the unmet and changed needs of the consumer and the identification of case managements responsible for the overall management. This is a necessary procedure when a consumer may have multiple providers. A package of service to meet client's needs is shared among other community providers. Communal knowledge of all services involved with the client helps reduce duplication and inappropriate servicing. Regular case review and forward planning helps to reduce the amount of crisis responses that agency personnel deal with. Regular communication between the agencies enables an increased knowledge of what services have to offer and generally broaden the knowledge base of local resources. If an agency is unable to meet a client's needs, a forum now exists where the situation can be discussed.

The issue of confidentiality may appear to raise problems with such a broad-based committee. It is recognized that information is shared at the meeting and that this may raise concerns about confidentiality. However, the committee participants are all experienced service providers who treat all information shared as confidential. The major success of this client-centred model of co-ordination is due to its deliberate sharing of information that has traditionally been viewed as completely confidential. It has been by putting the client's needs before the ideal of confidentiality that this committee has performed so well in actually meeting the identified needs.

Composition and criteria

Who is on this committee? The composition included members of the geriatric assessment team – geriatrician, social worker, senior nurses, physiotherapists and occupational therapists, home care, community nurses, meals on wheels co-ordination, two private nursing services and the day-care coordinator. The membership criteria stressed that a working knowledge or direct client involvement was necessary for participating committee members due to the fact that meetings are client-focused and all discussion is centred specifically on addressing the client's needs. A willingness to work with other agency personnel is very important. The multi-disciplinary membership of the committee ensures that the assessment, discussion and planned implementation of services view client's needs as primary.

In drawing up our criteria for acceptance on to the At Risk Register, we feel that it is not feasible that all clients receiving a service from a community-based agency are included on the register. Certain factors are considered prior to a client being accepted for review by the committee. These include (i) the person's medical, physical, mental and emotional status, (ii) frequency of admission to hospital, (iii) uncertainty regarding availability of informal support systems – the spouse, the family, the neighbours, the friends, (iv) ability of local resources to meet identified needs, (v) client's attitude and responses to actually using those resources and (vi) pending change in the person's circumstances.

The meetings are held once a fortnight. Due to the members' work commitments, a lunch time meeting was preferred and I feel that an important factor in the success of the meetings is that lunch is provided at these meetings by the hospital. A time limit of one hour is adhered to. The chairperson plays a key role in taking responsibility for maintaining the flow of discussion, keeping it on the topic and soliciting member contribution. The meeting is organized into two sections. The first half hour has two roles – new clients are discussed and a course of action to be decided upon and their client included on the register. Secondly, members discuss specific existing clients whose circumstances may have changed, thus warranting a renegotiation of existing services. The second half hour of the meeting is allocated to going through the actual client register. As each client's name is read out, if there is no change in that person's living arrangements, physical or mental status and social situation, we proceed immediately to the next person. The committee can not discuss each client at length if there is no change in their circumstances. When the client's name is read out and a service has information relevant to the care of their client in the community, then that change of circumstances is recorded on the register and services are remodified as necessary. The register is divided into three sections: (i) an active list – these people are mentioned at each meeting, (ii) those "on hold" – we review all the people every three months to see if the "on hold" group have changed in any way and (iii) the inactive list – either they have been placed in an institution or they are no longer with us.

Dynamics of the decision-making process

The committee uses the following sequence when addressing the individual needs of a person wishing to remain living in the community. An information base is gathered, using an holistic approach to a person's circumstances. Based upon the information gathered and resulting from multi-disciplinary discussion, service requirements that could meet the client's individual needs are stated. The discussion then focuses upon how these identified needs can be met, either through government-based community services, the non-government and voluntary services, neighbours, friends or purchasing of private services. Often a combination of the above is warranted. Details of how, by whom and when the package of service is to be delivered are then recorded. At each meeting, the appropriateness of service delivery is reviewed and adjusted as necessary. The committee may make a joint recommendation that because a client's needs surpass the availability of existing community resources, that the client may seek hostel or nursing home accommodation. The identified case manager will follow through this decision as a priority.

Conclusion

The At Risk Committee was established for the purpose of coordinating services provided by autonomous agencies. This model of coordinating services has been successful in improving the efficiency and effectiveness of service delivery to people wanting to remain at home. The client-centred approach to co-ordination has worked well for both the consumer and the agencies, by helping them to set priorities and redefine policy. The next step is a formal evaluation of the effect of At Risk Committees on nursing home admissions and use of agency resources in the area.

Carers, Professionals and Alzheimer's Disease. D O'Neill ed © 1991 John Libbey & Company Ltd

Chapter 30

NEUROPSYCHOLOGICAL TESTS AS A MEANS OF CORRECTING INAPPROPRIATE BEHAVIOUR OF CARE-GIVERS

D Ermini-Fünfschilling, A Monsch, HB Staehelin, *Gerontologische Beratungsstelle, "Memory Clinic", Felix Platter Spital, 4055 Basel, Switzerland*

Introduction

In 1986 a counselling centre for outpatients with memory problems or other signs of early senile dementia opened in Basel. This "memory clinic", has offered its services to more than 300 patients, their families and family doctors. The main objectives of the memory clinic are:

(i) to diagnose dementing illnesses as early as possible on the basis of medical, neuropsychological and laboratory tests. It is hoped that this will help us to learn more about the very early stages of dementia, to start treatment interventions before the cognitive deficits become too pronounced and to identify different courses of senile dementia by means of longitudinal follow-up examinations.

(ii) to evaluate and apply new methods of medical, neuropsychological and psychosocial assessment and treatment of early stages of senile dementias.

(iii) to give to patients and their families direct help by means of individual counselling. We also offer therapy groups for memory training, depressed patients and care-givers.

Research into carers

It is well known now that the burden of caring for a relative suffering from dementia is severe, and many articles have been written exploring various aspects of this problem (e.g. editorial by Steven Zarit, 1989). Further research is required into the factors which contribute to care-givers' stress, and into factors which alleviate it. In our memory clinic we have the opportunity to examine and follow patients from the early stage of the dementing process up to the time when patients become helpless and have to be cared for on a 24-hour basis. Thus we have learned a lot about the dynamics of a care-giver–patient relationship.

One aspect which we have examined is the tendency of care-givers to misjudge the mental status and abilities of their patients, expecting either too much or too little of them. The patient's resulting emotional reactions increase the care-giver's stress and frustration. Care-givers can also misinterpret a patient's mental deterioration as deliberate uncooperativeness or unwillingness to attempt tasks. This may in turn lead to negative reactions due to a lack of understanding, leading to further emotional reactions on the part of the patient. This vicious circle of negative emotions could perhaps be prevented if care-givers understood the nature of their patient's impairment.

Having observed these detrimental interactions, we decided to do a pilot study in which the care-givers would rate the cognitive abilities of their patients. Then we would compare the care-giver's ratings with the actual answers given by patients doing the same test. The discrepancy between the care-giver's rating and the actual test results could be discussed with and explained to the care-giver, leading to increased insight into their patient's difficulties and perhaps preventing inappropriate reactions.

Method

All participating patients were referred to us by family doctors and were given laboratory, medical and neuropsychological examinations. Care-givers were interviewed by a doctor and tested by a neuropsychologist. The test instrument we used was the Evaluation Rapide des Fonctions Cognitives (ERFC).[2] We preferred this instrument to the well known Folstein Mini-Mental State Examination by Folstein (MMSE)[3] because it covers more cognitive abilities relevant to the activities of daily living. It is easy to administer in about 10 minutes, and has a correlation coefficient of 0.91 in comparison with the MMSE.[4] The care-givers did the test themselves and then estimated the patients answers on the same test.

Results

Characteristics of patients and care-givers are outlined in Fig. 1. We found that all care-givers misjudged the cognitive deficits of their patients. Although each patient–care-giver relationship was unique, of course, we found that all care-

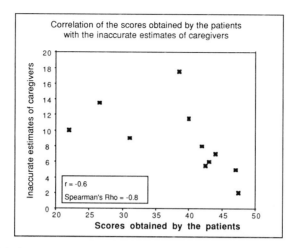

Fig. 1. Relationship between care-giver's inaccurate perception of patients' score on cognitive testing and the patients' actual score.

givers misjudged their patients' disabilities, with the main trend in this study being slightly towards underestimation.

Two examples will demonstrate this misjudgement.

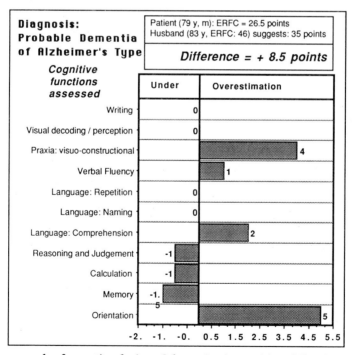

Fig. 2. An example of overstimulation of the patient's cognitive ability by the spouse.

Example 1, overestimation (Fig. 2)

This represents a couple with a close relationship. The husband refuses to accept his wife's cognitive decline and compensates for her difficulties by taking over all household duties so that neither of them faces the painful fact of her failures. She realizes this and reacts with anxiety and some depression. She also feels quite competent when she does attempt something. This constant pressure causes much tension in their relationship, and increases her helplessness. In the examination setting he also overestimated her results. In discussing this we were able to counsel him to keep his wife as active as possible within her capabilities.

Example 2, underestimation (Fig. 3)

This couple also had a close relationship. However the husband is very protective of his partner. Sensing her difficulties and uncertainly, he allows her to do very little, feeling that he is being kind by sparing her. She complains of feeling useless and worthless and inactive, sees herself as no longer having a reason to live. The husband underestimated his wife's abilities in the test situation. When the extent of her remaining cognitive potential was demonstrated to him, it was possible to advise him to allow her to remain as active in the household as possible. He was able to adjust his reactions; the patient is no longer depressed, and the couple is much happier.

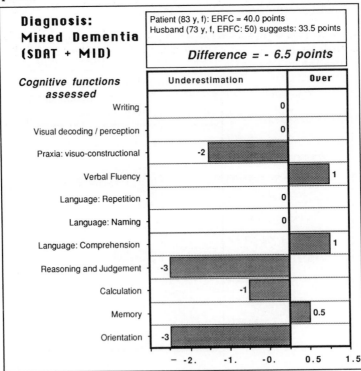

Fig. 3. An example of understimulation of the patient's cognitive ability by the spouse.

Summary

Much has been written about the emotional reactions of patients to increasing awareness of their difficulties in the early stages of dementia. A care-giver's recognition of a patient's daily problems also leads to a variety of emotional reactions, some of which could result in a deterioration in their relationship. We have shown that estimations of a patient's cognitive abilities are often incorrect, resulting in inappropriate expectations and reactions. We therefore suggest the inclusion of a care-giver's rating of the patient's mental status on neuropsychological tests in order to facilitate discussion of eventual expectations.

References

(1) Zarit, SH. Do we need another "Stress and Caregiving" Study? *The Gerontologist* **29(2)**, 147-148.

(2) Gil R, Toullat G, Plouchon C, Michenau D, Cariou B, Rivault L, Sicot I, Boissonnot L, Neau JP. Une méthode d' évaluation rapide des fonctions cognitives (ERFC). Son application à la démence sénile de type Alzheimer. *Sem Hôp Paris* 1986, **62(27)**, 2127-2133.

(3) Folstein MF, Folstein SE, McHugh PR. Mini Mental State – A practical method for grading the cognitive state of patients for the clinician. *J Psychiat Res* 1975, **12**, 189-198.

(4) Stæhelin HB, Ermini-Fünfschilling D, Grunder B, Krebs-Roubicek E, Monsch A, Spiegel R. Die Memory-Klinik. *Therapeutische Umschau* 1989, **46(1)**, 72-77.

Carers, Professionals and Alzheimer's Disease. D O'Neill ed © 1991 John Libbey & Company Ltd

Chapter 31

THE DEMENTED ELDERLY IN A GROUP

Eva Krebs-Roubicek, *Psychiatric Clinic, Wilhelm Klein Str. 27, CH-4025 Basel, Switzerland*

In the University Psychiatry Clinic in Basel we admit about 200 patients over the age of 65 years each year. About a third of these patients suffer from different forms of dementia with varying degrees of severity, others from depression, delusional disorders or dependence. During the assessment procedure, the patient takes part in different activities in the admission ward. Some of these patients, mostly the demented ones, cannot be discharged back to their original surroundings and must be transferred to the long-stay wards of the hospital. They also take part in activities on these wards. Most of these activities are carried out in different forms of groups. From a survey of the literature we know that group-work with the elderly has the following advantages:

(i) the elderly are less inhibited in a group;

(ii) other group members can provide support against a powerful leader;

(iii) the loneliness which is a special problem of the elderly can be decreased due to the experience of acceptance by the group members;

(iv) due to possible identification with the group leader or other members, emotional development can be supported.

Types of group work

In work with the demented elderly, we use modifications of the classical group therapy in different training groups, especially memory-training groups, focally-orientated groups, go-round groups, creative groups, self-help groups and activity groups for cooking and similar activities.

During the work with these groups we have observed the following changes in the groups. The group has an activating function, diminishing or slowing down the amount of cognitive losses as group members gradually show more interest in

199

each other and the amount of spontaneous interaction increases. This can also be observed in severely demented patients during a long-term stay in different institutions and especially during long-term hospitalization in a psychiatric clinic. During group therapy, we usually observe that affective factors will be better modulated, more lively and more appropriately expressed. The elderly also develop assertiveness in dealing with personal rights. These changes of behaviour were not confined to the group sessions alone, but could be observed as well outside of the group ambience.

Creative artistic activity

In our work with the elderly we learnt to place a high value on artistic and creative activities. Such activities can reduce various deficits in the elderly, especially by intensification of communication and also by strengthening and stabilizing identity and self-esteem. In the groups, we have observed an increase in contact attempts between the group members and their group leader. The difficulties in introducing art therapy into work with the elderly can be seen in their negative expression of their surroundings. It frequently expresses low esteem for this form of therapy. From a therapeutic point of view we emphasize that the non-verbal nature of this form of therapy enables the elderly to look back on their lives, to solve conflicts and to express their expectations of the future. Many of these creative products are full of symbols or aspirations.

As many elderly abolish previous experiences from their memory, especially painful and unpleasant ones, art therapy can be a meaningful way to reassess them. Art therapy represents a very useful approach in the therapy of depressive patients. The basis for this positive effect is based on the following points:

(i)   it is a means of self-control;

(ii) it provides evidence of existing vitality due to the creative artistic activity;

(iii) it enables the possibility of acceleration of positive transference;

(iv) the creative product can be seen as a means of sublimation.

Emphasis must not be placed on the production of a useful item corresponding to market values, but rather on the production process itself which provides experience with material and techniques, strengthens self confidence, supports the need for very good workmanship and enhances self-reliance and self-responsibility. Artistic activities in this sense have a therapeutic effect. They stimulate the ability to communicate and enhance self-esteem.

In addition to our in-patient work, we are also working with one out-patient group which I will describe in more detail. In this group we work partly with creative techniques using pencils, chalks and water colours. The group setting corresponds to the setting of an analytically orientated group therapy, such as that described by Foulkes. Frequently, we use techniques from the catathymic picture experience of Leuner. This group takes place once a week for 60 minutes in a slow and open form. During the first three to six months, the group members have difficulty in identifying themselves as a group. The group has now been running for over two years. At the beginning there was marked fluctuation in the attendance: however, in the following sixteen months, five to seven group members attended regularly. In the last three months, the fluctuation again increased after some of the group members left the group and the new members have difficulty in feeling that they belong to the group.

Group members

I would like to introduce you to some of the group members. The first is Mrs Alma. She is 74 years old, single and used to work as a teacher of German and art. Her hobby was travelling and painting. About 40 years ago, she wrote an autobiography which she is now reworking. For most of her life she lived with a sister who was mentally retarded and with her mother. After the death of her mother, her sister had to move to a nursing home. Mrs Alma herself has suffered for many years from different somatic disorders, mostly arthritis. Recently, after the death of a friend with whom she had travelled widely, she lost her interest in travelling and developed some depressive symptoms as well as cognitive symptoms – mainly loss of memory and concentration. At about this time she joined the group. She developed a virtually immediate relationship towards the group and especially enjoyed those sessions when we were drawing. She was a very important group member and we all perceived her as a lively person but she left the group after her hip operation as she was complaining she could not walk so far.

Mrs H, who is 64 and married, has one son who lives with his family in Brasilia, suffering from a psychotic disorder. The son is disabled and cannot work and his parents are supporting him and his family financially. Mrs H suffers from concentration and memory difficulties and is reacting in a depressive way to her cognitive disturbances. She finds support in a religious group that she visits once a week and she works part-time with elderly in the neighbourhood or in old peoples' homes. A Hungarian by birth, she still has problems with expressing herself properly in German. These language difficulties and various worries about her son and the cognitive disorder are causing her a lot of distress. In the group, she enjoys the feeling of security and the feeling of being accepted by the others. She especially enjoys the non-verbal medium for expressing feelings and memories from beloved holidays with her husband, which she would have difficulty in expressing verbally.

Mr L, 63 years old, is married with four children of whom three are married and one has died, apparently committing suicide as a drug addict. Mr L used to own a book shop but due to financial problems had to sell his shop and is working in a chemical factory in the publishing department. Due to chronic alcoholism, he has had multiple falls and a severe motor-cycle accident with brain injury and post-traumatic epilepsy. Despite all this, his cognitive decline is still limited: immediate memory is most affected. He seldom confabulates and his primary memory and abstract thinking are almost intact. His behaviour in the group was very quiet at the beginning, speaking only when spoken to. During the last few months, he has become much more active in the group and was able to talk about

201

his relationship with his wife and about the loss of his son. He and another group member realized that they have something in common and could express this feeling in the group. They both speak frequently about their problems in those group sessions when the women are missing or in the minority which partly reflects their problematic relationships with their wives. Mr L said he could not draw, but he expressed his admiration for abstract art, especially Paul Klee. His first drawings were quite accomplished, but he did not like them. About six months later, he was much more happy about his pictures. Recently, he painted a very fine picture dominated by a tree in the middle of the picture, giving it an expression of steadiness and hope.

The last patient is Mr D, who is 81 years old, married, has two daughters, both of whom are married. Mr D used to work in a paint shop and travelled a lot as a young man with a bicycle around Europe, and later with his wife all over the world. He suffers from a very severe form of Parkinson's disease and shows moderate cognitive losses. He enjoys the group a lot even though he is relatively slow in expressing his ideas: he can find his place in the group and is well accepted. It is possible for him to express himself and he has greatly improved emotionally since he joined the group.

Therapeutic benefit

The mixture of artistic activities allied with analytically-orientated group therapy in the specific combination of the group members in the group described above could help to achieve varying degrees of therapeutic benefit. In this group, we could observe a development of a strong interpersonal interest between group members. Members of the group frequently meet each other outside of the group for lunch, for short trips or visits. It seems that the demented members get most of the attention from the others.

The group leader in this group does not need to be as active as the group leader in our in-patient group, who has to be very active. The group members who were originally depressed are slowly assuming a very active role in the group work as they improve. The positive changes in the ability to relate to the others could be equally well observed in the creative artistic expressions of the group members.

Conclusion

In conclusion, group-work with the elderly is comparable to group-work with younger participants: but we must remember that even the slightest changes of setting can lead to confusion and even failure of the group. In group-work with in-patients with dementia, sessions of one hour seem to be too long. Therefore, we decided to introduce 30-minute sessions for three times a week, as frequently patients with agitation, depression or dementia are unable to tolerate longer sessions.

After evaluating our experiences, we think that group therapy with the demented elderly should be accorded the high priority which is its due.

Bibliography

Aissen-Crewett M. esthetische Erziehung alter Menschen – unter besonderer Be-rücksichtigung therapeutischer Effekte bildnerisch-kreativer Aktivit ten. *Z Gerontol.* 1987, **20**, 314-317.

Alpaugh PK, Birren JE. Variables affecting the adult life span. *Human Development 1977,* **20,** 240-248.

Hoffman D. Art programming for the elderly. *Educational Gerontology* 1978, **3,** 17-33.

Lazarus LW. A programme for the elderly at a private psychiatric hospital. *Gerontol* 1976, **16,** 125-131.

Lazarus LW. *Self psychology and psychotherapy with the elderly.* 1980, **13,** 69-88.

Miller S. Some thoughts on attitudes: a starting point for creative work for the elderly. *Educational Gerontology* 1982, **8,** 175-181.

Petzhold H. *Mit alten Menschen arbeiten. Bildungsarbeit, Psychotherapie, Soziotherapie.* Lebenlernen, Pfeiffer, München, 1985.

Puglisi JT, Park DC, Smith AD. Picture associations among old and young adults. *Exp Ageing Research* 1987, **13,** 115-116.

Rogers BL. Using the creative process with the terminally ill. In: Davidson GW, ed., *The Hospice* 1978, 123-126.

Sylcox K. Our elderly: creativities often overlooked. *Activities, Adaptation & Ageing* 1983, **3,** 27-38.

Carers, Professionals and Alzheimer's Disease. D O'Neill ed © 1991 John Libbey & Company Ltd

Chapter 32

INCONTINENCE AND DEMENTIA

JB Walsh *MB MRCP, Mercer's Institute for Research on Ageing and St James's Hospital, Dublin 8, Ireland*

Incontinence is not an illness: like chest pain, breathlessness or cough, it is a symptom complex. It is very often due to a combination of factors and like any other symptom it must be investigated and the cause(s) established. It is very common in elderly people, affecting 12 per cent of the population over the age of 65. There are two approaches to incontinence in patients with dementia. The first is that most patients with dementia are in the over-65 age group, and therefore are subject to the same high prevalence of incontinence. The second approach hinges on the fact that there may be aspects of incontinence in demented patients which relate to the dementing process, i.e. due to an apraxia or to forgetting where the toilet is. Illuminating this second approach is complicated by the paucity of dementia-specific research into incontinence. We can be reasonably certain that mild to moderate dementia is not associated with an increased prevalence of incontinence. Incontinence should be aggressively assessed in all dementia patients: it is important that we do not ascribe it to dementia until all other avenues have been exhausted.

Optimism is essential in the assessment and management of incontinence in patients with dementia. Like many other symptom complexes, incontinence can sometimes be cured, often significantly decreased and always managed more easily. There is no justifiable reason why a patient's clothes, chair and bedding should be the "collection point" for urine: with proper assessment, anticipatory management, continence aids and occasionally drug therapy, urinary continence can be easily contained without a patient's clothes becoming wet.

The ageing bladder

Normal bladder capacity is about a pint, and although some people can tolerate several litres in their bladder, it is normal to experience a desire to void at this capacity. In people with Alzheimer's disease and in people with what is known as the ageing bladder, there is a different pattern. Brocklehurst has shown an increased incidence of unstable bladders as people with normal cognitive function grow older. The bladder does not fully empty having a resting pressure and a slight residual volume. In the unstable bladder there are spastic contractions within the bladder. These cause a desire to void just before micturition: there is often insufficient time to get to the toilet and they get a leak of urine. In over 90 per cent of women and men without outflow tract obstruction the commonest cause of incontinence is due to a spastic bladder. In a demented patient this may be ascribed to laziness by ill-informed staff.

Other causes of incontinence

Other causes of persistent incontinence include pelvic floor weakness (usually causing urge incontinence), neurological causes (i.e. stroke , spinal injuries), overflow incontinence secondary to obstruction (e.g. prostatism in the male), autonomic neuropathy and atrophic vaginitis. Of particular interest to those working with demented patients is normal pressure hydrocephalus, which classically causes the triad of dementia, incontinence and gait apraxia: this condition is potentially remediable.

Several factors can cause transient incontinence or can aggravate pre-existing incontinence. These include acute illness of any kind, acute confusional states, urinary tract infections, acute stroke, drugs and psycho-social factors. I do not think people manipulate the environment by wetting themselves: if they do so, it is a very rare occurrence. It is productive to investigate for these factors that cause transient incontinence, as reversal of treatment of these factors usually ameliorates the incontinence, and may even cure it.

Assessment

When a person becomes incontinent of urine it is very important that a full medical history is taken. They must have a mental state examination and a full physical examination. If severely cognitively impaired, a supplementary history should be taken from the carer. In relation to incontinence the history should include information as to when it started and whether or not it was associated with some other illness, how it has progressed and whether it occurs by day and/or by night, how many times, whether pads are worn and if so, how many are used. It is worth trying to classify the pattern of incontinence into either stress incontinence, urge incontinence or unawareness of passing urine until wet. A review of environmental factors is important to ensure that incontinence is not due to inappropriate or inadequate toiletting facilities. Access to toilets and the length of time it takes to get to the toilet should be noted.

Drug review is essential. Professor Millard in St George's Hospital has likened the combined effect of sedatives and diuretic therapy to asking a person to drink six litres, putting them in plaster casts, placing the toilet 200 yards away and then asking them to remain continent! So drug review is very important to eliminate unnecessary sedation and unnecessary diuretic therapy. Other culprits include anticholinergic agents, e.g. some antiarrhythmic agent and tricyclic antidepressants which may precipitate retention with overflow incontinence in susceptible patients.

Particular points of interest in the physical examination include abdominal examination to exclude a distended bladder with overflow incontinence. Clinical assessment is usually adequate to make this diagnosis: if any doubt exists, measurement of residual volume by ultra-sonography or by insertion (and prompt removal) of a catheter will occasionally be required. A rectal examination is mandatory: particular attention is paid to the prostate in males and to constipation, although bladder obstruction by faecal impaction is often quoted but is relatively uncommon. I tend to restrict the vaginal examination for those cases where the incontinence does not settle down immediately. The mucosa of the urethra is oestrogen dependent and for that reason has the same appearances as the vagina. It is very important to have a healthy lining membrane at the base of the bladder: giving oestrogen can improve the quality of the endothelium.

Investigations

Simple investigations should include a mid-stream urine for microscopy and culture. Cystometry is only indicated if surgery is considered. Several methods are available for the measurement of incontinence. Weighing incontinence pads is a simple and useful quantitative tool.[1] Individual monitoring charts are very useful, not only for monitoring the frequency and pattern of incontinence, but also because it guarantees that the person is toiletted and ensures continuity when staff change over in institutional care. When we used the incontinence pad weighing device initially, nine out of ten patients referred to us for treatment of "intractable" incontinence became continent. Once the nurses made sure that the pads were weighed every two hours, the patients were guaranteed to be toiletted every two hours and became dry in 90 per cent of cases. Regular pad weighing is thus both diagnostic and therapeutic: we began to have great difficulty establishing incontinence because the pads were drying up so rapidly!

Diagnosis

On the basis of the history, examination and simple investigation outlined above, possible contributory factors should be listed and dealt with. Illness and infection should be treated, structural abnormalities corrected where possible and drug therapy rationalized. In the case of patients with dementia, strenuous efforts should be made to ensure optimal environmental management and provision of cues. For example, the provision of lighting at night-time, signs pointing to the toilet or the use of alarm systems to self-toilet.

Empirical treatment of the three main types of incontinence can be attempted. In the case of the unstable bladder and urge incontinence, bladder training and bladder drill may be of some assistance.[2] However, the training should not be persisted with beyond 3–4 weeks if there is no improvement. Toiletting regimes are the most important method of managing the unstable bladder: this means that the bladder is emptied before a leak occurs. Drug therapy has been found to be of little help in groups, but can help in individual cases. Anti-cholinergic agents, dicyclomine, low dose imipramine, propanthelin, propantheline and flavoxate are among the agents used.[3] Terodiline (miccurin) is a compound which has been more recently introduced and may be of value in some cases. Stress incontinence may be due to weakness of the pelvic floor muscles or due to detrusor instability, and may respond to pelvic floor exercises. This group of patients is the most likely to require formal cystometry and possible surgical review.

Incontinence of which the patient is unaware until wet is probably the commonest form of incontinence in patients with moderate to severe dementia. Although definite evidence for efficacy of timed-voiding regimes in this population is unavailable, it is accepted as the most appropriate form of therapy for managing this incontinence. Ideally the patient should be assessed by inspecting his/her pad at half-hourly intervals to find the shortest period between voidings. A regime of voiding is then instituted using intervals slightly shorter than the shortest period. An alternative approach is to use a two-hourly toiletting regime.

intractable incontinence

If the assessment, diagnosis and management outlined above are unsuccessful, the incontinence may need to be contained using pads or catheters. Catheterization is permissible in the acute phase of a stroke, or if essential in the management of a medical or surgical condition, but in these instances it should be removed as soon as possible. We use them in our wards for the acutely sick elderly for skin protection or acute high dependency: it is worth noting that 90 per cent of patients with strokes are incontinent on admission but only 10 per cent continue to be after six months. All catheters should be Teflon or silicone coated to avoid reaction and stricture formation. The balloon should contain no more than 5 ml: the old 30 ml balloon takes up a fair bit of the bladder volume and results in a continuous residual volume, which is a potential culture medium. Friction from the catheter tip against the bladder wall predisposes to haemorrhagic cystitis and recurrent septicaemias.

Other implications of long-term catheterization are trauma of catheter insertion, with resultant occasional severe gram negative septicaemia, urethral mucosa inflammation, catheter encrustation and obstruction, acute and chronic pyelone-phritis and renal failure. For those few in whom a catheter is unavoidable, leg bags should be used so that the patient does not have to have a catheter on view, and can thus preserve his/her dignity.

We do not use catheters in our long-stay wards: we recommend full all-in-one pads or else close-fitting plastic-backed pads. It is essential that the proper net pants supplied by the manufacturer are worn at all times with the pads to ensure a close fit. Otherwise there will be leakage of urine. Modern developments of pads have been tremendous: the advance in technology of disposable diapers for children has had a tremendous spin-off effect for adults. Many people do not realize that a pad is a very complex item: it is not just a little bit of wadding enclosed in plastic.

The inner layer is a hydrophobic dry layer which tends to let water pass through: it also acts as a barrier so that it does not immediately overflow. Then there is a cotton layer and an absorbent layer: this may be paper pulp, wood pulp and sometimes a plastic as well which becomes gel-like when wet. The advantage of the plastic gel is that the pads size can be reduced by up to 50 per cent and are therefore less bulky. Because of the bigger bladder of the adult, it is more important that they have more paper and wood pulp rather than the plastic and a smaller pad.

An alternative for men is the external catheter which is very useful. In the past there were problems with the ties leading to gangrene: this does not occur nowadays because the fixative is an expanding one. However some demented patients have great difficulties accepting condom catheters

Faecal incontinence

I have dealt with urinary continence almost exclusively as faecal incontinence is virtually always curable. Assessment should ensure that there is no faecal impaction giving rise to overflow diarrhoea or inappropriately leaking faecal matter. A person normally has a bowel movement once a day on average. The gastro-colic reflex is a reflex which occurs after the stomach fills after a meal: the controlled reflex spasm of the bowel will send a contraction down to the lower bowel within about half an hour. The person will then feel the desire to empty their bowel. Demented patients may not be able to inhibit this reflex, but carers can make use of it. If carers can understand that the patient tends to have a bowel movement after breakfast, lunch or any main meal, then it is much easier to anticipate. If they were taken and put on the toilet after meals then faecal incontinence should not occur: faecal incontinence is a non-drug management situation.

Conclusion

Prevention is also important: in planning a new day-care centre or hospital,[4,5] it is very important not to cut back on essentials, especially with regard to the provision of toilet and bathroom facilities. Incontinence is a symptom, accurate assessment is essential and the condition is always a manageable one.

References

(1) Walsh JB, Mills GL. Measurement of urinary loss in incontinent patients. *Lancet* 1981, i, 1130-1131.

(2) Rooney V. Bladder re-education and timed voiding programmes in measuring and managing incontinence. *Geriatr Med* 1989, **26(Supp)**, 26-27.

(3) Briggs RS, Castleden CM, Asher MJ. The effects of flavoxate on uninhibited detrusor contractions and urinary incontinence in the elderly. *J Urol* 1980, **123**, 665-66.

(4) Schroyer JA. Interior design and Alzheimer's disease. In O'Neill D (ed), *Carers, Professionals and Alzheimer's Disease*. London, John Libbey, 1991.

(5) Cohen U. Environments for people with dementia: new approaches, new solutions. In O'Neill D (ed), *Carers, Professionals and Alzheimer's Disease*. London, John Libbey, 1991.

Carers, Professionals and Alzheimer's Disease. D O'Neill ed © 1991 John Libbey & Company Ltd

Chapter 33

COPING WITH WANDERING

John Fleetwood *MB, FRCGP, Our Lady's Hospice, Dublin 6, Ireland*

My brief is to discuss the impact of an Alzheimer patient on the family from the general practitioner's point of view with particular reference to the problem of wandering. There would be very little point in my discussing detailed symptomatology and diagnosis which have been dealt with in other papers at this symposium. However I do feel justified in reinforcing my colleagues' pleas for thorough investigation and early recognition of this condition with particular emphasis on the importance of excluding depression, with its very real risk of suicide in certain cultures. In a recent survey of elderly suicides in London by Catell, 22 per cent had cerebral pathology while 77 per cent had had depressive symptoms before death. Some of the latter were certainly misdiagnosed and might have been successfully treated. It is of some relevance to this paper that several of the deaths were associated with wandering and occurred at some distance from the family home. Diminished perception, including poor vision and deafness, is a frequent complicating factor in making a diagnosis. This should be noted by the family doctor who is usually the first professional to be involved in investigating the possible diagnosis of Alzheimer's disease or other dementing diseases. In a recent survey, O'Connor found that general practitioners mistakenly rated several patients as demented who were suffering from functional psychiatric disorders, in particular depression.[1] This suggests that we should have a much higher index of suspicion when confronted with an elderly confused patient.

Problems rather than abnormalities

But to the family, or those immediately concerned with the individual patient's welfare, an accurate diagnosis may be of secondary importance. Confusion about place with resultant wandering is one of the most troubling of the many symptoms and problems common to all dementing diseases. This problem is often compounded by the fact that the patient may retain a very considerable degree of physical fitness: if this is combined with an element of aggressiveness, particularly in a powerfully built man, the other members of the family may come to the end of their tether and ask for some form of hospitalization.

211

Some years ago, I undertook a survey of the family reasons for admission of 300 patients (including many demented patients) to Our Lady's Hospice in Dublin. Contrary to what is sometimes claimed, families asked for admission as a last resort: in many cases they would have been happy to have continued family care, even with seriously confused patients, if some help at home were available. About 25 per cent of our admissions could have been delayed or avoided altogether if adequate provision of night-sitting and day-care services had been available. It is interesting to note that Kinier and Graycar in Australia also indicated that the families of demented older people were reluctant to hospitalize them despite the tensions which their presence in the home often caused.

Wandering

Wandering may involve three areas: the house, the immediate environment and further afield. The risks vary somewhat between each of these and deserve further assessment. Within the house, the effects of wandering can range from disturbance of other people during the night to much more serious hazards to the family as a whole: gas taps may be turned on, electrical appliances used improperly or household poisons mixed with foodstuffs. In the setting of a nursing home, wandering at night may be a major anxiety not so much because of safety but because of disturbance to other inmates, sometimes of the opposite sex. When the person disturbed is not demented, the incident may be described to visitors with embellishments which aggravate a simple disturbance to something barely short of sexual harassment or even assault. Unfortunately, there are visitors who will take at face value everything their relative says, with consequent difficulties for the nursing home proprietor.

In principle, there is nothing wrong with allowing a confused patient to walk in an enclosed garden: unfortunately in practice the carer must be as alert to danger as is the parent of a small child. It is easy enough to ensure that weed killers and garden tools are locked in a shed, to see that paths are safe and that the goldfish pond is covered with netting. However, visitors can leave gates unlocked or even wide open and an active octogenarian, just like the active three year old, can wander thoughtlessly into the path of danger. Sometimes retaining some semblance of normality, he may be successful in using public transport to reach some district with childhood or business associations. Possibly in Ireland this is even easier nowadays as senior citizens travel free on public transport which obviates the need for money on a bus. Sometimes even fragile patients may walk for long distances either aimlessly or in a confused effort to reach some known objective.

One morning at six o'clock our door bell was rung violently by a frail 85 year old woman wearing only a nightdress and an anorak who had walked some four kilometres in pouring rain. She was not a patient of ours and could give no explanation of why she had rung our doorbell except to say over and over again "You are doctors." She was already becoming hypothermic but her disappearance had been discovered and the police notified, so that a call to the local station resulted in quick reunion with her family. She was one of the lucky ones. In rural areas, the wandering demented patient encounters different dangers to those in the city. Slurry tanks, small streams, irascible bulls and farm-yard machinery have all claimed the lives of older people at some time. While it would be possible to quote many further instances of wandering, to do so would be a pointless academic exercise unless we can make some practical suggestions about how to reduce, or hopefully eliminate, danger to mentally confused and physically active elderly people.

Multi-disciplinary approach

In most cases, a multi-disciplinary approach is required. The spouse, the immediate family, the extended family, neighbours, the medical and welfare services all have a role to play. Intercommunication is essential and the Alzheimer Society of Ireland and similar bodies elsewhere provide a vital forum for discussion and dissemination of news about advances and particularly about available services. Education of the public is a most important element in the work of such a society.

The spouse and immediate family are the people on whom the burden of a patient's tendency to wander falls most heavily. What practical advice can we give them? Knowledge about the condition is vital to any effort at continuing positive home care. You will note that I stress the word "positive", for in most chronic cases a dynamic component to treatment is vital to prevent home care from degenerating into a custodial mode. In this respect I can thoroughly recommend Carmel Sheridan's book *Failure Free Activities for the Alzheimer Patient* which emphasises the need for an active approach to home care and gives many practical suggestions about how to occupy, utilize and stimulate what is left in the failing brain.[2]

It is important that the family should understand something of the pathology and prognosis of dementia. It must be explained to them that the body ages at different rates. They will then appreciate why in some cases the patient's night is disturbed or food is refused simply because the physically fit sufferer has had no physical exercise during the day, and is just not normally tired at bed time or hungry when meals are being served. Restlessness and wandering may also be due to frustration and if it appears that a confused patient wants to visit some place with happy though vague memories, I always advise that every effort be made to satisfy this want, even repeatedly, rather than bluntly refusing to do so or temporizing indefinitely.

Practical measures

Safety in the house is something which affects everyone from infancy to the senium. High on the list of hazards are open fires of all descriptions. Fixed fires should always have a guard which can only be removed by using two or more slightly difficult manoeuvres. Solid-fuel fires should have a small easily opened gate which will allow coal, turf or wood to be replenished without danger. The mesh should be wide enough to let heat out and portable naked electrical element fires of any type should never be used where a confused person may try to move them. A survey of accidents to elderly people (not all of them demented) demonstrated beyond any doubt than unguarded open fires were the cause of a huge number of serious injuries and deaths. "Curiosity killed the cat" is an old proverb but tragically more than cats have been killed when drawers and cupboards containing sharp instruments and household poisons including alcohol have been too easy to open. Child-proof catches which can be easily and cheaply fitted are equally effective in keeping units safe from senile interference. Improper installation of electrical fittings causes deaths every year. Advice should be sought from a qualified electrician, not only about the fitting of fail-safe devices, but also on the positive side about the installation of warning systems to alert the household of dangerous situations. These may range from a simple bell triggered by opening a door to sophisticated closed-circuit television.

What other steps can families take to protect confused senior members who are liable to wander? There are three elements in this form of total care. Familiarity, encouragement and clarity. Under the rubric of familiarity I mean essentially leaving things as they are: for example a familiar arm chair is always in the same place. Encouragement is part of positive home care: the patient should be encouraged to carry out familiar non-hazardous tasks. Examples could include vacuum cleaning, kitchen chores not involving hot objects, brushing paths, bringing in fuel, washing a car and raking up leaves. By clarity I mean such items as good lighting and measures like painting the lavatory door a strong contrasting colour. Further measures include ensuring that floors and corridors are lit by low intensity floor-level lamps at night which do not disturb sleep or dazzle a newly awakened person, but which give sufficient light to avoid falls while wandering around the house.

Particularly in the early stages of the disease, physical and mental activity is of prime importance and will help to induce normal hunger and fatigue which will be responded to in some cases in a normal way. Of course activity may have to be divided into several half-hour sessions because of the Alzheimer patient's reduced attention span. A positive approach in this area will reduce wandering tendencies in many cases.

Restraint

Should any form of restraint be used to curb a tendency to wander? I do not think there is anyone nowadays who would be happy to go back to physical restraint of the straight-jacket type. Unfortunately there will always be a hard core of cases who, because of their condition or lack of adequate supervision, will go through periods in which no treatment seems to reduce the wandering tendency. In these some form of restriction may be felt to be necessary for safety. The only form of body restraint that I would accept reluctantly is the safety harness of the Posie type which prevents bed-bound or chair-bound patients from falling forward or sideways. In the latter case a comfortable chair with a built in table is useful and has a more normal appearance.

214

The question of pharmacological restraint must be faced. Is one ever justified in using mind-altering drugs to control a patients activity? Reluctantly again, I must say "Yes" but always with a proviso that the patient has been thoroughly checked to rule out any factor, including medication, which may spark off restlessness or irritability. Too often, we still see patients on long-term medication of all types which is either unnecessary or positively harmful. I am unhappy about the present tendency to repeat prescriptions on a monthly basis without seeing the patient, particularly in elderly subjects on "chronic" medication. The British Geriatrics Society has recommended monthly visits as a minimum service to elderly patients on such medications.

Minimizing the risks of wandering

It may seem that I am the person who has been "wandering" far from my brief of discussing our subject in relation to Alzheimer's disease! My intention has been to show that this is a multi-faceted problem: straying away from home is only one aspect which requires extra measures to be taken. No matter how many safe-guards are made, individuals will occasionally wander far afield and practical steps to minimize the effects of this are worth using. The patient should constantly wear a card in a plastic cover around his/her neck with his/her name, address and contact telephone numbers. Carrying the card in a pocket will inevitably mean that it is not transferred when clothes are changed. Alternatively, an identity wrist band of the MedicAlert type may be worn. Care should be taken that the patient carries only a small amount of money: documents such as credit cards, cheque books or passports should never be carried. Where a woman patient insists on wearing expensive jewellery which may be lost or stolen, it is well worth while having a base metal imitation made. Many elderly women particularly insist on carrying their few treasures around with them in a mistaken belief that they are safer: it is a sad fact of modern life that even alert elderly people are prime targets for muggers and bag snatchers.

If the patient wanders despite all precautions, a systematic search must be instituted. The immediate vicinity should be checked and old haunts such as a favourite pub, church or other locality are worth investigating if a blank is drawn. Nearby friends or family members should be contacted and asked to be vigilant. If the police have been alerted and the wanderer is found without their help, do not forget to inform them so that they can cease their investigations. I have been told by the police that it is most useful to have some unwashed article of the person's clothing in the event that dogs have to be used in a search.

A phenomenon which is familiar to anyone involved in geriatric care is the mental deterioration which so often follows any traumatic event such as exposure, a fracture, or even trivial injuries. All of these may be relevant in the case of the wandering Alzheimer patient. In my opinion it is mandatory to examine them thoroughly after such incidents and to continue observation for several days. The family and associates should be warned that scolding grandad for wandering is a pointless and self defeating approach. Warm concern and expressions of relief are much more likely to produce the desired results.

Conclusion

It may seem that my suggestions about wandering have been overly facile or optimistic and I would be the first to agree that they will not be useful or effective in every case – but in what human endeavour do we enjoy 100 per cent success? In a chronic socially disruptive condition like Alzheimer's disease, even a modest relaxation of the stresses within a family is well worthwhile.

References

(1) O'Connor, DW *et al.* Do general practitioners miss dementia in elderly patients? *Brit Med J* 1988, **297**, 1107-1110.
(2) Sheridan C. *Failure Free Activities for the Older Patient.* Cottage Books, 1987.

For further reading

Fleetwood, JF. *As You Get Older.* Town House, Dublin, 1988.

Carers, Professionals and Alzheimer's Disease. D O'Neill ed © 1991 John Libbey & Company Ltd

Chapter 34

STRATEGIES FOR DRUG TREATMENT AND RESEARCH IN ALZHEIMER'S DISEASE

BE Leonard, *Pharmacology Department, University College, Galway, Ireland*

Introduction

Strategies for the development of drugs that may be used to treat dementing diseases may be considered from several points of view, namely from the point of view of the experimental psychopharmacologist, the clinical researcher and, most importantly, from the point of view of the psychogeriatrician.

Experimental studies in animals

The study and possible treatment of dementias may be approached from several angles. Firstly, diminution in regional blood flow within the brain may be utilized; the regional changes that result appear to reflect the degree of cerebral impairment, at least in animals. Secondly, it may be possible to change brain metabolism by experimental means. An example that might be relevant for understanding dementia is to try to change the structure of membranes in the ageing brain. There appears to be an increasing hardening of some of the membranes around nerve cells with ageing; enhancing the fluidity of these membranes may facilitate co-ordination between nerve cells and thereby attenuate the age-induced functional deficits. A typical candidate for this could be phosphatidyl serine which fluidizes the neuronal membranes in *in vitro* studies at least. This compound can enhance memory performance in aged animals but is without effect in young animals, thereby suggesting that it may correct some age-related deficit.

Lastly, it has been well established that in all ageing animals there seems to be a very good correlation between the deficit in choline-acetyl-transferase, which brings about the synthesis of acetyl-choline, and the degree of dementia. This suggests that the cholinergic system may be crucially involved in the causation of dementia. Drug induced defect models, which to some extent mirror this approach, have been used in man. Thus, when healthy young volunteers are treated with atropine or scopolamine, a reversible deficit in memory is produced which may be attributed to a reduction in central cholinergic transmission; these drugs act by blocking muscarinic cholinergic receptors. The interesting aspect about this approach is that many of the behavioural effects seen both in man and animals are rather similar to dementia.

The area of the brain believed to be involved in short term memory, termed the hippocampus, appears to be particularly affected by such drugs. However, such effects on memory cannot be specifically ascribed to a defect in cholinergic transmission alone. Thus if one takes too much diazepam (Valium) or chlordiazepoxide (Librium), amnesia is also produced, this effect being attributed to a facilitation of inhibitory transmission in those sub-cortical regions of the brain concerned with memory and emotion. These are the sort of models which pharmacologists working in the laboratory can study in an attempt to simulate some of the major symptoms seen in the dementias. Such models may then be used to test compounds which may eventually be of value as drugs to treat patients with dementia.

Table 1. Experimental approaches that have been used to detect putative anti-dementia drugs

1. **Use of neurotoxins** to lesion the cholinergic system, e.g. N-amino-deanol; aziridinium (AF-64M), ibotenic and kainic acids; trimethyltin. Lesions of basal forebrain cause cortical hypofunction e.g. impaired conditioned avoidance behaviour; disruption of cognitive performance.

2. **Electroconvulsive shock** induced retrograde amnesia in animals and man.

3. **Genetic models** – e.g. hippocampally deficient mice show impaired acquisition and retention behaviour; senescence accelerated mice show loss of cholinergic neurones and spontaneous age associated amyloidosis.

4. **Oxygen deficient models** – learning and memory disrupted by low oxygen tension in inspired air.

5. **Aged models** – regional changes in brain glucose reflect cognitive impairment in aged rats; age related deficits in complex maze behaviour correlated with defective choline acetyl-transferase activity.

6. **Drug induced defect models** – atropine and scopolamine induced amnesia similar to total hippocampalectomy; benzodiazepine induced amnesia.

Other animal models have been developed by using neurotoxins that are injected directly into the brain to produce specific lesions of neurotransmitters thought to be involved in Alzheimer's disease. Hemicholinium, for example, is a compound which blocks the transport of choline into the nerve terminal and thereby reduces the amount of acetylcholine available. In animal studies there are a number of compounds which might be useful in certain stages of dementia. Theoretically, it should be very easy to take these compounds straight to the patient and obtain positive results. However, despite the positive results obtained from animal studies, there has been little evidence that such compounds are active in patients. This raises the crucial question regarding the validity of the animal models which we are using to develop drugs for the treatment of the dementias.

Table 2. Reversal of selective neurotransmitter lesions by putative anti-dementia drugs

1. Ibotenic acid lesions reversed by :
Physostigmine, choline, piracetam, THA (tacrine), vincamine, arecholine, "Hydergine".

2. Behavioural defects in aged rodents reversed by :
Exifone (scavenger molecule!), clonidine, naloxone.

3. Trimethyltin lesions reversed by :
Neuropeptides, captopril, phencyclidine, piracetam.

4. Electroconvulsive shock amnesia reversed by :
Physostigmine.

5. Scopolamine/hemicholinium amnesia reversed by :
Physostigmine, piracetam.

Four points should be considered in evaluating animal models of dementia.

Firstly, the models may be valid but the major problem may arise with the nature of the chemical compounds that are being tested.

Secondly, many of the drugs which have been developed as a result of looking at their effects in these models have very serious side effects which limit their usefulness in the long-term treatment of a demented patient. We therefore need drugs with fewer side effects, longer duration of action and that act over broad dose ranges. Tetrahydroamino-acridine (THA), for example, is hepatotoxic and has a very narrow therapeutic dose range. Each patient has to have the dose individually titrated and even then the results are not very startling in terms of clinical response.

Thirdly, while it is easy to condemn and criticise the experimental psychopharmacologist who is working on animal models, we must accept that at a clinical level we have not yet developed sufficiently sophisticated diagnostic methods to detect and objectively assess patients adequately in the early stages of dementing diseases. This means that it is difficult to test drugs at a stage when there is still a reasonable amount of functioning brain tissue. Animal models may help us to try and bridge this gap.

Finally, we must ask ourselves whether symptoms such as cognitive impairment

219

are amenable to drug treatment at all. For example, research workers in the German Democratic Republic have been studying the cholinergic projections to the cortex of human brain and found that the way in which the cholinergic system is arranged in the cortex is quite different from any other neurotransmitter system. It appears that the neurones project to the cortex like a series of "fields" which don't overlap, so that when the nerve terminals die, the "fields" are lost. The particular "fields" may be extremely important in relating information from the external world to the cortex, to enable the cortex to appraise what is going on in the environment. Thus it seems likely that if a particular terminal "field" of the cholinergic system is lost, the function served by it is irretrievably lost. Attempts at cognitive improvement using drugs that facilitate the cholinergic system may therefore have only a very limited value! On a more light-hearted note, a working "ratologist", studying the action of esoteric chemicals on models of the dementias, has the following advantages:

(i)   He does not have to ask the animal for consent;

(ii)   He is mainly limited by money in the number of studies that can be undertaken;

(iii) He can produce a lot of scientific papers!

Perhaps the most important experimental aspect is the development of drugs for prophylactic use. In order to do this effectively we have to discover aetiological factors involved in the dementias, a method to prevent nerve cell loss and tangle formation, to prevent the inevitable progression of the disease. At present we have little understanding of what can affect any of those pathological parameters so the main strategy is to develop therapy in a fairly arbitrary way. One such approach, already mentioned, is to find ways of stimulating the cholinergic system in a patient with dementia. Secondly, to use so-called nootropic agents which I will be discussing later and thirdly, to look at other neurotransmitter systems which we know from animal experiments are involved in memory, learning mechanisms and cognition. In this respect, there is evidence from post-mortem brain analysis that the cholinergic, dopaminergic, serotonergic and peptidergic systems are defective in Alzheimer disease. Understanding the reasons for such defects may be a useful strategy for treating the dementias.

Study of the pathology of the Alzheimer's brain as a strategy for drug development

How far have these strategies advanced? If we consider the cholinergic system, we know that there is cell loss in the nucleus basalis of Meynert, the main region where the cholinergic cell bodies project to the cortex. This region of the brain is rich in tangles and the key enzyme which is involved in the synthesis of acetylcholine is defective in cortical regions. This deficit seems to correlate with the behavioural deficits and we know that the way in which the nerve cells transport choline (the precursor of acetyl choline) into the nerve terminals is also defective.

Thus, there is fairly good evidence of a cholinergic involvement in Alzheimer's disease, although it is uncertain as to whether it is causative or coincidental.

Table 3. Pathological changes in neurotransmitter systems in the brain of the Alzheimer patient

1. Cholinergic system	Cell loss in nucleus basalis Tangles occur in nucleus basalis Decreased choline-acetyltransferase activity and choline uptake
2. Noradrenergic system	Cell loss in locus coeruleus Tangles occur in locus coeruleus Decreased dopamine beta-oxidase and reduced noradrenaline synthesis
3. Serotonergic system	Cell loss in raphe nucleus Tangles occur in raphe nucleus Decreased serotonin synthesis

It would appear that the adrenergic system, which is not so popular in terms of research strategies, is also worthy of attention in patients with Alzheimer's disease. Indeed this system is probably just as important as the cholinergic system in terms of arousal states, alerting and so forth. We know that there is a cell loss in the local coeruleus which contains the cell bodies that provide most of the noradrenergic projections to the cortex. Such areas are rich in tangles and there is a decrease in the amount of noradrenaline being produced and the enzyme which synthesizes noradrenaline, dopamine beta-hydroxylase, is defective. The way in which noradrenaline is transported into the nerve terminals is also defective. Thus on pathological grounds, one could make a very good case for developing drugs that activate the noradrenergic system.

Another neurotransmitter system that is worthy of consideration is the serotonergic system; defects in the functioning of this system in patients with Alzheimer's disease have also been described. In the case of the serotonergic system, we are dealing with the cell bodies of Raphe which are responsible for providing the serotonergic stimulus to the cortex, the hippocampus and other regions of the brain. Any disturbance in the functioning of this transmitter could lead to an abnormality in the pattern of sleep, feeding, mood, sexual activity, etc. However, it may be argued that it is unlikely that the dementias will be completely cured merely by understanding these transmitters.

Thus an overview of the research into the possible causes of Alzheimer's disease shows there are many other potential aetiological factors. Aluminium silicate and the involvement of this metal with amyloid, circumstantial as it may be, has been highlighted by the scientific journals and in the media. The publication in the *Lancet* showing an imperfect correlation between the frequency of Alzheimer's disease and the distribution and amount of aluminium in drinking water was widely discussed by the media and caused a tremendous problem with the public perception of aluminium as a risk factor. If it were as simple as that then we would have solved the problem of dementia many years ago! We do know that such heavy metals accumulate in the brains of some patients but it is uncertain whether this is co-incidental or causal factor.

Cellular metabolism

When searching for the causes of Alzheimer's disease, it is probably more realistic to think in terms of cellular metabolism which somehow becomes defective in those individuals who are programmed to develop Alzheimer's disease. Changes in such factors as the brain ammonia concentration play a role; biopterin is a co-factor in dopamine and noradrenaline synthesis and may be defective in some of the dementias. At the more structural level of the brain cell, there is evidence that tubulin sequestration may occur and lead to early death in some brain cells. Vitamin deficiencies, particularly involving those of the B complex and vitamins C and E, are yet another source of debate among researchers regarding the cause of Alzheimer's disease.

Table 4. Some aetiological factors that have been implicated in Alzheimer's Disease

Aluminium silicate and calcium salts in amyloid protein

Disturbance in brain carbohydrate metabolism – due to a deficiency in glucose transport caused by altered insulin receptor?

Hyperammonaemia

Decreased somatostatin-like immunoreactivity in cortex

Decreased biopterin in CSF

Sequestration of tubulin in neurones

Hypothalamic mediated changes in endorphins

Vitamin deficiencies – particularly vitamin B complex and vitamin E

All these different strands of evidence emphasize that we have to have a very catholic approach to our research in this area: it would be foolish to rely on the possibility that one neurotransmitter system is primarily involved. All of the transmitter systems are interlocking and the basal metabolism of the brain is also affected. Thus the brain of the Alzheimer's patient shows gross biochemical and structural abnormalities that need to be unravelled before we can hope to make any real headway in preventing the rapid decline that follows the onset of the disease.

The clinical psychopharmacological strategy

The outcome of psychopharmacological research has been disappointing so far in clinical practice. A whole series of cerebral vasodilators are still prescribed in many countries in the world for the treatment of dementia. If one analyses the good double-blind controlled clinical trials, there is no convincing evidence at all that these compounds are of any use. A possible exception is "Hydergine", but with this drug there have not been enough good trials to say whether it is truly beneficial. The pharmacological principle behind the use of vasodilators is that there is insufficient blood getting to the brain and therefore if more blood is delivered by dilating the cerebral-vessels, then more oxygen and glucose will also be delivered to the brain cells so that those cells still functioning normally will benefit and compensate for the defective cells. This is an extremely crude approach to brain function. Thus dilating the vessels to the brain with such compounds may also dilate the vessels in the rest of the body, which could end by draining blood away from the brain rather than to it!

Furthermore, the vasodilator theory does not take into account what is called the "recruiting mechanism" in the brain. This is a mechanism whereby the brain compensates for reduced blood flow to one area by automatically increasing the blood supply to the region by increasing the blood carrying capacity of the vessels to that region, providing of course, the brain region is still able to function. Clearly there is no purpose in increasing blood supply to dead cells so the brain would automatically shut off blood supply to the dead part of the brain. Thus treating dementing patients with such drugs as the cerebral vasodilators is unlikely to benefit the patient and may be harmful!

Nootropic agents

Another group of drugs which are still prescribed widely are the metabolic enhancers, some of which started life as cerebral vasodilators. The strategy for using these agents is based on the hope that they might facilitate glucose transport and thereby improve brain metabolism. By and large these drugs, as exemplified by centrophenoxine, do not appear to have any worthwhile therapeutic benefit.

A further group are the "nootropic" agents (from the Greek words meaning "forward to the mind" or improving the mind). Examples of such drugs are piracetam and its analogues. These are substances which do not have sedative, antidepressant or antipsychotic properties. It is claimed that they specifically enhance learning and memory and in addition facilitate the transfer of information from one hemisphere of the brain to the other. Animal experiments show that they increase the brain's resistance to hypoxia and related assaults without having a noticeable effect on non-nervous tissue. However, if one looks at all of the double-blind trials that have been undertaken to date, there is no evidence that such drugs are therapeutically effective in patients with dementia.

223

Psychostimulants and neuropeptides

Similarly, the use of psychostimulants such as the amphetamines in dementia is not new. The rationale seems to be an empirical one, viewing such patients as very withdrawn, may be a little bit aggressive at times, anti-social, unmotivated and so forth. Administering psychostimulants might, therefore, help. Unfortunately, despite a plethora of drugs which have been used, none have been shown to have any benefit. Indeed, they can make the patient more aggressive and difficult to manage!

One of the most recent clinical approaches involves the neuropeptides. These neuropeptides are structurally based upon natural hormones, such as ACTH. In animal experiments, stable semi-synthetic analogues, when injected into old rats, give very impressive results regarding the ability of the animal to learn, acquire and retain new information. A further point in favour of such compounds is that they are non-toxic, so they are potentially ideal drugs. All of the clinical trials of vasopressin-like, ACTH-like, cholecystokinin-like or somatostatin-like peptides found in parts of the brain which might be important for learning, have so far shown no real effect in dementing illness.

Neurotransmitter enhancers

A further series of agents, and this is by no means a complete list, are the neurotransmitter enhancers, drugs which theoretically activate or facilitate central neurotransmission. Such substances have been used in patients to increase the activity of the dopaminergic system (e.g. L-dopa), facilitate the gabaminergic system (e.g. THIP), the serotonergic system (e.g. tryptophan) or cholinergic system (e.g. lecithin). Other substances such as 4-aminopyridine seem to increase acetylcholine synthesis and release, while pilocarpine is a muscarinic receptor agonist and thereby simulates the actions of acetylcholine. With the possible exception of the 4- aminopyridine, there is no evidence that any of these approaches is therapeutically beneficial. A miscellaneous group of substances includes "Gero-vital H3". This is a very weak, non-specific monoamine oxidase inhibitor, so it may have a minor effect on the brain but evidence for efficacy is negligible.

Table 5. Pharmacological agents that have been used to treat various types of dementia

DRUG CATEGORY	AGENT	BENEFIT TO PATIENT
Cerebral vasodilator	Papaverine	None
	Cyclandelate	None
	Isoxuprine	None
	Vincamine	?

DRUG CATEGORY	AGENT	BENEFIT TO PATIENT
Metabolic enhancers	Nafronyl	?
	Centrophenoxine	None
	Pyrithioxine	?
	Meclofenoxate	None
	Pyritinol	?
Nootropics	Piracetam	None
	Pramiracetam	None
	Aniracetam	None
	Oxiracetam	?
	Suloctidil	None
Psychostimulants	Methylphenidate	None
	Amphetamines	None
	Pipradol	None
Neuropeptides	Vasopressin-like	None
	ACTH-like	None
	CCK-like	?
	Somatotatin-like	?
	Naloxone	?
Neurotransmitter enhancers	Levodopa	None
	THIP	None
	Tryptophan	None
	Alaproclate	None
	Choline	None
	Pilocarpine	None
	4-Aminopyridine	?
Miscellaneous	Gerovital - H3	None
	Hyperbaric oxygen	None

In the table, 'none' indicates that placebo-controlled trials involving a reasonable number of properly diagnosed patients have not shown useful benefit of the agent to the patient. '?' indicates that insufficient clinical data is currently available to assess efficacy.

One may conclude that, so far, the psychopharmacologist has not made much of a contribution in developing effective drugs for the treatment of the dementias.

Potentially promising approaches

Despite such scepticism there are one or two other approaches which are potentially promising. The use of acetyl-carnitine is interesting in that there are now some double-blind controlled trials suggesting some marginal improvement in properly-diagnosed demented patients. However, the studies are small and need adequate replication. Studies involving the anticholinesterase, physostigmine, of which there are many, have also suggested that the cholinergic hypothesis is worth examining further. There are eight double-blind studies, four of which showed beneficial effects on memory performance and behavioural tests. These differences, a small improvement in memory without a generalized clinical improvement, were probably of marginal value but nevertheless deserve consideration.

The main problem with drugs like physostigmine is their variable absorption, the variable rate at which they are metabolized, and their difficulty of access to the brain. There seems to be a change in the permeability of the blood-brain barrier with age and such changes are even more pronounced in the patient with dementia. This means that the amount of drug crossing the blood-brain barrier cannot easily be standarized. It, therefore, has to be standarized on an individual patient basis and this is quite difficult to achieve. Such an approach has been used with the well publicized drug tetrahydroaminoacridine (THA), which in the first study published in the *New England Journal of Medicine* indicated that 16 out of 17 patients showed marked clinical improvement. However, more recently, scepticism has been cast on the value of THA. Most researchers are awaiting the outcome of a very large multicentre trial in the USA to see whether THA is as good as initially it appeared to be. Another problem with THA is that serious adverse effects may occur; the trial in the USA was temporarily suspended because the compound caused some liver toxicity! Thus the problems associated with drugs acting by facilitating the cholinergic system are due to their short half-life, lack of specificity, poor penetration into the brain and adverse reactions. These are just a few of the problems facing the clinical psychopharmacologist trying to develop drugs to treat Alzheimer's and related dementing diseases.

Strategies based on the pathology of multi-infarct dementia

Although Alzheimer's disease accounts for about 50 per cent or more of the dementia cases, it may also be possible to learn about dementing illnesses by looking at other forms of brain injury. Brain-cell loss can arise from head injury, stroke or birth defects; the behavioural consequences of vascular damage associated with multi-infarct dementia are somewhat similar to those occurring in the Alzheimer patient. In these progressive degenerative diseases, there is a common nerve cell loss. The brain itself is very vulnerable to the interruption of blood supply, even if that period is for a very short duration of a few seconds. The restoration of blood supply to the brain following a short hypoxic period can produce changes in brain chemistry, such as the formation of highly reactive free radicals. These are very highly active molecules which attack the lipids in the brain membranes, leading to lipid peroxidation and death of the cell. This has formed the basis of another approach to treatment by using free radical scavenger molecules. Such drugs have antioxidant properties which are therefore able to mop up any of the highly reactive peroxides which can occur in the brain.

There is experimental evidence to show that if the blood supply to the brain is temporarily impeded to produce a hypoxic state and then re-oxygenated, a sudden release of excitatory amino acids (such as glutamate) will occur. Such amino acids can act on specific excitatory amino acid receptors in the brain, the N-methyl-D-aspartate (NMDA) receptors. There is a connection between the stimulation of these receptors and the influx of calcium; over stimulation of these receptors by the release of glutamate which occurs following some hypoxic states leads to a dramatic mobilization of calcium and death of the cell. The rationale of intervention would be to try to reduce the effects of these excitatory amino acids immediately following a stroke. This strategy is being pursued experimentally in the hope that drugs that specifically block the NMDA receptors may be of some benefit in the prevention of multi-infarct dementia.

We know from studies in Alzheimer's disease that there are changes in the way in which glutamate can bind to receptors to produce its effects. It is also known that these receptors occur in the hippocampus and may be involved in short-term memory; this region of the brain is also known to be very rich in plaques and tangles in Alzheimer's disease. Thus, it is possible that there is an association between the altered amino-acid receptors and some of the defects that are seen in the dementias. Antagonists of the excitatory amino acid receptors may therefore be of potential value in attenuating the memory deficit found in the early stage of Alzheimer's disease.

Strategies based on changes in the immune system

Another approach hinges on the possibility that Alzheimer's disease might be an immunological disease. This is a concept which has not gained a great deal of support yet. However, AIDS has concentrated our attention on the immune system because of the enormous problem with AIDS associated dementia. By studying AIDS dementia we may gain insight into the relationship between the abnormalities in the immune system and brain function.

Ten years ago the brain and immune system were thought of as two separate entities. This is no longer acceptable: there is a two-way process, with a feed-back from the immune system to the brain and *vice-versa*. The possibility that Alzheimer's disease might be an immunological disease must now be considered. Focal accumulation of abnormal proteins, focal lesions, the production of neuritic plaques, the aggregation of lytic scavenger cells and the deterioration of the blood-brain barrier mean that the peripheral immune system has complete access to the brain in the demented patient. The production of specific anti-brain antibodies, which have been found in the cerebro-spinal fluid of patients with dementia may reflect this breach of the blood-brain barrier.

Among other aspects which warrant careful research is the way in which the body gets rid of invading micro-organisms and extraneous material. The brain microglia appear to play an important role in this defence, as do astrocytes and macrophages which can invade the brain. These cells may mediate the immune reactions in Alzheimer's disease. Recently, class II immunoreactive cells were found to co-localize with neuritic plaques in the Alzheimer brain. Antibodies to tangles and astrocytes have also been found in the Alzheimer brain but not in the normal ageing brain. This suggests that there is something abnormal in the immune system in the Alzheimer patient.

Immuno-psychiatry is a new discipline, promoted partly as a consequence of AIDS dementia. It may be a worthwhile strategy to examine deficiencies in neurotransmitters and also changes in the key immune cells (e.g. T cells, B cells, macrophages and stem cells) in Alzheimer's disease. We know that most of those neurotransmitter systems thought to be involved in modulating the immune system are, in one way or another, abnormal in the Alzheimer patient. It is possible that there is a relationship between the abnormality in the brain chemistry and the abnormality of the immune system so that the changes in brain function which could be a consequence of both, i.e. an interaction between the neurotransmitter system and the immune system. This is a difficult area to investigate at the moment but there does seem to be circumstantial evidence pointing towards a specific abnormality of the immune system in Alzheimer's disease.

The strategy of the psychogeriatrician

What practical advice have we for the clinician when the drugs developed so far show little evidence of benefit? The effects of most of these drugs on patients are of marginal value only. Despite thousands of papers published in the most learned journals we are left with "Hydergine" and some analogues. "Hydergine" is an interesting example of how drugs in the treatment of dementia are evaluated. It is stated in the United States that no alternative drug treatments have proved better than "Hydergine". However, this is mainly because none of them are of benefit! Hughes in 1976 examined 12 double-blind placebo-controlled trials involving "Hydergine" and concluded that these showed a consistent improvement in some of the symptoms of dementia. If this review article is carefully examined, however, the actual improvement was only relatively minor as far as the patient was concerned. It is worth remembering that changes on assessment scores and rating scales may have little relevance to the patient and the patient's relatives even though they may be considered to be evidence of efficacy to the researcher! The real measure of success of any drug treatment only occurs when the patient, and the patient's relatives, notice that the drug is beneficial! Clearly the pharmacologist has a long way to go to produce drugs that are effective and safe.

Conclusion

In considering drug therapy, the viewpoint of the patient and the carer are of fundamental importances. There are three points worth considering:

(i) Most patients and their carers want more practical assistance with daily living;

(ii) More public concern is needed regarding the problems of the aged. As yet there is little political pressure to ensure that these problems are faced. The public needs educating; it does not know a lot about the problems of ageing or, for example, the differences between ageing and dementia;

(iii) More research is needed to find useful drugs to improve the quality of life of patients with dementia. Clearly without research we are not going to get anywhere and it is abysmal that so little money is being spent on research in most European countries, particularly Ireland!

Finally, I would like to thank the Alzheimer's Society of Ireland for organizing this symposium that lead to the production of this book. For the first time we have an organization that is not only doing something for the patients but also campaigning for more research. Of course, without the political will we will not get very far. I am just hoping that the politicians will take notice of what is going on!

SECTION 8
The Nature of Alzheimer's Disease

Carers, Professionals and Alzheimer's Disease. D O'Neill ed © 1991 John Libbey & Company Ltd

Chapter 35

IS ALZHEIMER'S DISEASE ONE DISEASE?

GK Wilcock *DM, FRCP, Dept of Care of the Elderly, University of Bristol, UK*

Introduction

The issue that I have to address is one that I'm not sure that I have the answer to, but I would like to try to explore some of the more important evidence that points in the direction of the possibility that Alzheimer's disease may be a number of diseases, or else a disease with a variety of sub-conditions or sub-categories. There are many ways to approach this problem, and I have decided to pick out some areas of scientific and clinical research indicating that it is worthwhile pursuing the concept that Alzheimer's disease is heterogeneous, but will leave the reader to make up his or her own mind.

There are many fundamental questions that one could explore, but I think that there are three which are most important. The first of these is to examine whether Alzheimer's disease is, as is often claimed, merely an acceleration of the normal ageing process. It is important since if Alzheimer's disease is only an acceleration of normal ageing, it makes it very difficult to accept the concept of more than one type.

When considering the evidence that Alzheimer's disease may be more than one condition, it is essential to determine whether the clinical differences are reflected in other areas such as neuro-chemistry and neuropathology. Another vital question is whether the plaques and tangles and the other hallmarks of Alzheimer pathology are in fact specific for a single condition, or whether they represent the only way, or one of a limited number of ways, in which highly specialized cells, such as neurones, respond to a variety of external or internal insults.

Accelerated ageing or disease?

When we look at the question as to whether Alzheimer's disease represents accelerated ageing, it is apparent that most of the protagonists have conducted clinical studies and that they have examined the distribution of intellectual change in a cohort of subjects taken from a community setting, and sometimes from a hospital or other institutional setting.[1] What they discover is that when they measure the ability of elderly people to score on intellectual assessment schedules, instead of finding two discrete populations, i.e. one group scoring abnormally and the other group scoring normally, the spread of scores is part of a continuum and there is no discrete cut-off. This makes it very difficult not to entertain the notion that intellectual function in the elderly forms a continuum, and dementia is merely a part of this.

However the disadvantage of studies like this, which is often not addressed, is that they are cross-sectional, i.e. they look at the individuals at one point in time. There are very few studies that have followed up the subjects that they have studied for very long, and the natural history in the "normals" and the Alzheimer's disease patients has also not been adequately explored. In addition very few of the subjects come to post-mortem to confirm whether or not the diagnosis is Alzheimer's disease, which is important as we have no diagnostic marker for Alzheimer's disease during life.

So these studies, convincing though some of them may be and unconvincing as the majority are, need to be counter-balanced against the weight of evidence that can be derived from basic scientific examination of brain material taken from the people in whom Alzheimer's disease has been confirmed, both during life and at post-mortem. There is a wealth of evidence, both at the macroscopic level and at the histological level, examining the distribution and severity of neuropathological changes, which indicates that Alzheimer's disease is separate from normal ageing. Therefore for the rest of this paper I will adopt the standpoint that Alzheimer's disease is not accelerated normal ageing, but is a separate disease entity that may potentially be sub-divided into further groups. Whether these represent separate diseases or sub-divisions of the main disease I leave for the reader to decide.

Early and late onset

The most obvious starting point for a discussion of possible sub-groups of Alzheimer's disease is the difference between old and young people with the disease. It is often said that the disease in younger people is different from that in older people. Rossor et al [2] looked at the level of various markers of neurotransmitter systems in the brains of a large series of people who had died, both young and old, using the age of 79–80 as a cut-off point. There were very definite differences between these two groups of patients in the percentage loss of neurotransmitters compared to normal brains. There was much less choline-acetyl-transferase, a marker for the cholinergic system, in the younger patients than in the older group of patients. This age differential is maintained for other markers such as those for the noradrenergic and the somatostatin systems. These findings are mirrored by the histopathological changes, as the severity and the distribution of the pathology is different in the younger patients than in the older patients.

Macroscopic examination of the brain, as in the study of Hubbard and Anderson,[3] shows that the degenerative process in the younger patients is more widespread and involves most if not all of the lobes of the brain, whereas in older patients it seems to be concentrated mainly on the temporal lobe. The difference between younger and older sufferers has, of course, been studied in the clinical setting. The first of these studies that I would like to consider is that of Seltzer and Sherwin.[4] They studied 65 patients of whom approximately half were classified as "young" and half as "old", and followed them up over a period of several years, noting the way in which the disease presentation progressed. The young group had a much greater predominance of language disorder and a shorter survival time. This information led to the proposition that perhaps there might be a predominance of left-hemisphere dysfunction in young patients with Alzheimer's disease compared to the older patients.

A similar study by Filey[5] and colleagues also confirmed that the younger age group had greater difficulties with language functions, whereas the older group had greater difficulties with visuo-spatial function. They considered that this implied that the older people had predominant right-hemisphere dysfunction.

Other clinical sub-groups

(a) Clinical information

In describing evidence for the existence of sub-types defined by parameters other than age, I will refer to studies where the appropriate variables have been controlled for, and have omitted several studies where the information reported is inadequate. There is still room for controversy in all these clinical studies, but they nevertheless point in a similar direction. Bothwinick[6] and his colleagues studied a relatively small group of people with Alzheimer's disease for four years and they found that the majority of them progressed (as might be expected), but that five of them remained relatively static for a relatively long time. Most people with Alzheimer's disease go through the majority of the course of their disease in the space of four or five years, although this is correspondingly longer in older patients. They wondered if this group with an apparently static clinical picture constituted a sub-group. However this study is difficult to interpret because, like most of the studies in this area, the patients were not followed up long enough to obtain a post-mortem. These patients may not actually have had Alzheimer's disease or may have been a group who had extremely early dementia but appeared, because of the insensitivity of the assessment schedules, to be normal.

The study by Mayeux[7] and his colleagues is perhaps more interesting. They also studied a group of patients with Alzheimer's disease for four years, and picked out some very definite sub-groups, but again there is very little evidence about the post-mortem findings. It looks from the information in this very careful study that their subjects could be divided into four groups: a group with a rather benign course similar to that described by Bothwinick, a typical group, and two interesting but atypical groups who both displayed motor abnormalities, myoclonus in one and extra-pyramidal features in the other. Myoclonus consists of a rather strange type of jerky movement that occurs at random and is often associated with other dementing illnesses, and the extra-pyramidal features refer to changes similar to those in Parkinson's disease. This study has been replicated by several others and most clinical workers now know that if they come across a person who has Alzheimer's disease, and who also has motor disturbances of this sort, it is likely that their disease pattern will be different, and in particular more aggressive than it is in others who do not have this type of abnormality.

Friedland and colleagues[8] asked six patients with Alzheimer's disease to draw a picture of a house, and discovered that there are groups of people with a similar degree of Alzheimer's disease but who have markedly different graphic and visuo-spatial disabilities. They backed this up by looking at the way in which the brain was functioning at a simple level, in terms of its metabolism of glucose in these subjects using Positron Emission Tomography Scanning, i.e. PET scans. They found that the two groups showed different pictures on PET scanning: those with particular difficulties in visuo- spatial capabilities had abnormalities in the utilization of glucose particularly in the right hemisphere, and those with relatively preserved visuo-spatial capability were affected predominantly in the left hemisphere. This implies the presence of either sub-groups or else of two different types of disease. They also examined the symptoms in their patients who had motor disorders, and measured the concentration of a variety of different biochemical markers in the cerebro-spinal fluid which are thought to represent the degree of activity of various neuro- transmitter systems. The level of activity in those with myoclonus and extra-pyramidal disorders was significantly different when compared with that of "typical" Alzheimer's disease patients. This study showed that the clinical differences between the groups found some expression in the cerebro-spinal fluid markers, and possibly of brain neuro- transmitters if the lumbar cerebro-spinal fluid is representative of what is happening higher up in the nervous system.

(b) Neuronal and neurochemical changes

In most series of Alzheimer's patients in whom the level of marker enzymes for the cholinergic system is measured, there is always a sub-group in whom the level of these marker enzymes is normal. We examined a group of these subjects in whom the diagnosis of Alzheimer's disease had been made clinically, and confirmed histologically, and in whom there was no other alternative potential cause for their disorder. Not only was the marker enzyme for acetyl-choline normal in some, but there was also no reduction in the number of cells in the basal nucleus, that part of the brain that is responsible for synthesizing most of the acetyl-choline. In addition there was no increase in the number of neurofibrillary tangles in this area. There were however abnormalities in terms of loss of neurones and neurofibrillary tangle formation in the brain-stem sub-cortical nuclei responsible for the noradrenergic and serotoninergic input to the cortex.[9] In other words, there is a small group of elderly patients with Alzheimer's disease in whom there is no cholinergic deficit, but in whom the disease is definitely associated with other neurotransmitter abnormalities.

(c) Specificity of histological markers

I would like to move from the concept of potential sub-groups to consider the pathological features of Alzheimer's disease. The pathology of Alzheimer's disease is not specific. We find plaques and tangles in people who are normally aged, although in small numbers. We also find a similar picture in people with Down's syndrome, which is often thought of as a model for Alzheimer's disease. We know that tangles are present in the brains of some people who have been boxing and have become demented at a later date, so-called dementia pugilistica. We know that patients with Alzheimer's disease may have a brain which shows many plaques but very few tangles. Head trauma has often been linked and is increasingly being linked to the development of Alzheimer's disease in at least a few patients.

The trouble with most of these studies is that the majority of the patients were elderly and it is difficult to be sure whether there is any pathologically relevant connection. There is one striking case in the literature of a man of 22 who had a very severe head injury, and subsequently died of Alzheimer's disease (clinically and proven histologically) at the age of 32, despite the absence of a family history of Alzheimer's disease or any other form of dementia.[10] It may be that trauma itself has a role in producing plaques and tangles.

More interestingly, tangles can occur outside the central nervous system, totally unassociated with Alzheimer's disease. A relatively recent paper from Japan described a single 76-year-old man without dementia who was found to have tangles in the upper cervical ganglion, a collection of nerve cells at the top of the neck.[11] Yet when his brain was examined there was no evidence of more than a very small number of neuro-fibrillary tangles and plaques within the brain itself, despite the large number of tangles within the upper cervical ganglion. It might be argued that these are totally different to the Alzheimer's disease tangles, but many of their staining properties were similar to those seen when the neurofibrillary tangles of Alzheimer's disease are examined using the same stains.

Conclusion

I would like to conclude by saying that I cannot help thinking that everyone over the age of fifty falls into one of two groups, and that each of these groups has two separate sub-groups, a total of four categories. On the one hand there are those who are not demented, a proportion of whom have no evidence of plaques or tangles, and they are clearly quite normal. The second sub-group within this non-demented category consists of those who are judged to be not demented, and who have a few plaques and tangles, particularly in medial temporal structures, and who are thought to be normal, despite this histological picture. (They may not be normal.) On the other hand there are those with dementia, some of whom have no plaques or tangles, and clearly have a dementia that is caused by a different condition.

The final category are those who have dementia, and in whose brains one can find plaques and tangles. It is this group which I consider to be of the most importance at the moment. It is in this group that there is so much diversity of clinical and histological presentation and also biochemical abnormality, that heterogeneity cannot be easily discounted. We must seriously consider whether Alzheimer's disease is either a single disease with many different presentations or is in fact a constellation of different conditions. Perhaps the brain is so specialized that it can only react to exogenous influences in a very limited number of ways.

References

(1) Brayne C, Calloway P. Normal ageing, impaired cognitive function, and senile dementia of the Alzheimer's type: A continuum? *Lancet* 1988, **ii**, 1265-67.

(2) Rossor MN, Iverson LL, Reynolds GP, Mountjoy CQ, Roth M. Neurochemical characteristics of early and late onset types of Alzheimer's disease. *British Medical Journal* 1984, **288**, 961-64.

(3) Hubbard BM, Anderson JM. A quantitative study of cerebral atrophy in old age and senile dementia. *J Neurol Sci* 1981, **50**, 135-45.

(4) Seltzer B, Sherwin I. A comparison of clinical features in early- and late-onset primary degenerative dementia. One entity or two? *Arch Neurol* 1983, **40**, 143-46.

(5) Filley CM, Kelly J, Heaton RK. Neuropsychologic features of early- and late-onset Alzheimer's disease. *Arch Neurol* 1986, **43**, 574-76.

(6) Botwinick J, Storandt M, Berg L. A longitudinal, behavioural study of senile dementia of the Alzheimer type. *Arch Neurol* 1986, **43**, 1124-27.

(7) Mayeux R, Stern Y, Spanton S. Heterogeneity in dementia of the Alzheimer type: evidence of subgroups. *Neurology* 1985, **35**,453-61.

(8) Friedland RP, Koss E, Haxby JV, Grady CL, Luxenberg J, Schapiro MB, Kaye J. Alzheimer's disease: clinical and biological heterogeneity. *Annals of Internal Medicine* 1988, **109**, 298-311.

(9) Wilcock GK, Esiri MM, Bowen DM, Hughes AO. The differential involvement of sub-cortical nuclei in senile dementia of Alzheimer's type. *Journal of Neurology, Neurosurgery and Psychiatry* 1988, **51**, 842-49.

(10) Rudelli R, Strom JO, Welch PT, Ambler MW. Post traumatic premature Alzheimer's disease. Neuropathologic findings and pathogenetic considerations. *Arch Neurol* 1982, **39**(9), 570-75.

(11) Kawasaki N, Murayma S, Tomonaga M, Izumiyama N, Shimada H. Neurofibrillary tangles in human upper cervical ganglia. Morphological study with immunohistochemistry and electron microscopy. *Acta Neuropathol* 1987, **75**(2), 156-59.

Carers, Professionals and Alzheimer's Disease. D O'Neill ed © 1991 John Libbey & Company Ltd

Chapter 36

MOLECULAR NEUROPATHOLOGY OF ALZHEIMER'S DISEASE

Claude M. Wischik *BA, MBBS, PhD, Cambridge Brain Bank Laboratory, Department of Psychiatry, University of Cambridge Clinical School, MRC Centre, Hills Road, Cambridge CB2 2QQ, UK*

The need for a molecular approach

This paper reports progress with our attempts to understand the pathology of Alzheimer's disease at the molecular level. Although Alzheimer's disease is defined in traditional terms by the histological lesions, such as those described by Alzheimer and Perusini in 1907, our understanding of these lesions remained unchanged until quite recently. Despite numerous attempts to draw various kinds of correlation between dementia and findings in the light microscope, our understanding and all our theories must remain provisional until they can be expressed in terms of molecular processes.

This is not a matter merely of scientific curiosity, but a very practical matter. Drugs do not work at the whole cell level, but at the level of the single molecule. Until we can understand a disease process in terms of the relevant molecular processes, it is not possible to develop a rational therapeutic approach. Diabetes provides a useful illustration of this theoretical approach. Knowing that there is damage to the pancreas is only a stepping stone on the way to reaching a useful understanding of diabetes. Until we came to understand diabetes in terms of deficiency of the molecule insulin, it was not possible to intervene usefully in the disease process. In Alzheimer's disease, we have been able to see the pathology for almost a century, but we are approaching it almost as if we were gazing at a diabetic without any concept of insulin. Until we can see through the pathology down into the molecular processes that cause the changes which are visible in the light microscope, we can have no hope of developing a drug, except by accident.

Replacement therapies?

Psychiatry has made great strides by accident. To take the analogy of diabetes further, is there just a neurotransmitter deficit in Alzheimer's disease? Could we perhaps hit on just the right neurotransmitter replacement which would slow down the process of dementia? Some people today think that by boosting cholinergic function, or by screening for other "cognitive enhancers", we could make a significant impact on cognitive deficit. I do not think that this is likely. As I will try to make clear, there is progressive destruction of neurones in this disease, neurones which we know to be critical for information processing in the cortex. The cognitive enhancers may enhance the capacity to use residual function more effectively for a short time, but they cannot slow down the process of accelerated neuronal destruction, whose hallmarks are the tangle and the neuritic plaque. The challenge, as I see it, is to reach such an understanding of the basic disease mechanism that we can devise a rational treatment which slows the actual pathology. This would be a marvellous thing: for the first time in psychiatry to devise a rational mechanistic treatment for a mental illness.

Molecular approach focused on neurofibrillary tangle

How does one begin to attack this sort of problem? Traditional pathology has defined plaques and tangles as the hallmark features of this disease. There has been considerable recent progress in the understanding of plaques at the molecular level, in terms of abnormal deposits of amyloid protein. It has recently become possible to measure amyloid protein accumulation in the brain biochemically. Unfortunately, it does not appear that the extent of amyloid deposition predicts dementia. Indeed, recent work is starting to suggest that amyloid accumulation is much more closely related to the ageing process than to the specific changes which are associated with dementia. Nevertheless, work on abnormal processing of the amyloid precursor protein is now progressing very rapidly in many laboratories around the world.

The task that we have set ourselves in our laboratory is to try to understand the neurofibrillary tangle. Among the reasons for focusing on the tangle is the clear evidence that numbers of neurofibrillary tangles correlate with the degree of cognitive deficit. The tangles form in a class of cortical and hippocampal neurones, called pyramidal cells, known to be critical for higher associative function. Furthermore, it has been known for some time that there is a close relationship between the abnormality occurring in tangles, and that occurring in the abnormal nerve terminals found in the neuritic plaques. As I hope to show, we are now beginning to understand the functional implications of tangle formation at the molecular level.

Structural studies of neurofibrillary tangles

We set about the problem by first learning how to isolate tangles in a form suitable for further study. When isolated tangles could be visualised by electron microscopy, it was possible to study their inner molecular architecture. The tangle consists of a dense array of filaments called paired helical filaments (PHFs) which are all identical to one another, and which accumulate in vast numbers within the cortical pyramidal cells affected by this disease process. Their numbers become such as as to predominate over all the other cellular organelles which are required for normal neuronal function. At higher power it becomes possible to see that these filaments have very characteristic and regular features. They have wide to narrow modulations every 80 nm, and it is because of this twisted appearance that they are called paired helical filaments (PHFs).

By using various imaging techniques and by careful observation of the way the paired helical filament untwist, we showed that the PHF is in fact a rather flattened ribbon-like structure (Fig. 1). From further careful structural analysis it was possible to build up a model of the inner architecture of each filament. Each filament represents a double helical stack of sub-units, and each of these sub-units has three domains distributed in the form of a "C". So in cross-section, the PHF appears as 2 C-shaped subunits, arranged back to back. We were able to verify this model using very sophisticated image analysis techniques developed in Cambridge, and it is possible to see that the structure predicted from analysis of fragmentation patterns agrees very well with the calculated distribution of matter in the PHF. So the PHF is a double-helical stack of C shaped sub-units twisted into a ribbon-like structure (Fig. 2).

Theoretical implications of structural analysis

Although this may all seem rather technical, it is in fact a very important statement about the basic pathology of Alzheimer's disease. When Alzheimer first saw neurofibrillary tangles, he considered them to be some abnormal form of neurofibres, that is an abnormal form of the fibres which are normally found inside neurones. Various modern theories are not very different from the idea first put forward by Alzheimer, and implicit in his term "neurofibrillary tangle". For example, many workers in the field think that the tangle is simply made up of normal intracellular fibres which have somehow got stuck together to form a tangle. What our work on the structure of the PHF tells us is that this is absolutely not the case.

The normal neurone contains within it three kinds of fibres: microtubules, neuro-filaments and actin filaments. The paired helical filament which forms in Alzheimer's disease is different from any of these normal fibres. It is a completely new fibre and structure which is produced as a result of some quite specific molecular abnormality. It is also likely that PHFs found in Alzheimer's disease are different from the abnormal filaments that are found in other kinds of tangle-forming disease. Although a number of disease processes can produce tangle-like pathology inside cells, recent careful immunochemical analysis shows differences at the molecular level. This is a point not widely understood in this field today, particularly by those who regard the tangle as a non-specific neuronal

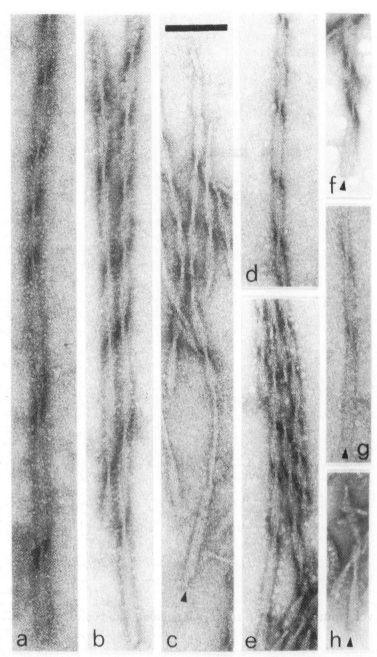

Fig. 1. Electron micrographs of individual paired helical filaments, showing their twisted ribbon-like structure. In c a single PHF can be seen to have split in half, showing that they have paired internal structure. The flattened ends show complete untwisting to produce completely flat PHFs.

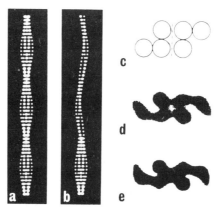

Fig, 2. Schematic representations of internal structure of the PHF. In c, d and e, the PHF is shown in cross-section, schematically in c, and in d and e according to the actual computed cross-sectional density map. The PHF is a double helical stack of C-shaped subunits. Schematic representations of longitudinal views of PHFs are shown in a and b.

response to injury. The over-all shape of the tangle at the light microscope level is fairly non-specific, but at the ultrastructural, and as we have recently found, at the molecular/biochemical level, the Alzheimer PHF is a unique pathological molecular structure. So, an important characteristic of Alzheimer's disease is that where there ought to be normal neuro-fibres, these are completely replaced by paired helical filaments which have the characteristic structure I have described.

The structure of the PHF also gives us some idea about how this sort of thing might come about. We postulate that there is some pre-existing normal gene. The gene is programmed to produce some normal cell product, but as a result of some disease-specific modification, which we do not as yet understand, that normal molecule is changed. The nature of that change is the main focus of our research at the moment. What we can say from the structural analysis of the PHF is the following: as a result of that change, the modified precursor is unable to remain free in the cell, but instead polymerises into a highly resilient filamentous structure, which eventually accumulates within the cell to such an extent that it kills the cell. In other words, the PHFs in Alzheimer's disease are formed as a result of the pathological polymerisation of some precursor molecule which has been modified in a very precise and disease specific manner. We can deduce from the regularity of the PHF that the underlying molecular change affects a single molecular complex in a very regular and reproducible manner.

This is analogous to the situation in sickle cell disease. In sickle-cell anaemia there is a very minor change in the ß-haemoglobin molecule. As a result of that change, the heamoglobin molecule cannot function properly to transport oxygen in the blood. Instead, it forms fibres inside red cells by a process of abnormal polymerisation, and these become the sickle fibres. These sickle fibres are quite different in structure from the paired helical filament, but the process is the same – some molecule has gone wrong and has acquired the capacity to polymerise and

243

to damage cells secondarily. In the way that sickle fibres damage red cells in sickle cell disease, so the PHF polymers damage neurons in Alzheimer's disease.

PHF core proteins vs fuzzy coat proteins

What is this abnormal molecule which polymerises to form the PHF? To get this information, we had to learn how to produce very pure biochemical preparations of PHFs. This in itself is a very difficult problem, and indeed the preparation we developed has now been patented. In the process of getting to this point, we tried a number of proteases (proteases are enzymes which digest protein) and it turned out that it was possible to purify PHFs by virtue of the fact that they are highly resistant to proteases. The filaments resist digestion with wide range of powerful proteases: this is a very important point which I will come back to later on when discussing potential therapeutic approaches. In the process of digestion we found that the filaments were stripped of a fuzzy outer coat, leaving behind the core material, i.e. the core structure of the filament. It appears that the filament is made up of two parts: a fuzzy coat on the outside which can be stripped away with proteases, and the basic core structure of the filament which consist of the 3-domained sub-unit I described earlier, and which is resistant to attack with proteases.

We were able to discover that antibody markers which recognised sites located in the fuzzy coat of the filament weren't necessarily present in the inner core after it had been digested. This suggests that a lot of the arguments about the nature of tangles which have been based on histological antibody staining may be misleading, as the antibodies may be reacting with the material which is on the outside of the PHFs, and not necessarily part of the basic core. Cell components that look close together in the light microscope, even when antibodies are used to identify them, may actually be in significantly different locations when the matter is analysed at the molecular level. This is because the change in scale required in passing from the level of the cell seen in the light microscope is about 1000-fold. This is the same change in scale needed to pass from the level of, say, my fingertip, to the level of the cells which make up my finger. A good deal of the debate about the molecular nature of the tangle has ignored the simple fact that observations made with the light microscope, even with the aid of highly specific molecular probes in the form of monoclonal antibodies, give very imprecise information about the underlying molecular architecture of the structures we are attempting to study. From this work it is clear that if we are trying to understand how the PHF arises at the molecular level, it makes a great deal of difference whether the molecule we find in the tangle is actually in the fuzzy coat of the PHF, or if it is in the core structure. It may, for example, become trapped in the fuzzy coat long after the PHF has formed, and give very little useful information about the sequence of events giving rise to the PHF.

Characterization of part of the inner core of the PHF

Our next step was to use the protease-treated preparations of PHFs to raise our own antibodies against the inner digested core of the PHF. We screened these antibodies and found that those which labelled isolated PHFs in the electron microscope, consistently labelled a single protein band in our purified PHF extract from Alzheimer brain. This electrophoretic gel band could not be found in identical preparations from normal brain tissues. This means that the antibodies which label the filaments also label a protein which is uniquely present in the Alzheimer brain extract for PHFs. It follows therefore that this protein band must come from the PHF.

We were able to prepare this protein in sufficient purity to enable us to sequence it at the level of individual amino acids. An amino-acid sequence is the key to the gene: it is the key to discovering the identity of the molecule. From this sequence we are able fairly quickly to work out from which normal protein the fragment that we had extracted from the PHF had come. Indeed, the fragment extracted from the inner core of the PHF amounts to about 1/3 of the whole parent molecule.

The normal parent molecule is called tau protein. I will outline the normal function of tau protein a little later. The first question is why there is only part of the tau molecule in the PHF. The portion of tau found in the protease resistant core of the PHF corresponds to a distinct functional domain of tau protein. It corresponds to a stretch of the molecule which contains exactly 3 tandem repeats each of exactly 32 amino acids. Indeed, this is called the repeat region of the tau molecule. Protein molecules are linear sequences of amino acids, which are described from the N-terminus (amino) to the C-terminus (carboxy). The tau molecule consists of 200 amino acids at the amino end, next, the repeat region of about 100 amino acids, and finally a short C-terminal segment of about 80 amino acids. The tau molecule is thus attached very tightly via its repeat region to the inner core of the PHF, whereas the rest of the molecule projects from the PHF into the fuzzy coat. So, when we do the protease digestion step, we remove only the portions of the tau molecule that project from the PHF, but not the tightly bound repeat region (Fig. 3).

The work I have outlined represented the first definitive biochemical, structural and immunological demonstration that tau protein is intrinsic to the protease-resistant core structure of the PHF. It also showed that tau is bound via the repeat region to the PHF. These results have helped to shed a good deal of light on certain aspects of the pathology which can be studied in the light microscope. This is in general the correct order of things in research of this kind. Once we have unravelled relationships at the molecular level, it becomes possible to understand phenomena at the level of histology better.

Intracellular vs extracellular tangles

The presence of a certain portion of tau protein in the fuzzy coat, and another portion in the protease-resistant core makes it possible to understand some of the

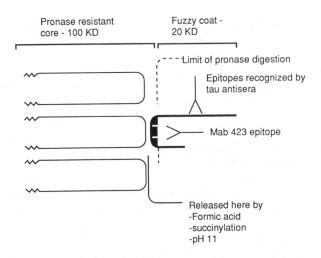

Fig. 3. Diagram of distribution of tau protein in the PHF. The dark hair-pin structure is tau. It consists of a 200 amino acid residue segment which projects from the core filament, and is lost after protease (pronase) digestion. The same applies to the C-terminal end of the molecule. One the 3-repeat region is left behind after protease digestion, and this is firmly bound to the inner core of the PHF. Antibody 423 is selective for this part of the molecule. The whole cross-sectional mass of the PHF is 120 kD (kilodaltons) per subunit. Of this, 20 kD per subunit is lost after pronase digestion. The remaining part of tau contributes only about 10 kD per subunit, leaving about 90 kD per subunit unaccounted for. We are currently working to characterize this inner core of the filament.

differences between intracellular and extracellular tangles. Depending on whether we use monoclonal antibodies directed against the repeat region of tau, or against the N-terminus, it is possible to distinguish quite clearly between tangles which are still inside living cells, and tangles left behind in the extracellular space by cells which have already died. Extracellular tangles cannot be labelled by N-terminal tau markers, but retain reactivity with markers for the repeat region.

It is possible to understand this in terms of the structural and biochemical work I have outlined. While PHFs remain inside cells, they retain the fuzzy coat. Once the cell dies, PHFs are attacked by proteases in the extracellular space which remove the fuzzy coat. In other words, what we have done to PHFs with proteases in the test-tube is very similar to what happens once the cell dies in the brain. But even the proteases available in the extracellular space are limited by the fundamental resilience of the PHF. Only the fuzzy coat is digested, at least for a considerable period after the death of the cell. This also tells us that for some reason, and despite that fact that the PHF is a highly abnormal structure, the cell fails to degrade even portions of the PHF which are accessible to proteases. This is an intriguing finding. Normally, when the healthy cell produces proteins which are abnormal in some way, it is able to degrade abnormal proteins before they do any damage. In the case of the fully assembled PHF, even portions of the structure which could be degraded are not attacked while they remain within the cell. The reason for this is unclear at the present time.

Abnormal tau protein in the PHF

Another important result of this work derives from the properties of the mono-clonal antibodies we have raised against the protease-resistant core PHF preparations. We have found recently that several of the antibodies which recognise the tau extracted from PHFs do not cross-react with normal tau proteins. Indeed, we have used these antibodies to develop the first biochemical assay for neurofibrillary pathology in Alzheimer's disease. For the first time, we are able to measure the severity of the disease process biochemically, simply by measuring the quantity of PHF-specific tau protein. We are able to distinguish unambiguously between normal tau and PHF-specific tau, and we have been able to show that there is a clear transfer of abnormal tau protein from axons to cell bodies as the disease progresses. We are now engaged in a large study which seeks to establish whether it is the quantity of abnormal tau protein which determines clinical dementia, or whether it is the number of extracellular tangles which determine dementia. In other words, it is now possible, with the tools we have developed, to answer the question whether the earliest stages of cognitive deficit are the result of a functional abnormality in tau protein, or whether there is no clinical abnormality until neurones have actually been destroyed. Our preliminary data is starting to show that the biochemical abnormality is more important, but that extensive cell death only occurs at the end-stages of the disease. This has very important therapeutic implications, since it implies that we could delay the symptoms by dealing with the molecular changes before they appear in the form of gross pathological changes.

Theory of molecular pathogenesis of dementia

We can now consider the normal role of tau protein in the brain. Tau protein is one of a class of proteins known as microtubule-associated proteins. One of their most important functions is their role in maintaining the stability of microtubules. Tau protein is the only protein which maintains the stability of microtubules in axons. To understand the importance of this, it is necessary to understand that the axon represents the part of the neurone which establishes connections with other neurones. In simple terms, all information processing by the brain depends on the viability of axonal transport systems, which in turn depend on microtubules, which in turn depend on tau protein.

We have recently shown that the tau protein which is found in the core of the PHF is not only abnormal immunologically, in that it can be recognised selectively by certain antibodies, but also that it is abnormal functionally. It is possible to measure tau function in the test-tube by its ability to cause microtubules to form out of tubulin, the protein which normally polymerizes to form microtubules. The tau protein extracted from PHFs fails to cause microtubule assembly in the test-tube, and fails even to bind to assembled microtubules. This is very surprising, since the repeat region of tau, the region described in some detail above, is in fact the microtubule-binding domain. It is possible with this data to begin to put forward a molecular theory of dementia.

Before doing so, it is first necessary to describe a little of the neuroanatomy of the cells which are particularly vulnerable to tangle formation in Alzheimer's disease. As I mentioned earlier, these are the pyramidal cells. The human cortex is arranged into columnar units or modules, each the depth of the grey matter in extent, and about 0.3 mm in diameter. Each column functions as an integrated unit, with inputs from other columns, or from sensory projections, and outputs to other columns in the cortex, or to other brain regions. A column is like a single chip, or integrated circuit. Information processing by the cortex depends on patterns of activity set up between these modules. The bulk of communication between modules is mediated precisely by pyramidal cells. These are in fact the projection cells, which fire at the completion of a certain computation, and project the result to other columns for further processing. The column is composed predominantly of small inter-neurones, which are part of the internal circuitry of the column. But all associative processing between columns, whether in the same brain hemisphere, or in the contralateral hemisphere, is mediated by the axons of pyramidal cells. These axons, which are maintained by the pyramidal cells, are referred to as the cortico-cortical association pathways (Fig. 4).

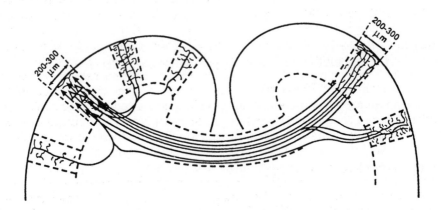

Fig. 4. Cortico-cortical association fibres in the cortex. These fibres are the axons of pyramidal cells which are particularly vulnerable to neurofibrillary pathology of the Alzheimer type. These fibres mediate the bulk of associative processing in the cortex. In Alzheimer's disease, tau protein, which ought to be in the axons, is modified, and sequestered with PHFs which accumulate in the cell body. It is hypothesized that this leads to functional disconnection in the cortex, which shows itself as dementia.

So it is now possible to bring these various facts together. Higher cortical function depends on the cortico-cortical association pathways, which are in fact the axons of pyramidal cells. These pyramidal cells are the prime casualties of neurofibrillary pathology in Alzheimer's disease. Specifically, tau protein is required to maintain the integrity of the microtubules on which the viability of the pyramidal cell axons depends. However, in Alzheimer's disease, axonal tau protein is modified in such a way as to be non-functional as regards microtubules, and in fact is entirely relocated out of axons, and into the cell body in the form of protease-resistant aberrant polymers, namely the paired helical filaments. The net effect of this in the early stages would be dysfunction in cortico-cortical association pathways, and eventual complete disconnection as a result of cell death. In other words, it is possible to visualise dementia in Alzheimer's disease as a consequence of cortico-cortical disconnection, caused by an abnormality in tau protein, associated with the aberrant polymerisation of PHFs.

Further analysis of the molecular pathogenesis of the PHF

Although we have shown that an abnormal form of tau protein is bound up within the core of the PHF, we have so far managed to analyse only 10 per cent of the molecular mass of the PHF core. Work now in progress aims to characterise the remainder of the inner core, to understand how it is put together, and what other molecular species are involved. We have recently managed to identify a novel protein in preparations from the PHF core, and we are currently attempting to characterise this further.

Other recent work has shown that amyloid protein may also be implicated at some stage in the process of tangle formation. For example, we have recently prepared a series of antibodies which show that granular inclusions appear in cells prior to PHF formation, and that the same proteins that are found in tangles can also be found in these granular inclusions. In particular, there is recent evidence that the intracellular domain of the amyloid precursor protein may be caught up within these structures. However, as I have said earlier, one must beware of data that is only histological. It is necessary to back this up at the molecular/biochemical/ultrastructural level, and to discover the precise nature of the association between precursor structures to the PHF and the amyloid precursor protein.

Therapeutic implications

I would like to conclude by considering potential therapeutic applications of a molecular understanding of PHF formation. I have presented a hypothesis in which dementia might be comprehensible in terms of a fundamental molecular abnormality which expresses itself by aberrant polymerisation of an as yet incompletely described molecular complex, to give rise to the PHF. This complex includes modified, dysfunctional tau protein, and other species we are only beginning to characterize. The net effect of the polymerisation of this complex is that it is highly resistant to proteolytic attack in the assembled form.

There may be an important clue in this. It is possible to speculate that the reason we see PHF accumulation is precisely that it has escaped proteolytic degradation. As I mentioned earlier, the healthy cell has means of disposing of wrongly folded proteins. However, if a partial degradation product of a wrongly folded protein had the propensity to form regular polymers, it would escape complete degradation, and would accumulate indefinitely. Indeed, we have shown that while the inner core of the PHF is extremely resistant to proteolytic attack in the assembled state, the constituents of the inner core, including abnormal tau protein, are quite susceptible to proteases once the structural regularity of the PHF is disrupted. The polymerisation and accumulation of the PHFs within neurones may represent a system which has escaped degradation, and which the cell may come eventually to treat the aberrant polymer as though it were a normal cell constituent. Unfortunately, the PHF is far from normal, and its accumulation eventually proves lethal to the cell.

If this kind of model were true, there would be very important therapeutic hope. One could argue that degradation might have gone to completion had polymerization not occurred. This would suggest that if one could block the assembly of the PHF, one might save the cell from the lethal consequences of PHF accumulation. Alternatively, it may be possible to discover the reason behind the primary abnormality in the molecules which eventually give rise to the PHF, and somehow to block this.

Ultimately, the hope for rational approaches to treatment depends on capturing relevant steps in the disease process at the molecular level, and using these as test systems to discover compounds which block critical steps in the disease pathway. For example, we have recently found compounds which disrupt PHF structure, and which permit PHF degradation by proteases. We have found other compounds which bind with very high affinity to isolated PHFs. We do not as yet know if these will prove useful therapeutic leads, but findings such as these indicate that it is possible to target the PHF pharmacologically with some specificity. It may also be possible to develop compounds which permit specific visualisation of plaque and tangle pathology by brain imaging techniques.

From what I have said, it is clear that the steps resulting in the formation of the PHF are quite complicated, and one can say with reasonable confidence that it is extremely unlikely that we will find a way to block the disease process by accident. In science, there is always an element of luck, but the luck is only comprehensible in a framework of painstaking analysis. I believe that the molecular analysis of the PHF is now approaching a point where it will become feasible in the foreseeable future for us to discover therapeutic approaches to Alzheimer's disease which aim to block PHF formation.

Bibliography

Roth M, Wischik CM. The heterogeneity of Alzheimer's disease and its implications for scientific investigations of the disorder. In Airie T (ed), *Recent Advances in Psychogeriatrics*. London, Churchill Livingstone, 1985, Ch.6, 71-79.

Wischik CM, Crowther RA. (1986) Sub-unit structure of the Alzheimer tangle. *Br Med Bull* 1986, **42(1)**, 51-56.

Crowther RA, Goedert M, Wischik CM. The repeat region of microtubule-associated protein tau forms part of the core of the paired helical filament of Alzheimer's disease. *Ann Med* 1989, **21**,127-132.

Wischik CM. Cell biology of the Alzheimer tangle. *Current Opinion in Cell Biology* 1989, **1**, 115-122.

Wischik CM. Molecular neuropathology of Alzheimer's disease. In Katona C (ed) *Dementia Disorders: Advances and Prospects*. London, Chapman and Hall, 1989, Chap. 3, pp.44-70.

Carers, Professionals and Alzheimer's Disease. D O'Neill ed © 1991 John Libbey & Company Ltd

Chapter 37

MOLECULAR GENETICS OF ALZHEIMER'S DISEASE

AM Goate, *Dept of Biochemistry & Molecular Genetics, St Mary's Hospital Medical School, Imperial College of Science, Technology and Medicine, Norfolk Place, London W2 1PG, United Kingdom*

Introduction

The clinical and pathological manifestations of the disease called Alzheimer's disease (AD) were first described by a German doctor, Alois Alzheimer, in 1906. He described a patient in middle age (55 years) who had shown a progressive decline in mental abilities over several years, ultimately leading to death. Post-mortem examination of her brain revealed a smaller than average brain due to massive cell death and the presence of numerous protein deposits, amyloid plaques and neurofibrillary tangles.

Alzheimer's disease is now recognized to be the most common form of dementia, accounting for more than half of all cases of dementia reported. In Britain alone, more than 500,000 people are affected by AD. The disease is most common in the elderly with an incidence of 10 per cent amongst those over the age of 65 years, rising to 20 per cent of those over the age of 80 years.

Several causal models have been proposed for AD including: (i) the build-up of toxic substances in brain cells (e.g. aluminium) over many years. When a critical level of cell death has occurred the clinical signs of dementia are observed; (ii) a slow virus disease similar to that postulated for other neurodegenerative diseases of late onset. However, no infectious agent has ever been recovered from diseased brains; (iii) a genetic disease. Many epidemiological surveys have been carried out to try to identify risk factors (other than age) associated with the development of the disease. Although a high level of aluminium in the diet or head trauma have been suggested as possible risk factors, the only consistent risk factor observed in these studies was a positive family history of AD.

Positive family history

Although most cases of AD are sporadic, approximately one third of cases have a positive family history of disease in a first degree relative, particularly pre-senile AD (age of onset less than 65 years). The most striking evidence suggesting the importance of genetic factors in the aetiology of the disease is the existence of a number of large multiply-affected families (Fig. 1). In these pedigrees the illness appears to be inherited in a manner consistent with autosomal dominant transmission, i.e. approximately 50 per cent of the offspring of an affected individual become affected regardless of the gender of the affected parent. This tells us two things about the disease gene: (i) that only one copy of the mutant gene is required for an individual to develop the disease since we receive one copy of each gene from each of our parents; and (ii) that the disease gene does not lie on either of the sex chromosomes since both male and female offspring have an equal chance of inheriting the disease whether the affected parent is their mother or father. The disease in such families has an onset in mid-life (before 65 years) but does not seem atypical in other ways from the more common senile onset form of the disease. Within a family the age of onset of disease is very tightly clustered (x years ± 10 per cent) but can vary greatly from family to family. Two plausible explanations for the fact that only one third of AD cases have a positive family history have been suggested: (i) that the disease is heterogeneous: some cases are genetic and others are non-genetic or, (ii) that, due to the late onset of disease, other predisposed relatives may die of other causes before manifesting the disease.

Genetic strategies

The existence of large multiply-affected families allows the use of genetic strategies to determine the cause of disease in these families. It has been observed that virtually all individuals with Down's syndrome who survive to the fourth decade of life develop a pathology in the brain typical of that seen in AD. These individuals have inherited three copies rather than two of chromosome 21 from their parents. This observation led workers to suggest that the gene causing AD in the large pedigrees may lie upon chromosome 21. This was first tested by Peter St. George-Hyslop et al in 1987 using four pedigrees with early onset AD. They reported linkage between AD and several DNA markers on the long arm of chromosome 21 (Fig. 2). Genetic linkage is a statistical observation: a particular genetic marker is observed to co-inherit with the disease phenotype more often than the 50 per cent expected by chance. If markers lie close together on a chromosome then they will frequently be co-inherited whereas those markers far apart on a chromosome or on different chromosomes will frequently be separated during meiosis (the special type of cell division which occurs in sperm and eggs which results in only one copy of each of the parental chromosomes being present, the diploid number being restored after fusion of the sperm and egg at fertilization). Therefore, the number of times two markers become separated by recombination at meiosis reflects the distance between them on the chromosome.

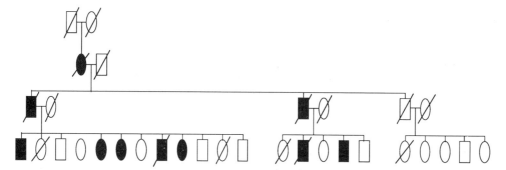

Fig. 1. Diagram of an Alzheimer's disease pedigree. Black symbols denote affected individuals. Oblique lines indicate individuals who are deceased. The average age of onset in this pedigree is 55 years ± 5 years.

At about the same time that linkage was reported in these families, the gene encoding the protein deposited in the plaques was cloned and localized to the same region of chromosome 21. This led to the suggestion that the amyloid gene might be the site of the genetic defect in familial AD. Subsequent analysis of the inheritance of polymorphisms in the amyloid gene in large pedigrees has indicated that there are recombinations between the disease and the amyloid gene. The amyloid gene cannot therefore be the mutated gene in these families.

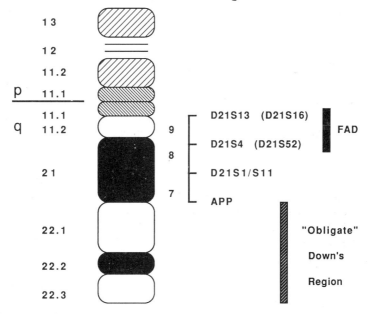

Fig. 2. Diagram of human chromosome 21 showing the position of DNA markers linked to the Familial Alzheimer's Disease (FAD) locus, amyloid precursor protein gene (APP) and the "obligate" Down's syndrome region. p indicates the short arm of the chromosome and q the long arm. The region where they join is called the centromere.

Attempts to replicate the linkage between AD and markers on chromosome 21 in different families has met with mixed results. Two groups, including our own, have replicated the results in families with early onset disease. In addition, we narrowed down the region of tight linkage to the region of the long arm of the chromosome just below the centromere (Fig. 2). In two other studies they were unable to detect linkage to this region in their families. One study used samples from families of Volga German descent. In this population there is known to be a high incidence of AD leading to an increased risk of both parents carrying the disease chromosome and therefore an increased risk of individuals carrying two copies of the disease gene. There are, therefore, two possible explanations for their results: either AD is a genetically-heterogeneous disease, i.e. there is more than one gene capable of causing AD when mutated, or that difficulties in the analysis of these families caused by inbreeding may have prevented the detection of linkage.

Several groups have failed to detect linkage between AD and markers on chromosome 21 in families with late onset disease. This could be for several reasons: (i) that there is another genetic locus predisposing to late onset disease; (ii) that the markers thought to be closest to the gene were uninformative in many families; or (iii) that not all cases of late onset AD are genetic. AD is very common in the elderly and modelling the disease based upon population risks shows that 1 in 16 cases would show familial clustering even if the disease was wholly non-genetic.

Detection of linkage to markers of chromosome 21 in families with early onset AD means that a genetic approach similar to that used for cystic fibrosis (CF) and Duchenne muscular dystrophy (DMD) may be used to isolate new markers closer to the disease gene and ultimately to clone the disease gene itself. It must be emphasized that this is a slow and painstaking process: however, the fact that it has been accomplished for CF and DMD gives hope for the future. In addition, an understanding of the pathological processes in the brain may lead to the identification of candidate genes for the AD locus which may be tested in the multiply-affected families in the same way as the amyloid gene.

Conclusion

Determination of the gene and mutation causing AD and the subsequent understanding of the function of the protein encoded by this gene will lead to a greater understanding of the disease process in both early and late onset AD. It is anticipated that when we understand what goes wrong in AD that we will be able to develop strategies which will prevent or delay the onset of disease beyond the average life expectancy of the population.

Bibliography

DC Davies (ed). *Alzheimer's Disease: Towards an Understanding of the Aetiology and Pathogenesis. Current Problems in Neurology: 11.* London: John Libbey, 1989.

Fowler CJ, Carlson LA, Gottfries CG, Winblad B. *Biological Markers in dementia of Alzheimer type.* Proceedings of the Stiftelsen Gamla Tjanarinnor Symposium on Aging and Aging Disorders No 1. London: Smith-Gordon, Nishimura, 1990.

Sinet PM, Lamour Y, Christen Y. *Genetics and Alzheimer's Disease. Research and Perspectives in Alzheimer's disease.* Berlin: Springer-Verlag, 1988.

Hardy JA, Rossor MN. Facts Sheet: *Genetics of Alzheimer's disease.* Available from the Alzheimer's Disease Society of Great Britain.

Chapter 38

THE REVERSED GENETIC APPROACH TO FAMILIAL ALZHEIMER'S DISEASE

Antoon Vandenberghe[1] *PhD, Goedele De Winter*[1,2] *Social worker,* **Mark Bruyland**[3] *MD,* **Jan Gheuens**[4] *MD,* **Jean-Jacques Martin**[4] *MD and* **Christine Van Broeckhoven**[1] *PhD, Department of Biochemistry*[1]*, University of Antwerp (UIA), Universiteitsplein 1, B-2610 Antwerpen; Innogenetics Inc*[2]*, Industriepark Zwijnaarde 7, Box 4, B-9710 Gent; Dept. Neurology*[3]*, City Hospital of Ronse, B-9600 Ronse; and Department of Neurology and Born-Bunge foundation*[4]*, University of Antwerp (UIA), Universiteitsplein 1, B-2610 Antwerpen, Belgium*

The application of reversed genetic techniques to understand the origin of Alzheimer's disease (AD) is a very topical issue. In our study, we did not take the risk of confusing the issue by combining data obtained from families linked to chromosome 21 and those who were not.[1] As long as the question of genetic heterogeneity remains, it is our aim to establish genetic linkage evidence for the AD locus within one single family.[2] We can reasonably accept that all patients within one AD family expressing similar clinical and pathological hallmarks have inherited the same molecular mutation.

Information and co-operation of Alzheimer families.

In Belgium, we were "lucky" to find two exceptionally large AD families co-operating in our research.[3,4] From one of the families we collected data on almost three hundred people, including 39 AD patients of whom 11 had a pathological brain examination. On paper the pedigree is very impressive, but listing the individuals available for linkage analysis study gives a rather poor result. Mostly, sampling of the first and youngest generation is complete but at this age the disease is not yet expressed. In the second generation only a few samples of AD

259

patients are available, but many are missing since many of the AD patients are deceased. We can rarely speak of a third generation.

The ideal starting position for genetic linkage analysis studies between an autosomal dominant disease trait and DNA-markers is to have access to large families with at least two, and ideally three, affected generations. The families need to be large since we want to avoid problems associated with genetic hete-rogeneity by establishing genetic linkage in a single family. However this situation is never found in AD families. Sometimes one can reconstruct information for a deceased AD patient. For example, in one branch of the pedigree, we have blood samples of the healthy spouse and six of his children allowing us to reconstruct part of the genetic information of the deceased AD patient for the particular DNA marker analysed.

In both families studied, the AD patients have a mean age at onset of 35 years with a mean duration of the disease of 7 years. In most cases the healthy parent of the AD patient is still alive: therefore these early onset AD families can provide more genetic information than late onset AD families and thus are more valuable for genetic research. In order to supplement our evidence for linkage with DNA markers of chromosome 21, there are several ways to enlarge the initial information content of the AD families who co-operate with this research.

Genealogy and pedigree

First, we can carefully re-inspect the genealogy of the pedigree. For example, on one occasion we came across an unmarried woman, recorded as a deceased AD patient. By rechecking the pedigree we discovered that she was also the mother of two illegitimate children, both of whom were affected with AD and who also had had children themselves. This simple manoeuvre resulted in five additional subjects, including one definite AD patient.

A second method to obtain additional samples is to extend the pedigree by going back one generation, looking for other relatives and to scrutinize their offspring, using age at death as a guideline (assuming that early death occurs virtually exclusively in AD patients). This is not absolutely specific but is a useful aid in enlarging the pedigree of the disease. In one of the AD families it was easy to go back to the end of the 18th century since the civil records are well documented back to the French Revolution. Gathering information about earlier generations requires an ever-increasing investment of work and time the further one goes back. In our second family, the situation is somewhat different because the disease entered the family by means of an illegitimate child: the mother died at the age of 74 years and her parents died at the age of 56 and 68 years. Keeping the mean age at death of 42 years in mind, we can reasonably assume that the unknown father introduced the disease gene in the family. Although enlarging of this pedigree seems hopeless, we found that an unmarried man lived in the same house at the time of conception! We are now tracing his relatives and their offspring looking for AD patients. Again, this is very laborious.

Family links

Probably the best way to enlarge the families would be proof that both families are mutually related. Indeed, the occurrence of two large AD families with the same characteristic symptoms in such a small country as Belgium would not be expected. We examined church and civil records back to the year 1750, but were unable to connect both families. Furthermore, the location of one family is around Antwerp, the other in a region called the Flemish Ardennes. Both clusters are separated from each other by about 100 kilometres. We have a highly speculative theory for this geographical separation. Around the year 1500 severe climatological and geological disturbances frightened the people living in the Flemish Ardennes region, resulting in the migration of a high number of people to the North of the country. Perhaps in this period both families became separated. This hypothesis, although scientifically unproven, is very intriguing: small differences occur in the brain pathology of both families possibly resulting from a small divergent evolution due to environmental factors.

A third way to expand the information content of the families is simply to wait. The majority of the children in the first generation are too young to express the disease, but some of them are now reaching the characteristic age of onset. A few are thought to show the first disease symptoms already. This information is growing steadily and will be added to the linkage study. The follow-up depends on careful contact with the families.[5]

The availability of DNA-markers

Where the availability of large families is an essential "tool" in our approach, this is also true for DNA markers. The DNA markers D21S16 and D21S1/11 which initially showed linkage with an AD gene on chromosome 21 (6) proved either not to be linked at a close distance or were not informative in our families. Another DNA marker from the same region on chromosome 21, D21S13, was tested in our families. Our results are expressed in LOD scores: an LOD score is a logarithmic measure for the likelihood of linkage: +1.0 means a likelihood of 10 against 1, +2.0 of 100 against 1. We found a small positive LOD score of + 1.5 at a recombination distance of about 10 per cent. This means a maximal evidence for linkage at a genetic distance of 10 centiMorgan away from the mutation point. By September 1988, by adding additional family information and samples, the LOD score reached + 2.0. Special sequence signals tell us that D21S13 is a transcribed gene. However, taking the linkage results into account, this gene is not a candidate for an Alzheimer's disease gene. We estimate that the genetic distance between the D21S13 marker and the disease locus is about 10 centiMorgan. For an accurate localization of the mutation, additional markers need to be analysed. We have generated new DNA markers from the suspected region and isolated some interesting ones. However, a lot of technical work needs to be done before these markers will be suitable for testing in the families.

Finally, an important source of family material became recently useful by the development of the PCR (polymerase chain reaction) amplification technique. One of the AD families was initially studied by L Van Bogaert in 1940.[7] Eight brain specimens belonging to this family were collected. Although the DNA in formalin-treated brains is severely degraded, it is feasible to apply the amplification-method and to recover DNA marker information from these samples.

Conclusion

Extending pedigrees, generating new DNA markers and making markers suitable for PCR amplification are approaches which require an often underestimated amount of work and time, but will finally prove or disprove the existence of a mutant sequence on chromosome 21 underlying the origin of AD in these families.

References

(1) Barnes DM. Troubles encountered in gene linkage land. *Science* 1989, **243,** 313-314.

(2) Van Broeckhoven C. Molecular genetic analysis of early onset familial Alzheimer's disease. *Neurobiology of Aging* 1989, **10,** 437-438.

(3) Martin JJ, Gheuens J, Bruyland M et al. Familial Alzheimer disease. *Neurology* 1990, submitted.

(4) Van Broeckhoven C, Genthe AM, Vandenberghe A, et al. Failure of familial Alzheimer's disease to segregate with the A4-amyloid gene in several European families. *Nature* 1987, **329,** 153-155.

(5) De Winter G, Vandenberghe A, Gheuens J, Martin JJ, Van Broeckhoven C. Social impact on Alzheimer's disease families co-operating in a scientific research program. In O'Neill, D , ed, *Carers, Professionals and Alzheimer's Disease* 1991; John Libbey, London.

(6) St George-Hyslop PH, Tanzi RE, Polinsky RJ et al. The genetic defect causing familial Alzheimer's disease maps on chromosome 21. *Science* 1987, **235,** 885-890.

(7) Van Bogaert L, Maere M, De Smedt E. Sur les formes familiales précoces de la maladie d'Alzheimer. *Monatsschrift Psychiat Neurol* 1940, **102,** 249-301.

Carers, Professionals and Alzheimer's Disease. D O'Neill ed © 1991 John Libbey & Company Ltd

Chapter 39

ENVIRONMENTAL FACTORS IN THE PATHOGENESIS OF ALZHEIMER'S DISEASE

L Liss MD, *Division of Neuropathology, Department of Pathology and Cognitive Disorders Clinic, Office of Geriatrics, Ohio State University, College of Medicine, Ohio, USA*

A brief summary in an attempt to discuss the aetiological factors considered to be modifiers of Alzheimer's disease will of necessity be very condensed. This may lead to a fragmentary discussion of only a few aspects. Any investigation of aetiology should include a review of risk factors: considering the multifactorial aetiology of Alzheimer's disease, variability of expression is fully expected. We might even be dealing with an Alzheimer syndrome rather than with a specific disease. The separate subdivisions of this syndrome may be represented as; (i) the autosomal dominant variant of Alzheimer's disease, a hereditary form with a 50 per cent of risk factor which is uncommon; (ii) the group with Down Syndrome which has a 100 per cent risk factor and a number of unique characteristics which make it a distinct subdivision; and (iii) those who are over 80 years old, the group which concerns us most as it represents the majority of Alzheimer's disease sufferers. The multifactorial hypothesis of Alzheimer's disease postulates multiple aetiological factors, many of which can be modified by extrinsic factors.

Plaques and tangles

The correlation between the anatomical substrate of Alzheimer's disease, the plaques and tangles, and the severity of clinical symptomatology has been shown to be a valid criterion in various studies. We generally accept that the diagnostic criteria for Alzheimer's disease are the presence of *in vivo* clinical findings of dementia and post mortem pathological findings of plaques and tangles. Although the correlation between these two pathological structures in dementia remains largely unknown, despite a number of hypotheses, it is generally accepted that we are dealing with a morphological substrate of a disease and not an epiphenomenon. The involvement of specific areas by plaques and tangles, or only one of these components, is of considerable interest since it indicates that these two hallmarks of the disease are likely to be the result of different pathophysiological processes, which further substantiates the multifactorial aetiology of Alzheimer's disease.

Olfactory bulb

Recently we studied the olfactory bulb which appears to be a good marker for severity of dementia. The nucleus centralis of the olfactory bulb shows considerable pathological change which correlates with the severity of changes in other areas of the brain, and in many cases with the severity of the clinical dementia. The changes in the nucleus centralis of the olfactory bulb are predominantly neurofibrillary tangles. They were present in 100 per cent of our 75 cases of Alzheimer's disease in which the olfactory bulbs were examined. By contrast, plaques were present in only 28 per cent of cases and were always accompanied by neurofibrillary tangles. Apparently the development of both neurofibrillary tangles and plaques is possible in the nucleus centralis, yet neurofibrillary tangles predominate while plaques are present in only slightly over one-quarter of all the examined cases. One possible explanation for this apparent pathophysiological dichotomy may be the influence of extrinsic factors which have nothing to do with the aetiology of the disease *per se,* but which can influence either the early development or suppression of plaque or tangle formation.

Hypoxic encephalopathy

An example of how an extrinsic factor, which is not connected with the pathogenesis of Alzheimer's disease, can influence the pathological picture and possibly the clinical course of Alzheimer's disease is demonstrated by hypoxia of the watershed area in the brain. In Alzheimer's disease, especially in individuals who have orthostatic hypotension, there is a dramatic difference between the density of plaques and tangles in the tips of the gyri and the valleys of the sulci. The latter show very high concentration of pathological changes while over the tips of the gyri there is usually a minimal degree of pathology or even total lack of pathological change. We have not found this density gradient of pathological changes in young and healthy individuals who died in either moderately or severely advanced stages of Alzheimer's disease. This particular finding suggests that mild hypoxic changes represent a process which injures neurons, produces changes in tissue on submicroscopic level and creates a *locus minoris resistantiae* where the changes of the Alzheimer-type occur much earlier.

Conversely one can also postulate that good perfusion of tissue with maintenance of tissue integrity represents a defensive factor against the disease by delaying the formation of the pathological changes. If one extrapolates these findings from the topographical difference within a single brain to differences between individuals with good and poor circulation in the brain, a hypothesis seems likely that individuals with good circulation are at lower risk of developing clinical dementia, although they might have been genetically preprogrammed to develop Alzheimer's disease pathology at the same time. This hypothesis is, of course, valid only if we accept the significance of the plaques and tangles as the true expression of the pathogenic mechanism causing dementia and not as an epiphenomenon which does not correlate with clinical symptomatology.

Alcoholic encephalopathy

A role for alcoholic encephalopathy as a modifier for the clinical expression is suggested by the relatively high incidence of Alzheimer's disease among individuals with Wernicke's encephalopathy. Pathological studies show an unequivocal difference between Alzheimer's disease in alcoholic encephalopathy and ordinary cases of Alzheimer's disease. The most important difference is the early and severe involvement of the mammillary bodies, predominantly by plaques, but also by neurofibrillary tangles. The mammillary bodies in Alzheimer's disease are involved late in the course of disease and in very advanced cases as a rule. This is in contrast with cases of Alzheimer's disease with Wernicke's encephalopathy, where we found the earliest changes to be in the mammillary bodies.

These changes are also found in individuals who were not profoundly demented, were younger, and who had been diagnosed as suffering predominantly from an alcoholic encephalopathy/dementia of Wernicke type. In these people we find definite evidence of neuroaxonal plaques in the mammillary bodies. Changes in other areas of the brain such as hippocampus and temporal lobe may be very early and mild. We are again dealing with a *locus minoris resistentiae* created by the pre-existing pathological process unrelated to aetiology of Alzheimer's disease.

Aluminium neurotoxicity

There is also an interesting relationship between alcohol and aluminium neurotoxicity. Ubiquitous aluminium is neurotoxic and yet is effectively prevented from entering the brain. We found evidence of elevated aluminium in the cerebellar vermis as well as mammillary bodies of alcoholics. This apparently represents a secondary event, related to pre-existing damage, which allows aluminium to be deposited. It appears that pre-existing pathology is a requirement for aluminium entry to the brain, and aluminium deposition will also occur in cases of pathology unrelated to Alzheimer's disease such as alcoholic damage to cerebellum. It has also been shown that ingestion of alcohol greatly accelerates absorption of aluminium, although it has not been demonstrated that it affects the deposition of aluminium in the brain tissue of experimental animals.

The ability of aluminium to produce experimental neurofibrillary tangles, and some instances which indicate that alteration of the aluminium protective barrier has resulted in formation of neurofibrillary tangles in man represents compelling circumstantial evidence that aluminium is the factor participating in, or responsible for, formation of neurofibrillary tangles. If we assume that these pathological structures represent a morphological substrate rather than an epiphenomenon, then aluminium has to be considered as part of the aetiological chain of events leading to development of Alzheimer's disease. The significance of the environmental overload as suggested by Norwegian and British studies is more difficult to prove, although increased amounts might conceivably result in an acceleration of the pathological process in a damaged brain deprived of its natural protection against aluminium.

Positive and negative modifiers

We have to consider, therefore, that hypoxia, alcoholic encephalopathy and possibly other environmental factors represent extrinsic modifiers which can result in acceleration or delay of the onset of the clinical symptoms of the disease. They also may affect the severity and rapidity of progression of symptoms. With Alzheimer's disease we are dealing with a condition which is apparently genetically determined to a certain extent and which occurs in the majority of the cases toward the end of life. Therefore, modifiers which accelerate the onset can result in a dramatic increase in the number of cases. Equally modifiers of the disease which tend to delay the onset by several decades can result in practical elimination of the majority of cases of this disease with today's life expectancy. Further concentration on these factors is therefore not only justified but imperative.

Carers, Professionals and Alzheimer's Disease. D O'Neill ed © 1991 John Libbey & Company Ltd

Chapter 40

ANIMAL MODELS OF MEMORY – AN ELECTROPHYSIOLOGICAL APPROACH

MJ Rowan *PhD, Department of Pharmacology and Therapeutics, Trinity College, Dublin, Ireland*

Long-term potentiation is the phenomenon whereby synaptic transmission between neurones in the brain is enhanced for long periods following electrical stimulation. No other phenomenon has aroused such great interest as a possible neurophysiological basis for certain types of memory.[1,2] This paper is divided into three main sections. First of all I will focus on the possibility that long-term potentiation provides a good model for the formation and maintenance of certain types of memory. Secondly, I will examine the possible mechanisms of long-term potentiation with special reference to pharmacological ways of interfering with its generation. This should provide a means of determining possible causes of memory deficit that occur in dementias and ageing. Thirdly, I will review possible pharmacological strategies that might enhance long-term potentiation: for example, by interfering with calcium or biogenic amines, in particular 5-hydroxytryptamine (5-HT).

The hippocampus

The experiments to be described were carried out on rat brain hippocampus. This region is one of the largest areas lying below the neocortex in the central nervous system. Damage to this region can produce marked deficits in a wide range of learning tasks in the rat, particularly those involving spatial memory function. In patients with Alzheimer's disease disruption of intrinsic hippocampal circuits and their inputs is believed to account for the loss of ability to remember recent discrete events.[3,4]

The hippocampus is composed of three main regions: the dentate, CA3 and CA1 regions (Fig. 1A). There is strong evidence that the main pathway for transmission through this brain structure comes primarily from the entorhinal cortex and related areas, via the perforant path on to the granule cells in the dentate region. These neurones form synapses with CA3 neurones which then go on to form synapses with CA1 neurones. The main output from the hippocampus is from the CA1 neurones. We can monitor transmission through the trisynaptic pathway using electrophysiological techniques.

Hippocampus proper

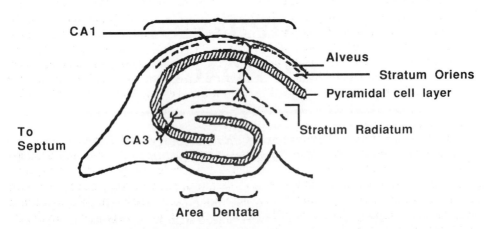

Fig. 1 A (above). Schematic diagram of a transverse section through the hippocampus. B (below). Highlighted pyramidal cell body and its dendrites. Stimulation and recording was carried out in the CA1 region of the stratum radiatum. The inset shows the pre-synaptic nerve volley followed by an excitatory post-synaptic potential (EPSP).

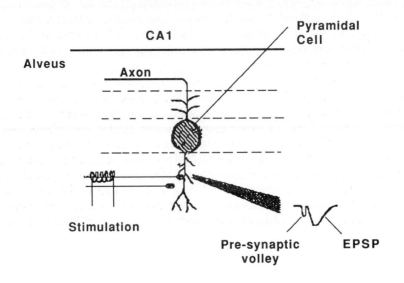

If one places microelectrodes in different layers of the hippocampus, one can record synaptic potentials in response to electrical stimulation (Fig. 1B). A stimulating electrode can evoke a pre-synaptic nerve volley which is due to the grouped firing of afferent neurones. Following this there is a post-synaptic response, the excitatory post-synaptic potential (EPSP), in the dendrites of pyramidal and granule cells. The relationship between the pre-synaptic input and the post-synaptic output gives one an indication of the strength of synaptic transmission. One can induce a long-term potentiation of transmission through these hippocampal pathways by applying what is called a tetanus; that is, a train of high-frequency bursts of stimuli to the afferent paths.[5] For example, the tetanus might be composed of ten bursts of stimuli, with each burst containing ten stimuli at 200 Hertz. Long-term potentiation is characterized by an increase in synaptic strength such that the amplitude of the EPSP evoked by stimulation of the afferent fibres at a fixed intensity is increased for periods greater than about fifteen minutes. In brain slices the duration of long-term potentiation is usually up to about eight hours whereas in the intact animal it may last for several weeks.

Long-term potentiation and memory

What is the evidence that long-term potentiation may provide a neurophysiological basis for memory in the hippocampus? An increase in synaptic strength in hippocampal pathways, which is very similar to long-term potentiation, has been shown to occur in a large number of learning and memory models including classical conditioning of the nictitating membrane,[6] bar-press operant conditioning,[2] active avoidance learning in a shuttle box[2] and spatial learning in a maze.[7] The latter two are particularly interesting: in the active-avoidance learning task high-frequency stimulation of the perforant path was used as a conditioning stimulus. They showed that the animals that didn't learn very well, that is, had poor memory, showed long-term depression rather than long-term potentiation of transmission. In the case of the spatial learning experiments, there was a strong inverse correlation between the ability to recall the task and the rate of decay of electrically induced long-term potentiation of transmission in the hippocampus of aged rats.

One would expect that interventions that impair memory should also impair long-term potentiation if it has a role in memory mechanisms. Electroconvulsive shock treatment is known to produce marked temporary amnesia in both animals and man. We carried out an experiment in which electro-convulsive treatment was applied to animals in ten sessions over a period of twenty days.[8] We monitored the ability of the rat's hippocampus to generate long-term potentiation *in vitro* in terms of the amplitude of the excitatory post-synaptic potential and of the firing which is generated in the cell bodies of the pyramidal cells. We found that 24 hours after the last electroconvulsive treatment session there was a great reduction in the ability to generate long-term potentiation at both of these levels.

Long-term potentiation and dementia

Of particular interest with Alzheimer's disease is the study of the effects on long-term potentiation of factors that have been associated with dementia-like states in man. Aluminium is of particular interest. A single intra-ventricular injection of aluminium in rats was shown by Crapper-McLachlan et al to inhibit the generation of long-term potentiation and the population spike 15 days later.[9] This was at a stage before any sign of neurofibrillary damage was apparent. A large number of interventions that impair the functioning of the brain's aminergic systems (acetylcholine,[10, 11] noradrenaline,[12, 13] 5-hydroxytryptamine[12]) – as occurs in Alzheimer's disease – can in certain circumstances inhibit the ability to generate long-term potentiation. The possibility that benzodiazepines may mimic certain aspects of the memory loss in dementias has been proposed. Long-term potentiation has been shown to be blocked by midazolam.[14]

Ageing is a well recognized predisposing factor for dementias. Aged animals have been shown to display disrupted functioning of the hippocampus including impaired retention of long-term potentiation.[7, 15]

Lastly I would like to focus on the N-Methyl-D-aspartate (NMDA) receptor. It is one of the receptors for the excitatory amino-acid transmitter glutamate. There is evidence for dysfunction of these receptors in Alzheimer's disease.[16] Antagonists that block the NMDA receptor or its associated channel can greatly inhibit long-term potentiation in certain pathways in the hippocampus.[17] It would appear that the receptor doesn't normally play much of a role in synaptic transmission because a block of the NMDA receptor linked channel occurs when physiological levels of magnesium are in the solution. However, when one applies high-frequency stimulation of sufficient intensity, one can produce a depolarization of the neurone that removes the magnesium block. Thereby one gets a selective involvement of NMDA receptors during the high-frequency burst. An interesting aspect of NMDA channels is that they allow calcium through the membrane: it is thought that this calcium entry is crucial for the generation of long-term potentiation. Calcium triggers a variety of intracellular processes including activation of calmodulin kinase and protein kinase C.[18]

Long-term potentiation and calcium

We have focused as stated on calcium in order to investigate possible means of enhancing long-term potentiation. Figure 2 is a plot of the relationship between the concentration of calcium in the medium and the ability to generate long-term potentiation.[19] Note that there is a very steep jump between 0.8 mmol and 1 mmol calcium in the extracellular medium. This is a far bigger increase than occurs in normal synaptic transmission for such a small change in external calcium. This demonstrates the crucial role of calcium. It seems that there is a co-operative interaction that causes this steep concentration-response relationship, presumably at some intracellular calcium binding site.

We have looked at possible ways of modifying calcium entry. The compound

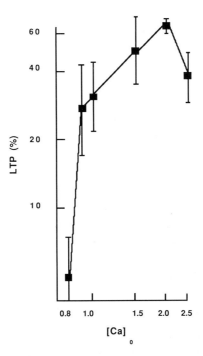

Fig. 2 Relationship between the amplitude of long-term potentiation and the extracellular calcium concentration.

4-aminopyridine is of both practical and theoretical interest. Preliminary studies showed that it might of some use in Alzheimer's disease but this was not confirmed by a subsequent report. It blocks voltage-dependent potassium currents and thereby increases calcium entry through voltage-dependent calcium channels. We found that the ability to generate maximal long-term potentiation was greatly increased in 10 micro-molar 4-aminopyridine (20, Fig. 3). This was blocked by pre-treating the tissue with the NMDA receptor antagonist APV. This indicates that if one can enhance calcium entry one can also enhance long-term potentiation.

A further study examined the role of calcium in a different way using the compound Bayer K 8644.[21] This compound has the opposite effect of the nifedepine type compounds on calcium entry, in that it promotes the opening of voltage dependent calcium channels instead of closing them or promoting their closure. We found that when we applied Bayer K 8644 in the presence of ethanol (in order to get the compound to dissolve in the physiological solution) there was a dramatic increase in the ability to generate long-term potentiation. The enhancement of long-term potentiation was blocked by the calcium channel blocker verapamil, which on its own had no significant effect. This means that long-term potentiation does not involve voltage-dependent channels necessarily, but that activation of these L-type channels, as they are now known, can modulate the process. We are not suggesting that these drugs will be of definite benefit in the

271

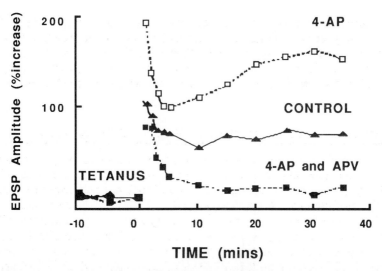

*Fig. 3 Effect of 4-aminopyridine (4-AP) on long-term potentiation. A (above). EPSP ampli-
tude plotted as a function of time, before and after tetanic stimulation (arrow) in control
media, in 10 micro mol 4-AP and in 4-AP plus 20 micro mol APV. B (below). Individual
EPSPs before and after the tetanus.*

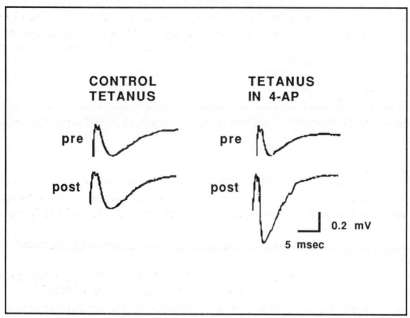

therapy of Alzheimer's disease, but they, or related compounds, should be of
interest from the point of view of the development of new therapeutic strategies
for dementias.

The aminergic system is also of some interest: if one enhances the cholinergic system by septal stimulation[22] or anticholinesterase drug treatment,[23,24] one can promote long-term potentiation. Stimulation of the adrenergic system in conjunction with stimulation of the perforant path input to the dentate in particular, but also in the CA3 region, has been found to promote long-term potentiation. This is thought to be a beta-adrenoceptor mediated phenomen-on.[25-27]

Long-term potentiation and the serotonergic system

Finally I will briefly mention some of our work on the serotonergic system. We have investigated the response of the hippocampus to application of 5-HT *in vitro*.[28] The predominant effect of 5-HT is to inhibit transmission when it is present in the perfusing solution: however, when the drug is washed out, there is a residual long-term enhancement of the transmission in approximately 25 per cent of our slices. This would imply that 5-HT is having a dual effect. We have analysed this pharmacologically and have shown that the inhibitory effect is mediated by a 5-HT 1A receptor type and compounds such as the 5-HT 1A receptor agonist, buspirone, have a relatively pure inhibitory action.[29] The nature of the receptor mediating the enhancement of transmission has not been characterized.

To conclude, I would like to describe an approach which, instead of looking in the literature for drugs or treatments that affect memory and then testing whether they can alter long-term potentiation, tested the idea that drugs which inhibit transmission through the hippocampus and thus long-term potentiation, like buspirone, can impair memory in a rat spatial memory test (the Morris water maze). This was positive.[30]

Acknowledgements

I am indebted to Dr Roger Anwyl. This work was supported by the Health Research Board of Ireland.

References

(1) McNaughton B, Morris R. Hippocampal synaptic enhancement and information storage within a distributed memory system. *Trends Neurosci* 1987, **10**, 408-415.

(2) Matthies H. In search of cellular mechanisms of memory. *Prog Neurobiol* 1989, **32**, *277-344*

(3) De Leon M, George A, Stytopolous L, Smith G, Miller D. Early marker for Alzheimer's disease: the atrophic hippocampus. *Lancet* 1989, ii, 672-673.

(4) Squire L, Zola-Morgan S. Memory: brain systems and behaviour. *Trends Neurosci* 1988, **11**, 170-175.

(5) Bliss TVP, Lomo T. Long-lasting potentiation of synaptic transmission in the dentate area of the anaesthetised rabbit following stimulation of the perforate path. *J Physiol (Lond)* 1973, **232**, 331-356.

(6) Berger TW, Sclabassi RJ. Long-term potentiation and its relation to hippocampal pyramidal cell activity and behavioural learning during classical conditioning. In *Long-term Potentiation: from Biophysics to Behaviour*. New York, Alan R Liss, 1988, 467-497.

(7) Barnes C. Ageing and the physiology of spatial memory. *Neurobiol Ageing* 1988, **9,** 563-568.

(8) Anwyl R, Walshe J, Rowan M. Electroconvulsive treatment reduces long-term potentiation in rat hippocampus. *Brain Res* 1987, **435,** 377-379.

(9) Farnell B, de Boni U, Crapper-McLachlan D. Aluminium neurotoxicity in the absence of neurofibrillary degeneration in the CA1 hippocampal pyramidal neurons in vitro. *Exp Neurol* 1982, **78,** 241-258.

(10) Baker G, Reynolds G. Biogenic amines and their metabolites in Alzheimer's disease: noradrenaline, 5-hydroxytryptamine and 5- hydroxyindole-acetic acid depleted in hippocampus but not in substantia innominata. *Neurosci Lett* 1989, **100,** 335-339.

(11) Hirotsu I, Hori N, Katsuda N, Ishihara T. Effect of anticholinergic drug on long-term potentiation in rat hippocampal slices. *Brain Res* 1989, **482,** 194-197.

(12) Bliss T, Goddard G, Riives M. Reduction of long-term potentiation in the dentate gyrus of the rat following selective depletion of monoamines. *J Physiol* 1983, **334,** 475-491.

(13) Stanton P, Sarvey J. Norepinephrine regulates long-term potentiation of both the population spike and the dendritic EPSP in hippocampal dentate gyrus. *Brain Res Bull* 1986, **18,** 115-119.

(14) Satoh M, Ishihara T, Iwama T, Takagi H. Aniracetam augments, and midazolam inhibits, the long-term potentiation in guinea-pig hippocampal slices. *Neurosci Lett* 1986, **68,** 216-220

(15) Landfield P. Hippocampal neurobiological mechanisms of age-related memory dysfunction. *Neurobiol Ageing* 1986, **68,** 517-579.

(16) Proctor AW, Wogn EHF, Stratmann GC, Lowe SC, Bower DM. Reduced glycine stimulation of [^{3}H]MK-801 binding in Alzheimer's disease. *J Neurochem* 1989, **53,** 604-605.

(17) Collingridge G. The role of NMDA receptors in learning and memory. *Nature* 1987, **330,** 698-704.

(18) Anwyl R. Protein kinase C and long-term potentiation in the hippocampus. *Trends Pharmacol Sci* 1989, **10,** 236-239.

(19) Mulkeen D, Anwyl R, Rowan MJ. The effects of external calcium on long-term potentiation in the rat hippocampal slice. *Brain Res* 1988, **447,** 234-238.

(20) Lee WL, Anwyl R, Rowan MJ. 4-aminopyridine mediated increase in long-term potentiation in CA1 of the rat hippocampus. *Neurosci Lett* 1986, **70,** 106-109.

(21) Mulkeen D, Anwyl R, Rowan MJ. Enhancement of long-term potentiation by the calcium channel agonist Bayer K8644 in CA1 of the rat hippocampus in vitro. *Neurosci Lett* 1987, **80,** 351-355.

(22) Robinson GV. Enhanced long-term potentiation induced in rat dentate gyrus by coactivation of septal and entorhinal inputs: temporal constraints. *Brain Res* 1986, **379,** 56-62.

(23) Ho T, Miura Y, Kadokawa T. Effects of physostigmine and scopolamine on long-term potentiation of hippocampal population spikes in rats. *Can J Physiol Pharmacol* 1988, **66**, 1010-1016.

(24) Ito T, Miura Y, Kadokawa T. Physostigmine induces in rats a phenomenon resembling long-term potentiation. *Eur J Pharmacol* 1988, **156**, 351-359.

(25) Hopkins W, Johnston D. Noradrenergic enhancement of long-term potentiation at mossy fiber synapses in the hippocampus. *J Neurophysiol* 1988, **59**, 667-687.

(26) Harley CW. A role for norepinephrine in arousal, emotion and learning? Limbic modulation by norepinephrine and the Kety hypothesis. *Prog Neuro-Psychopharmacol & Biol Psychiat* 1987, **11**, 419-458.

(27) Sarvey JM. Protein synthesis in long-term potentiation and norepinephrine-induced long-lasting potentiation in hippocampus. In *Long-term Potentiation: from Biophysics to Behaviour.* New York, Alan R Liss, 1988, 467-497.

(28) Rowan MJ, Anwyl R. The effect of prolonged treatment with tricyclic antidepressants on the actions of 5-hydroxytrytamine in the hippocampal slice of the rat. *Neuropharmacology* 1985, **24**, 131-137.

(29) Rowan MJ, Anwyl R. Neurophysiological effects of buspirone and isapirone in the hippocampus: comparison with 5-hydroxytrytamine. *Eur J Pharmacol* 1986, **132**, 93-96.

(30) Rowan MJ, Cullen WK, Moulton B. Buspirone impairment of performance of passive avoidance and spatial learning tasks in the rat. *Psychopharmacology* 1990, **100**, 393-398.

SECTION 9
Diagnosis and Assessment

Chapter 41

EYE MOVEMENTS AND FIXATIONS IN THE EVALUATION OF ALZHEIMER'S DISEASE

JT Hutton *MD, PhD, Director, Neurology Research and Education, St. Mary of the Plains Hospital, 4014 22nd Place, Suite 2, Lubbock, Texas 79410; Clinical Professor, Neurology, Texas Tech University Health Sciences Center, Lubbock, Texas, USA*

This book addresses several research approaches to the evaluation of persons with Alzheimer's disease. The technique which I will present concerns the potential of eye movements and eye fixations as a possible approach to testing and evaluating persons with suspected Alzheimer's disease. The first reference that I could find that connected eye movements and mental processes was that of Andreas Laurentius who wrote in 1599 that the eyes were..."wholly given to follow the motions of the minde, they doe alter and conforme themselves unto it in such manner, as they Blemor the Arabian, and Syreneus the Phisition of Cypres, thought it no absurdite to affirme that the soul dwelt in the eyes." While poetic, this passage also suggests that Laurentius appreciated that the eyes quickly reflect thought processes.

Visual tracking studies

In our research we used infrared reflection techniques to monitor eye movements. If slow visual pursuit of a person with Alzheimer's disease is contrasted to the visual pursuit of a normal person, small catch-up eye movements are noticed with Alzheimer's disease. Catch-up saccades are commonly observed by clinicians when examining Alzheimer patients. For example, the Alzheimer disease patient

279

cannot smoothly pursue or track with the eyes the motion of the examiner's finger as it is moved from side to side. This phenomenon suggested one of the measures that we evaluated in Alzheimer patients. We had several questions at the outset of our smooth pursuit research.

(i) Was our clinical observation that demented patients track differently from normal controls correct?

(ii) Is this visual tracking difference specific to Alzheimer's disease?

(iii) What is the relationship between the number of tracking errors and the severity of behavioural changes in Alzheimer's disease; that is, do the number of errors reflect the severity of the dementia syndrome?

(iv) Do Alzheimer patients track differently from persons with pseudodementia or depression?

(v) Do Alzheimer patients track differently from patients with Pick's disease?

Tracking errors

An experiment compared age-matched normal subjects to Alzheimer patients, stroke patients, persons who had dementia syndrome secondary to space occupying lesions and to persons with Parkinson's disease. All of the patient groups had significantly increased numbers of tracking errors when compared to elderly normal controls suggesting that this was a test sensitive for brain dysfunction, but not specific for Alzheimer's disease.

Table 1. Catch-up saccades during pursuit

	Normals	Alzheimer dementia	Stroke	Space-occupying lesions	Parkinson's disease
N	8	6	10	6	5
Mean	16.5	37.5	73.8	44.6	66.7
SD	11.26	16.41	30.71	19.76	40.11
p value	1	<.02	<.01	<.01	<.02

Each patient group was compared with normals using the rank sum test. All tests were one tailed.

We next addressed how this particular measure of tracking dysfunction related to severity of the dementia syndrome. Using an inverted Folstein Mini-Mental State score plotted against the number of catch-up saccades, we found a strongly positive correlation between increasing severity of dementia and increasing numbers of catch-up saccades ($r = .79$, $p < .001$). This correlation also holds by using a functional rating scale score, i.e. how care-givers rate the behaviour of

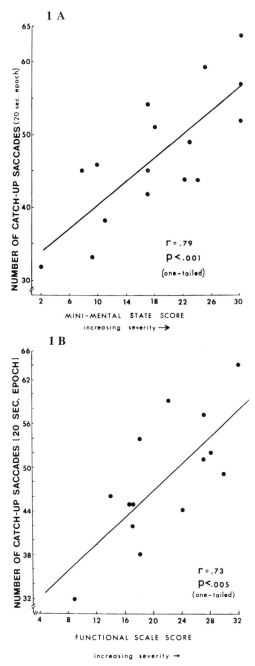

Fig. 1 a,b. Dementia severity as measured by the Mini-Mental State Exam (Fig. 1a) and the Functional Rating Scale (Fig. 1b) is plotted against eye tracking dysfunction as measured by a catch-up saccade index. The tracking speed was 18.4 deg/sec.

281

the Alzheimer family member, versus the number of catch-up saccades ($r = .73$, $p < .005$).

The next question dealt with possible group differences that might exist for this task among Alzheimer patients when compared to elderly normal subjects and elderly depressed persons. A statistically significant difference was found between the group of Alzheimer's patients and the normal controls as well as between the Alzheimer's patients and the elderly depressed persons ($p < .0001$). This suggests that quantified study of eye movements may be of benefit for differential diagnosis of Alzheimer's disease and pseudodementia.

Pick's disease

Comparing patients with Pick's disease and Alzheimer patients is problematic as it is difficult to find clinically diagnosed Pick's disease patients and later confirm the diagnosis by autopsy. The visual tracking performance of a Pick patient, subsequently confirmed pathologically as having Pick's disease, was quite normal, as compared to normal controls. It was, in fact, almost hypernormal apart from the patient's distractibility, common in Pick's patients. In contrast, Alzheimer patients of the same degree of severity of dementia as the Pick's patient had grossly abnormal visual tracking. A possible reason for this difference is the visual tracking areas of the brain located in the parieto-occipital region are affected by plaques and tangles in Alzheimer's disease, but are spared by the pathology of Pick's disease.

We conclude that Alzheimer patients have increased numbers of tracking errors during visual pursuit when compared to normal controls. Secondly, the number of tracking errors does not differentiate Alzheimer's disease from certain other neurological diseases. Thirdly, the number of tracking errors tends to reflect the severity of the behavioural decompensation. Fourthly, significant group differences were found between Alzheimer's and elderly depressed patients and between Alzheimer's and elderly controls. Finally, preliminary evidence suggests that visual tracking performance in Pick's disease is normal until an advanced stage is reached. This is in contrast to the impaired tracking performance found in Alzheimer's disease.

Cross-correlation coefficients

Visual tracking is not, however, a perfect measure and we have looked for more precise measures. One approach is to look at cross-correlation coefficients between eye and target location. Several questions arose regarding use of cross correlation coefficients:

(i) What happens to this measure of visual tracking performance in Alzheimer's patients over time?

(ii) How do cross-correlation coefficients compare to catch-up saccades with progression of the disease?

(iii) Does a cross-correlation coefficient discriminate among groups of Alzheimer patients, depressed patients and elderly normal controls?

(iv) Does a cross-correlation coefficient relate meaningfully to dementia severity in Alzheimer's disease?

We evaluated Alzheimer's patients with advancing severity of the disease serially over time. In the early stages, catch-up saccade index increases but beyond moderate degrees of dementia, it seems paradoxically to decrease. This apparent paradox loses validity if we look at tracking performance *per se*. The short catch-up saccades seen in tracking in the earliest stage are clearly abnormal. As an Alzheimer patient becomes more advanced, the saccades become fewer but longer. Finally, in the poor tracking performance of the most advanced patients, these catch-up saccades are fewer but longer still.

A more satisfactory approach is to look at a computer comparison of the location of the cursor and that of the eye following and to correct for the phase lag (the cross-correlation mean alluded to above). There is a reasonably good cross correlation mean early on, but as the disease advances the cross-correlation coefficient diminishes. Comparing cross-correlation coefficient for normals, depressed and Alzheimer patients, we found that the Alzheimer's patients have a mean cross-correlation coefficient of 0.88 compared with 0.97 for normals. The performance of the elderly depressed patients is similar to that of the elderly normal subjects. There are, however, statistically significant group differences between the depressed patients and the Alzheimer's patients ($p < .01$), and between the normal subjects and the Alzheimer's patients ($p < .01$).

The relationship of cross-correlation coefficients to dementia syndrome for different tracking speeds of .4 and .8 Hertz is maintained. For both the Mini-Mental State Exam and the Functional Rating Scale there are statistically significant correlations with reduced cross-correlation coefficient tracking measure as compared to dementia severity. Alzheimer patients' performance shows performance variability increases substantially over time, but on the average, performance for this visual task decreases over a one-year period. We conclude, therefore, that cross-correlation coefficients are a better performance index for Alzheimer's disease, particularly for advanced patients, than are catch-up saccades.

Scan path studies

A different measure still is that of the scan path. The scan path is the sum total of all saccades that a person makes when looking at an informative scene. Several questions regarding scan paths and dementia need to be answered.

(i) Do scan paths of patients with dementia differ from those of normal controls?

(ii) Are scan path differences specific either for Alzheimer's disease or for dementia caused by mass lesions?

(iii) What is the relationship between scan path differences and the severity of the dementia?

In an experiment we compared the performance of three normal controls and six dementia patients, three of whom had frontal lobe masses and three who had Alzheimer's disease. One of the scenes used was the "Country Farm Scene" from the Thematic Apperception Test. Infrared eye monitoring recorded the movements of the patient's gaze as he/she looked at the picture. The patients' scan paths differed depending on the task questions. We started with a free scan, that is the subjects looked at the picture without any instructions. Then they were asked how the people in the picture might be related. The controls seemed to have a preponderance of eye movements over the areas of the faces of the people in the picture, looking back and forth between the individuals. Next the subjects were asked what the man in the picture was doing. With controls there seemed to be a preponderance of eye movements in the central part of the picture, where the man is following a plough. Finally the subjects were asked the mood of the woman holding the books. There was a preponderance of eye movements over the woman's face trying to discern her mood. These are logical scan paths; one could look at these scan paths in controls and predict the questions that were asked.

When Alzheimer patients were asked how the people in the picture were related, there seemed to be much less focusing of the gaze on the relevant parts of the pictures. For the questions "What is the woman wearing?", there was not the preponderance of scanning on the lateral aspects were the woman's clothing is located. When Alzheimer patients were asked to look at the picture while pondering the mood of the woman, there did not seem to be the focusing of gaze to the appropriate part of the picture. These examples suggest that in Alzheimer's there is either visual distractibility or poor regulation of gaze.

Ocular motor programming perseveration

The second task was designed to elicit "ocular motor programming perseveration". Persons were asked to trace with their eyes a square. They were then asked to look back and forth between two dots. During this simple task the eye movements are measured. A group of normals can manage this task easily, tracing the figures in both tasks repeatedly. However, patients with Alzheimer's disease tended to continue the eye movements of the square task when the two dots are presented and vice versa. Although they were capable of tracing the figure, there was perseveration present which we refer to as "ocular motor programming perseveration."

We attempted to assess performance by severity of the dementia syndrome. A ten word learning task was used as a measure of cognitive ability. Normal persons were able to master the task quite well. Demented patients without ocular motor programming perseveration performed only moderately well and demented subjects with ocular motor programming perseveration had the most difficulty with this ten word learning task. The Porteus Maze test gives similar results. Those Alzheimer patients without ocular motor programming perseveration performed the task moderately well, but those with ocular motor programming perseveration performed poorly.

We concluded from this research on scan paths and dementia that poorly regu-

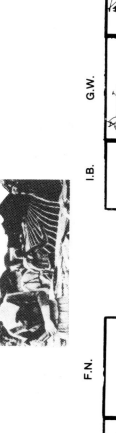

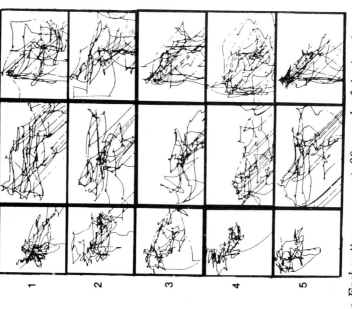

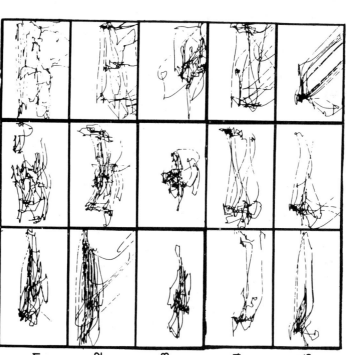

Fig. 2 (a,b). Effect of varying instructions while viewing a thematic picture. Each pattern represents 30 seconds of viewing time. Instructions preceding each exposure of the scene were as follows: 1. Look at this picture; 2. Try to decide how the people in the picture are related; 3. See if you can tell what the man is doing; 4. Study what the women are wearing; 5. Determine what the mood is of the woman holding the books. Fig. 2a. Note the different areas of gaze concentration as the instructions change and the consistency and similarity of these changes across the normal subjects. Fig. 2b. Illustration of the effect of varying instructions in three demented subjects. Patient I.B. had a focal frontal mass lesion; patients G.W. and L.P. had Alzheimer's disease. Note the difference between these scan-paths of demented subjects and those obtained from normal subjects (Fig. 2a). With demented subjects the changing instructions do not alter gaze location to the same extent as they do for normal subjects.

lated and perseverative scan paths can been seen in demented subjects. These scan paths differences can be seen in Alzheimer's disease as well as in persons with dementia secondary to frontally located mass lesions. We found that a continuum may exist with poorly regulated gaze being seen in milder forms of dementia, perseverative gaze in moderate and severe dementia and very strikingly akinetic gaze in some of the most severely demented persons.

Eye fixation durations

Clearly it is difficult to quantify scan paths and relate the abnormality observed in the scan paths to the severity of the dementia syndrome. In an attempt to quantitate, we looked at eye fixation durations during these scan paths. We investigated whether average eye fixation durations during visual scanning differed for groups of Alzheimer, mass lesion dementia and depressive pseudo-dementia patients and elderly normal controls. These groups looked at the same picture for 20 seconds in response to a particular question. On average, the Alzheimer group had longer eye fixation durations than did the other groups. In contrast, the group with the frontal lobe lesions had on average shorter eye fixation durations that either the normals or the pseudodementia patients. The pseudodementia patients and the normal subjects performed in a very similar fashion. We suggest that this was probably a compensatory prolongation of eye fixations in Alzheimer patients in order to maximize the amount of visual information. The frontal lobe patients were clinically quite impulsive and had brief eye fixations. This may reflect impulsive visual scanning which is insufficient to input the essential information.

Restricted upgaze

A final observation made was that conjugate vertical gaze limitations are really quite common in Alzheimer patients. Is this common neurological finding of limitation of upgaze of any functional significance? This was the cheapest experiment that I ever did. I bought a three dollar piece of wood: it was about eight feet tall and I attached large lettered cards at one foot intervals. Fifty persons in a nursing home sat in their bedside chairs and simply read what was written on each of the cards beginning at the bottom and reading the cards serially up to the ceiling. We found that 10 per cent of these persons could not read the top words despite unrestricted head movements. We found of those who had restricted upgaze, the vast majority had 15 degrees or less vertical conjugate eye movements in combination with a complicating factor such as mechanical neck problems or kyphosis (forward head position). These factors prevented them from compensating for their limited vertical upgaze. Normally a person can extend the neck to look vertically. A person with limited upgaze and stiffness of the neck has this angle restricted, so that he cannot compensate by using extension of the neck.

Televisions, room numbers and directional signs in institutions are frequently elevated. For the 10 per cent of persons with limited vertical upgaze this can be confusing. Such vertically placed information would be quite indistinct because once visual information is a degree or two off the fovea (that portion of the retina of the eye where vision is most distinct) it becomes quite blurred. This finding has implications for environmental design.

Conclusion

Abnormal visual tracking, abnormal visual scanning, and restricted visual access to vertically placed information may relate to visual confusion and even to falling and tripping in Alzheimer patients. The visual abnormalities probably contribute to environmental misperceptions. One approach to reducing confusion is to reduce competing and ambiguous visual stimuli. Empirically it is suggested that the environment for an Alzheimer patient should be depleted of both the amount and the complexity of visual information. Also effective communication and visual recognition are more likely to be successful for stationary targets than for moving targets because catch-up saccades may cause visual blurring. Extra time to look may benefit visual scanning in Alzheimer's disease and allow for completion of scan paths with compensatory prolongation of visual fixations. When functionally impaired upgaze exists, visual information should be lowered.

Abnormalities in eye movements and eye fixations alter visual input to a physiologically impaired brain. Complaints of visual disturbance with Alzheimer's disease relate to a problem with looking as well as seeing.

Bibliography

Antes JR. The time course of picture viewing. *J Exp Psychol* 1974, **103**, 62-70.

Chamberlin W. Restrictions of upward gaze with advancing age. *Am J Opthalmol* 1971, **71**, 341-346.

Fletcher WA, Sharpe JA. Smooth pursuit dysfunction in Alzheimer's disease. *Neurology* 1988, **38**, 272-277.

Hartje W, Steinhauser D, Kerschensteiner M. Diagnostic value of saccadic pursuit eye movements in screening for organic cerebral dysfunction. *J Neurol* 1978, **217**, 253-260.

Hutton JT. Eye movements and Alzheimer's disease: significance and relationship to visuospatial confusion. In, Hutton JT, Kenny AD (eds). *Senile Dementia of the Alzheimer Type*. New York, Alan R. Liss, 1985, 3-33.

Hutton JT, Nagel JA, Loewenson RB. Eye tracking dysfunction in Alzheimer-type dementia. *Neurology(Clev)* 1983, **34**, 99-102.

Hutton JT, Shapiro I, Loewenson RB, Christian BL, Nagel JA. Abnormal eye movements in dementia and aging. *Trans Am Neurol Assoc* 1981, **106**, 320-323.

Carers, Professionals and Alzheimer's Disease. D O'Neill ed © 1991 John Libbey & Company Ltd

Chapter 42

FRONTAL LOBE DEFICITS IN ALZHEIMER'S DISEASE

MR Sulway,* WA Longley,* GA Broe,* H Creasey,* EA McCusker,* AS Henderson, A Jorm, A Korten, H Bennett,*
*Australian National University, Canberra: *Aged and Extended Care Department, Repatriation General Hospital, Concord, NSW 2139, Australia*

This paper examines the neuropsychological findings, especially frontal lobe deficits of 35 Alzheimer's disease patients and 35 age-matched controls. These groups constitute part of a total of 172 cases and age-matched controls from a large-scale study carried out in two hospitals in Sydney. The purpose of the main study was to investigate risk-factors for Alzheimer's disease in an Australian setting. A detailed assessment was made of patients and controls. Cases were selected from referrals to dementia assessment clinics at Concord and Lidcombe Hospitals in Sydney. They were referred from general practitioners in the catchment areas. To make up the numbers, a number of veterans were included, as well as a number of patients from outside the catchment area. Rather than using hospital and community control groups, the controls were selected by the novel and more appropriate approach of matching the medical bias of the case selection. Accordingly, the controls came from the same general practitioner practices as the cases, selected in a random manner. Controls were matched for gender and age. To make up the numbers, it was necessary to recruit some controls from neighbouring practices.

Assessment

All cases received a full neurological examination. The standard evaluation included a Neurology of Ageing schedule and the Mini-Mental State Examination. Various screening examinations including blood tests, computerized tomography scans and electro-encephalograms were also carried out. Full neuropsychological assessment was carried out on all cases. The criteria for Alzheimer's disease were those of "probable" and "possible" Alzheimer's disease using the NINCDS-ADRDA criteria. Exclusions included those who were unable to undergo neurological or neuropsychological assessment in English, or those who lacked an informant. The randomly matched and selected controls were seen at home by a neurologist. A brief examination was carried out which included blood pressure measurement, the Mini-Mental State Examination and the shortened Neurology of Ageing schedule. Controls were accepted if they had a Mini-Mental State Examination score of 26 or more, were able to be interviewed in English and had a suitable informant. They were asked if they would be prepared to attend at the hospital for a more detailed neuropsychological assessment. Thirty-five controls agreed to this and were examined using the same battery of tests as the Alzheimer's disease patients. Informants for both cases and controls participated in a detailed risk-factor interview which was specially developed for this study. This completed the data collection for the first stage of the main study: results are still being analysed and will be reported elsewhere. One year follow-up of all cases is almost complete. The 35 controls who agreed to the full assessment were matched with 35 of the cases and I will present these results.

Results

There were no significant differences between the two groups in age, sex-ratio or educational achievement: nor were there any significant differences between the cases selected and the total Alzheimer's disease group, suggesting that these 35 cases were representative of the larger group. There was a significant difference in the MMSE score between patients and controls. The test battery was selected to include a wide range of psychological functions which clinical experience and research have shown to be affected in Alzheimer's disease. The battery included parts from well-known and frequently-used standardized tests. The theoretical approach underlying the test selection was that of Luria and Walsh, but we also included some normed tests. In addition to the formal test battery, each person was rated by the psychologists on a number of behavioural variables. This was aimed at obtaining information not available from formal testing: how people approached the tasks and responded to their own performance, and how they presented themselves at the assessment. The test battery took up to two hours to complete. This may seem very lengthy for elderly people, but most people tolerated this very well. For the few people who became fatigued, a brief tea-break enabled completion of the test-battery. In a few instances we had to call on all our charm and persuasive skills to get the best performances from our patients!

Analysis

Statistical analysis of our data was by analysis of variance and by the chi-square test. Our very detailed assessment yielded a very considerable amount of data. We will present a summary of our findings and discuss in detail only some of these to highlight the functional difficulties of our cases. Our findings confirmed the usual difficulties with orientation, memory and learning. We found deficits in language skills only at a higher level such as word and sentence generation. Our subjects did not show diminution of visuo-spatial abilities, but were handicapped in the areas of planning, abstraction and problem solving. Although our subjects still retained some insight into their condition, the following general behavioural deficits were seen: inertia, decreased productivity and aspontaneity. Self-control was significantly affected in the cases also. Frontal lobe functions were considered under five sub-headings: (i) attention and information processing, (ii) self-control, (iii) drive; (iv) flexibility; and (v) planning, and will be considered in more detail.

Frontal lobe function

The test results showed that the cases had difficulty in attention and information processing. The digit-span test showed significant differences in the digits-backward mode, but no difference in the digits-forward mode. As soon as processing was required, they faltered in their performance. The second difference was a prolonged reaction time. Our cases had problems with attention and were also much slower. Self-control was considered under several headings; poor self-monitoring on simple response tests such as the tapping test; poor self-monitoring of errors in tests, e.g. poor performance on verbal fluency and Porteus mazes. Problems in self-monitoring were manifest in the difficulties cases had in simple response tests such as the tapping tests where they were unable to inhibit errors.

In the more complex test of verbal fluency, our cases made a number of intrusive and other errors, for example including words beginning with a letter other than the one that they were supposed to be working with. On the Porteus mazes, the cases were unable to inhibit errors and were more impulsive as well. Thus, deficits in self-control tended to make the patient react in a more distractable, restless and less concentrated way. In terms of drive, we found that the cases needed significantly more prompting to start tests. An example is the Mental Control Test on the Wechsler Memory Scale which asks the person to count backwards from twenty to one: we found that they needed much more prompting to get started on that test. The cases also had much more difficulty in generating ideas, e.g. in the verbal fluency test where they were able to generate significantly fewer numbers of words than our controls.

Flexibility deficits can be considered in two ways: perseveration of elements and perseveration of concepts. Perseveration of elements in visual reproduction was tested by analysing different serial drawings by the cases. Perseveration of elements of the first drawing can be seen throughout following drawings. This can also be seen using the Visual Reproduction subset of the Wechsler Memory Scale: the patient is shown a shape for ten seconds and then is asked to draw it from memory. A perseveration of elements of the first drawing will be seen to intrude through the subsequent drawings. Perseveration can also be demonstrated in recall of verbal data, as was seen with the Word Recognition Test. This test involves learning a total of seven words over five trials. Thirty minutes later the subject is asked to recall the words, and if not successful is asked to recognize the seven words from a longer list. Our cases tended to repeat errors in learning

291

words and tended to make intrusive errors in recall, i.e. they included words from previous tests.

Perseveration of concepts can be demonstrated on the Colour-Form Sort Test. This test involves presenting the person with 12 blocks which are in four colours and three shapes. The person is asked to sort the blocks into groups, and having sorted on a certain basis (e.g. colour), is asked to name the basis of his sort. He is then is asked to sort another way (e.g. shape): if he is successful he is asked to repeat the first sort. Only 8 per cent of cases could manage the whole test, whereas 57 per cent of controls could do it. The fact that less than two-thirds of the controls could fully perform this test shows that they too have problems at this level of functioning, but not to the same extent as the cases. Our cases tended to sort one way, such as on the basis of shape, but when asked to sort another way, sorted on shape yet again instead of moving on to colour.

Planning deficits were assessed using, among other tests, level twelve of the Porteus mazes. This test requires the subject to comprehend a problem, work out the steps necessary to solve it and to carry out the steps without error. Level twelve was the highest level given. Our controls also had difficulty with this task, with only 68 per cent passing this task, compared with 20 per cent of cases. Our cases were also significantly slower and more impulsive on this task.

Summary

Frontal lobe deficits in Alzheimer's disease may be summarized as follows: the person with Alzheimer's disease tends to be inefficient in basic information-processing, deficient in self-monitoring, adynamic, perseverative (lacks flexibility) and has poor planning ability. Our reason for emphasizing frontal lobe deficits is that when we say that Alzheimer's disease patients are difficult to live with, we do not mean difficult to live with because their frontal lobe deficits make them disinhibited, irresponsible or facetious like those with frontal lobe deficits secondary to head-injury. Rather it is the apathy, inertia and reduced output that is so uncharacteristic in a person who was once energetic, busy and well-organized. Secondly, increasing frontal lobe deficits in the person with dementia reduce his/her independence. A person with a memory problem, but who is otherwise cognitively intact, can develop strategies to compensate for the memory problem. A person with frontal lobe deficits is far less able, and eventually totally unable, to compensate. We hope that an appreciation of these frontal lobe deficits will help family and carers to understand more clearly the nature of the difficulties of the sufferer.

Finally, in emphasizing the frontal lobe deficits, we are not denying the importance of memory, orientation and visuo-spatial problems, nor are we arguing for a strict localizing approach. We want rather to draw attention to the special functional difficulties which are often quite subtle initially and which have been somewhat underemphasized in past research. We believe that these particular problems are very disabling for the patient, and very difficult for family and carers to comprehend.

Carers, Professionals and Alzheimer's Disease. D O'Neill ed © 1991 John Libbey & Company Ltd

Chapter 43

EARLY DETECTION OF DEMENTIA OF THE ALZHEIMER TYPE AN INFORMATION PROCESSING APPROACH TO MEMORY DYSFUNCTION

L Wens[1], F Baro[2], and G d'Ydewalle[3], *NFWO Research Assistant[1], Department of Brain and Behavior Research[2]; Faculty of Medicine; Laboratory of Experimental Psychology[3], Department of Psychology, Katholieke Universiteit Leuven, Belgium*

Introduction

This paper presents an ongoing research project on memory dysfunction in the initial phase of Dementia of the Alzheimer Type (DAT). The article is limited to DAT as it is the primary form of dementia in old age. Central to our experimental memory research is that it is conducted with patients in the initial phase of the dementia process. What, in particular, is the specific nature and course of pathological memory functioning in the initial phase of dementia? The literature cites many examples of retained learning capacity in amnesic patients. On the basis of a comparison between various indirect and direct memory tasks, we have attempted to investigate the presence of such facilitation effects in DAT. The delineation of these facilitation effects and the determination of their integrity in an incipient dementia process will give insight into the nature of memory dysfunction in DAT.

Memory research

One of the first questions to be answered is why concentrate on memory research? Clinically, memory problems are one of the first symptoms of dementia. Despite the fact that there is still no complete consensus on the diagnostic criteria for dementia and DAT in spite of work by groups such as the NINCDS-ADRDA Work Group, the Symposium on Consensus Development in the Diagnosis of Alzheimer's Disease, World Health Organization, Geneva, March 1987, and the Symposium on Consensus Development in the Diagnosis of Alzheimer's Disease, the Nederlandse Vereniging voor Neurologie, 4 November 1988, there is general agreement that memory disturbances are one of the primary disturbances in the symptomatology. They occur early in the disease process: we also know from pathophysiological research that the critical structures and substrata involved in learning ability and memory are affected in a striking manner in DAT.

Benign and malignant senescent forgetfulness

In clinical practice, it is often not easy to make a good differential diagnosis between dementia and other organic brain diseases (primarily delirium) and non-organic or functional disturbances (primarily depression). At the same time, the difference between early dementia and the normal ageing process is not easy to define. Therefore the object of experimental memory research is to identify not only quantitative but also qualitative differences in information processing in both mentally healthy and demented elderly, with special attention to the changes in the early stage of DAT. Insights gained from experimental research are valuable not only for testing the value of current working hypotheses but also have relevance for clinical practice.

Early detection of dementia

The delineation of specific memory deficits in early DAT can also contribute to the entire research area of the early detection of dementia. Indeed, we know that there are treatable and potentially curable forms of dementia. Treatment may also consist of psychosocial support of family members and interventions that promote the autonomy of the patient. Any investigation into the nature of memory deficits in early dementia presumes a "case-finding" research design. The detection of these patients is problematic because of the difficulty of diagnosing early dementia and because the patients with dementia generally only encounter medical practitioners at a more advanced stage of the disease. Collaboration with general practitioners is thus essential: in general practice, short cognitive screening tests such as the Mini-Mental State Examination or the Short Portable Mental Status Questionnaire can be administered to elderly patients who are at increased risk for developing dementia. The "at-risk" patients who are thus detected may then be examined in detail, using instruments such as the CAMDEX. We also use groups of volunteers who are invited to participate in our memory research: our subjects are elderly nuns and people over 75 years of age from a particular town.

CAMDEX

The CAMDEX (Cambridge Mental Disorders of the Elderly Examination) of Roth and colleagues[1] is a recently developed standardized instrument for the diagnosis of mental disturbances of the elderly. Special emphasis is placed on the early detection of DAT. The following components are central to its use:

(i) a structured clinical interview to acquire information on the patient's present and past medical condition, and the family history of the patient. This interview is conducted with the patient as well as with a relative of the patient in order to obtain a better picture of the premorbid intellectual capacities, the personal and social functioning, the current behavioural pattern, and the capabilities of the patient;

(ii) a systematic investigation of mental function on the basis of testing a variety of cognitive functions, and a structured assessment of behaviour;

(iii) a short neurological examination;

(iv) laboratory tests; and

(v) neuroradiological examinations (EEG, CT-SCAN, SPECT, etc.).

The CAMDEX consists of a collection of previously existing approaches and methods in the diagnosis of mental disturbances in the elderly together with some important additions. The diagnosis itself must be made on the basis of operational criteria comparable to DSM-III-R and ICD-10 criteria.

Longitudinal research

The diagnosis of DAT can only be made with certainty post mortem. Clinical diagnosis on the basis of CAMDEX is supplemented with laboratory and radiological data. At the same time, a clinical estimate is made of the severity of dementia (minimal, light, moderate and severe) and, on the basis of the convergence between the various scales and measurements in the CAMDEX, a judgement is made on the certainty of the diagnosis (possible, probable, definite). We defined three diagnostic groups: a mentally healthy group, an at-risk group for DAT (minimal form), and a DAT group with mild severity. We observed these groups for a period of time with the aid of the CAMDEX in order to verify the diagnosis and to follow the evolution of the mental functioning. On the basis of the results of this longitudinal research, which was started in 1987, our groups now consist of 75 normal elderly people (normals), 15 patients with minimal DAT (DAT minimal), and 7 mild to moderately severe DAT patients (DAT mild).

Aspects of memory

The contrast between implicit and explicit memory is of interest. In *Measures of Memory*, Richardson-Klavehn and Bjork[2] discuss the "new" set of measurements in memory research, the indirect memory measurements. These differ from the traditional direct memory measurements primarily in the task instructions and the measurement criteria. In the direct memory tasks (free recall, cued recall, recognition), the task instructions explicitly call upon the knowledge of a well-defined event in the personal life of the individual. A typical event is the learning of a list of words. A recognition task is then used to determine whether the person can discriminate between items on and off the list. A free-recall task involves retrieving the learned words, with or without the help of cues.

In an indirect memory task, the individual executes a particular task without reference to a specific previous event. The measurement criterion investigates specifically whether there is a change (generally facilitation) in the task performance as a result of that previous event. In normal subjects, experimentally manipulated dissociations can be found between such indirect and direct memory tasks. Several examples of retained learning capacity in amnesia patients are described in the literature. They can be divided into the following two major groups:

(i) skill-learning: the ability to acquire and retain a variety of motor, perceptual, and cognitive skills, in spite of limited memory for the learning episode itself.

(ii) priming or facilitation effects: a facilitation in the performance of certain perceptual or lexical tasks (for example, perceptual identification, word completion, word association) because of previous exposure to the stimulus material (direct or repetition priming) or to associated material (indirect or associative priming), in spite of impaired recall or recognition of this material.

On the basis of the dissociations between the direct and the indirect memory measurements, hypotheses and theories are formulated about the existence of different memory systems and memory processes that are differentially affected in amnesia. Indirect memory tasks reflect the implicit memory on the basis of performance facilitation in the absence of conscious recollection. Direct memory tasks call upon the explicit memory, which is characterized by conscious awareness of the learning episode during successful performance. Implicit and explicit memories are collective terms for different, generally dichotomous, interpretations of the memory organization.

Implicit and explicit memory

Implicit memory flows from a temporary modification in abstract lexical, semantic, or procedural knowledge structures in which priming is ascribed to the procedural memory. Explicit memory is dependent on the formation and recollection of memory traces of specific events (declarative memory with two subcomponents: semantic memory and episodic memory). Graf and Mandler (1984) propose two processes that affect mental representations – activation and elaboration –

which they compare with the distinction between the procedural and the declarative memory. In the dissociations between the different memory systems and memory processes, a parallel is often drawn with the distinction between automatic and controlled processes that play a role in the levels and stages of information processing. The most important criticism of this postulated family of memory systems and memory processes is that the jump from indirect/direct memory tasks to implicit/explicit memory processes and systems is probably too simplistic.

Opposing viewpoints

Jacoby radically opposes the postulating of different memory systems and hypothesizes that perception, recognition, and free recall all rely on episodic memory (the non-abstractionist position).[3] Indeed, next to dissociations, there are many parallel effects between direct and indirect memory tasks. Implicit and explicit memory phenomena reflect different aspects of the memory for previous processing episodes. Rather than ascribing awareness of remembering to a particular memory system as an inherent characteristic, it is also related to differences in information from the test cues, differences in the nature of the retrieval processes, and the degree of correspondence between the processing required during the study test and the memory test. The difference between data-driven processing and conceptually-driven processing seems essential in this.[3, 4] But, as in the traditional analytical view, these processes are mostly posited *a posteriori*, and they cannot satisfactorily explain the multiplicity of data.

On the basis of a review of the literature, complex patterns of dissociation and parallel effects are found between direct and indirect tasks. In view of this enormous diversity of implicit memory phenomena, a dual approach appears to be the most feasible at this time.[2, 3, 5]

Forms of implicit memory

The first type is the automatic and short-duration priming resulting from the activation of existing, abstract representations. Examples include: (i) the perceptual identification task where there is no priming of non-words in amnesia patients but priming does occur with controls. This shows the need for the previous existence of linguistic units; and (ii) the word completion task with normal and amnesic patients where priming due to activation is independent of the nature of the level of processing during the study task (semantic versus non-semantic): the recognition task is sensitive, however, to the degree of semantic processing.

Secondly, longer duration priming effects of specific components of the formed episodic representations. These facilitation effects can be elaboration dependent, so equivalent findings are not always obtained in amnesia patients and normals. Examples include: (i) the fragment completion task by normals where facilitation effects are still present after seven days, despite a sharp drop in recognition accuracy; (ii) priming of newly learned associations: in normals this seems to be clearly elaboration dependent whereas amnesia patients manifest less and only short-duration priming in comparison with normals; and (iii) specificity of priming effects in a multiplicity of tasks: priming effects are modality specific and item specific.

Direct and indirect memory tasks are relevant to the understanding of the differences between tasks and forms of measurement procedures. At the same time, they can contribute to the construction or reconstruction of theories of different cognitive subdomains. However, they do not refer unequivocally to the opposition of explicit and implicit memory. A comparison of different indirect memory measurements is necessary to study further the phenomenon of facilitation effects. The theoretical foundation of the multiplicity of data must also be developed further.

Facilitation effects with DAT

By comparing the different indirect and direct memory tasks, we are trying to investigate the specific entity of such facilitation effects with DAT. The delineation of facilitation and investigating its intactness in an initial phase of the dementia will provide a deeper insight into the nature of memory dysfunctioning in DAT. In contrast with the extended study on retained learning ability in amnesia patients, particularly with Korsakoff's syndrome, research into facilitation effects in demented patients is still scarce. To a degree, the small patient numbers are probably at the root of the conflicts in the results obtained and their interpretations. In the following review, we summarize the few studies that have investigated facilitation effects in DAT patients, generally in comparison with amnesia patients.

Direct or repetition priming

In the word completion task, controls and all patients with Huntington's disease, Korsakoff's syndrome display priming effects but Alzheimer patients with mild to moderately severe disease do not. This may be due to a specific disturbance: the DAT patients could execute the word completion task as such because they had reached the same base level as the others. A similar lack of priming or a decreased priming effect in DAT patients has been shown with the word completion task and free association task, while the word association task also shows decreased priming effect in DAT patients of moderate severity. Estimation of frequency of occurrence of words in a study list is considered as a prototype of automatic processing, and the Alzheimer patients perform less well in this as well as in the controlled processes. When the word completion task is applied with the perceptual identification task, mild to moderately severe DAT patients show clear deficits on the traditional memory tasks (free recall, cued recall and recognition) but show clear priming effects in the indirect memory tasks.

The lexical decision task and reading task in a small study showed a repetition priming effect in the lexical decision task in spite of a poor recognition task among DAT patients. A clear dissociation was also found between improvement in reading speed and recognition of repeated sentences.

Indirect or associative priming

One of the dominant models of the structure of semantic memory describes the semantic memory as a network of conceptual nodes.[6] The representation of a word activates not only the node of that concept but also the related nodes, defined, for example, in terms of semantic or functional relations. This activation of related nodes improves processing accessibility. In a semantic facilitation task, the time a person needs to process a stimulus is measured under two conditions: when the stimulus is preceded by a semantically associated or by a semantically non-associated stimulus. A reduction in processing time is considered a facilitation resulting from the automatic activation by the semantically associated item that preceded it. Such facilitation is found, for example, in lexical decision tasks in younger as well as elderly people, while age differences were, indeed, found in controlled memory tasks like free recall and recognition.

Nebes *et al* used a naming task to investigate the intactness of the semantic network in mild to moderate DAT patients: 80 tachistoscopically presented words had to be named as quickly as possible.[7] In fact, they were offered in pairs, with and without semantic association. After this task came an incidental free-recall task and a recognition task. In contrast with the poor performance on the direct recognition tasks, there was a clear facilitation in the word-naming task. The authors use these and other semantic tasks to demonstrate that automatic forms of semantic processing are intact in Alzheimer patients. The many deficits in semantic tasks in Alzheimer patients are related to a specific disturbance in the semantic knowledge, namely, a preservation of general category information as opposed to a loss of specific characteristics in the semantic lexicon. These are generally tasks that demand attention and effort: making decisions on semantic characteristics of stimuli, the organizing of items in function of their semantic relationship, or the active searching for semantic processing. It is in this controlled semantic processing that Alzheimer patients fail.

Continuous recognition task

A recognition task is traditionally considered a direct memory task: in our study, we use a continuous recognition task as an example of a direct memory task. The continuous recognition task is a paradigm that measures the speed and accuracy of word recognition in the short-term and long-term memory. A sequence of words is offered consecutively, each word appearing twice within the sequence. The subject has to judge whether the word is presented for the first time (a new word) or the second time (an old word). The interval between the first and second presentation of a word is manipulated. Thus, for a number of words, the second presentation is situated in the short-term memory (intervals of one to seven words) and for other words it is situated in the long-term memory (intervals of more than seven words). The traditional distinction between these different "capacity memories" offers an interesting differentiation between normal and demented elderly people in the sense that the demented group already manifests disturbances in the immediate memory. The question that arises is whether these disturbances are already operative in the initial phase of dementia.[8]

Stimuli and procedure used in continuous recognition task

(i) Stimuli

The continuous recognition task consists of high and low frequency words in the Dutch spoken and written language with four to eight characters per word.[9,10] All the words have high visual imagery-values.[11] There are three possible exercise phases (four words in each phase presented twice). The test phase consists of two blocks of 50 trials each (25 words presented twice). The interval between the first and second presentation is manipulated with five interstimulus interval (ISI) conditions: 1, 2, 4, 8, and 16 words between first and second presentation of the same word. Each ISI condition has ten trials (five new/five old). A break is scheduled between the two blocks. There are three lists of words which are presented at random over the various subjects. In this way, repeated testing is possible.

(ii) Procedure

The words are shown on a screen, one at a time, and each word is presented twice. We instructed the subjects to judge whether the presented word is a "new" word (presented for the first time) or an "old" word (shown the second time). Therefore, the subject holds two buttons, one in the right hand and one in the left. The righthanded patients press the left button as a "new" word and the right button for an "old" word; the lefthanded patients do the opposite. The words remain on the screen until the subject pushes a button. There is a response time limit of 10 seconds for each time. The interval between pushing the button and the next stimulus is three seconds.

Lexical decision task

In a lexical decision task, series of letters are presented, and the subject must decide as quickly as possible whether this series forms a word or not. Traditionally, this test was used to specify the structures and processes of permanent knowledge stored in the semantic memory. We use this semantic task as an indirect memory task in order to investigate both indirect and direct facilitation effects.

For indirect facilitation effects, in view of the literature on amnesia patients and the scarce research on associative priming in demented patients, we expect a facilitation effect both in the healthy and in the demented elderly people: this facilitation is then ascribed to the automatic and short-duration activation of existing, abstract representations.[8]

For direct facilitation effects, the fact that each target word occurs three times in the same task permits the study of facilitation in the decision speed with the repeated words. This facilitation can then be understood on the basis of the temporary activation during the preceding presentation, but longer-duration facilitation resulting from episodic memory traces can also be given as an interpretation. Moreover, one cannot rule out that conscious recognition processes may be involved. We expect that the elderly will be sensitive in the continuous recognition task for the delay between the first and the second presentation of a word, while they will manifest facilitation in the lexical decision speed of previously seen words irrespective of the delay between the first, second and third presentation (the word pairs are presented randomly for each subject, the interval between the first, second and third presentation thus being arbitrary). When automatic processes are still intact in demented patients, the difference between the continuous recognition task and facilitation in the lexical decision speed will be still more pronounced. In the line of the scanty research on direct priming in DAT patients, we hypothesize that this facilitation is still present in the initial phase of dementia but is disturbed in mild to moderate dementia.

Stimuli and procedure used in lexical decision task

(i) Stimuli

An exercise 15 "word" pairs are presented, which can be repeated. The test is composed of 50 continuous "word" pairs (100 words). There are three lists, which are randomized over the subjects. The words are low frequency nouns in spoken and written Dutch consisting of three to seven characters.[9, 10] All the words have high visual imagery-values.[11] The pseudo-words are defined as having the same characteristics as the words, except that either the first or the last character is replaced by a "wrong" character. A non-word is a senseless recomposition of the vowels and consonants of a word. The subject receives feedback after each decision (high tone = correct; low tone = incorrect). The response time limit is 10 seconds; the interstimulus interval within word pairs is 250 msec, between word pairs three seconds.

(2) Procedure

A string of characters is presented to the subjects; they have to decide as quickly as possible whether the string is a word by pressing the "yes" button with the dominant hand (right hand for the righthanded); if the answer is no they push the "no" button with the non-dominant hand (left hand for the righthanded). The stimuli are composed of pairs of words, pseudo-words, and non-words, the first element being prime and the second the target stimulus. We use five types of word pairs: in the first three pairs, the same word is preceded by a semantically associated word, a semantically unrelated word, or a non-word; for the other two pairs a pseudo-word is preceded by, a word or a non-word. The semantic related-ness of the words is based on the work of De Groot (1980).

Results and discussion

An ANOVA performed on the accuracy of the recognition task showed a significant main effect of the diagnostic groups, of the new versus old words, and of the delay between the first and the second presentation of a word as well as a significant interaction effect of new/old and diagnostic group, new/old and delay, of diagnostic group and delay, and of new/old, delay, and diagnostic group ($p < 0.01$). In view of the hypotheses of this article and for reasons of simplification, we will not discuss the analysis of the frequency of the words and the difference between the first and second blocks. In fact, there are no diagnostic differences in the recog-nition of the new words (average accuracy in normals = 4.9; DAT minimal = 4.8, and DAT mild = 4.4) nor any differences in function of delay with the new words (average accuracy delay 1 word = 4.7; 2 words = 4.8, 4 words = 4.7; 8 words = 4.8, and 16 words = 4.7). Table 1 shows that the main and interaction effects can be ascribed to the recognition of the old words.

Table 1. Continuous recognition task: mean accuracy of old words in diagnostic groups in function of delay

Delay	Normal	DAT minimal	DAT mild	Mean
1	4.60	4.26	3.35	4.07
2	4.05	3.40	3.71	3.72
4	3.40	2.23	2.07	2.57
8	3.60	2.93	2.13	2.89
16	3.20	2.10	1.50	2.27
Mean	3.77	2.98	2.55	3.10

The average accuracy of the old words differs in the diagnostic groups with the highest score in the normals (3.77), then in the DAT minimals (2.98), and finally in the DAT mild (2.55). The recognition of old words is sensitive to the delay between the first and second presentation of a word with a clear difference in accuracy between short and long term memory in all of the groups. It is striking that accuracy in all groups declines in the transition from the 2 to 4-word delay instead of from the 4 to 8-word delay. The interaction between diagnostic groups and delay demonstrates that the patients with mild DAT have clear disturbances in both short- and long-term memory. The group with minimal DAT already show slight difficulties in short-term memory as well as in long-term memory in comparison with the control group.

The results of the average reaction times of the correct answers are similar: a significant main effect of the diagnostic groups, of the new versus old words and of the delay between the first and the second presentation of a word as well as a significant interaction effect of new/old and diagnostic group, new/old and delay, of diagnostic group and delay, and of new/old, delay, and diagnostic group. Table 2 gives the most interesting results of the average reaction times for old words.

Table 2 . Continuous recognition task : mean reaction time (msec) of old words in diagnostic groups and delay.

Delay	Normals	DAT minimal	DAT mild	Mean
1	889.750	1098.750	1572.000	1186.83
2	1086.750	1387.000	2208.000	1560.58
4	1159.750	1401.000	3451.250	2004.00
8	1155.500	1611.750	2671.500	1812.92
16	1251.500	1602.250	3486.750	2113.50
mean	1108.650	1420.150	2677.900	1735.50

In general, we can state that reaction times in all groups increase with the delay and that this is even more pronounced with mildly demented subjects. The minimally demented are somewhat slower than the control group both in short and long-term memory.

In line with our hypotheses, we have demonstrated clear disturbances in the mildly demented in both short and long-term memory by means of this recognition task as a prototype of a direct memory task. The minimal DAT group showed slight difficulties in short as well as long-term memory.

Results and discussion

In the lexical decision task, the accuracy of the decision is measured for the probe and the target words as well as the decision time of the target. ANOVA of the accuracy data shows a significant main effect of the groups, probe/target, pair type, and a significant interaction effect of probe/target and pair type. The high level of performance in all the groups (average accuracy: normals = 9.65, DAT minimal = 9.48, and DAT mild = 8.98) was noteworthy. Table 3 shows that there was less accuracy for pseudowords in all groups.

ANOVA of average reaction times of the target-hits gives a significant main effect of the groups, of the pair type, and a significant interaction effect of groups and pair type. Two important aspects can be deduced from Table 4. In comparison with the reduced accuracy for the pseudo-words, all the groups are slower in decision time with a pseudo-word, irrespective of whether it was preceded by a word (pair type 4) or a non-word (pair type 5). On the basis of the interaction between the groups and the pair type, we see that this slowing is more pronounced in the minimally demented group and certainly in the mildly demented group. In association with similar findings in previous research, we may hypothesize that the identification of pseudo-words (or pronounceable non-words) presumes controlled search processes in the semantic memory and that it is precisely these processes that are disturbed in DAT.[8] The demented groups ultimately achieved a high level of accuracy in the identification of pseudo-words.

Table 3 : Lexical decision task: mean accuracy in diagnostic groups as a function of pair type*

Pair type	Probe	Target	Mean
1	9.70	9.90	9.80
2	9.70	9.80	9.75
3	9.90	9.80	9.85
4	9.70	8.70	9.20
5	9.70	8.60	9.15
Mean	9.74	9.36	9.55

*Pair types: 1 = semantic related words; 2 = non-related words; 3 = non-word/word; 4 = word/pseudoword; 5 = non-word/pseudoword.

Table 4 : Lexical Decision Task: Mean reaction time (msec) of target-hits in diagnostic groups in function of pair type.

Pair type	Normals	DAT minimal	DAT mild	Mean
1	696	820	1254	923
2	730	863	1379	991
3	804	920	1440	1055
4	1268	1677	2659	1868

5	1342	1723	2718	1928
Mean	968	122.6	1890	1353

Another aspect is the facilitation effect in semantically associated word pairs. In all the groups, reaction time in non-associated word pairs is greater than in semantically associated word pairs. Further, *a posteriori* testing is needed to determine whether these differences are significant. This facilitation effect in both healthy and demented elderly people is ascribed to the automatic and short-duration activation of existing representations in semantic memory by the hypothesis.

Alongside this indirect facilitation, which is still intact in mild forms of dementia, the lexical decision task permits investigation of direct facilitation effects. Each target word occurs three times, which makes facilitation possible in the decision speed for repeated words. The ANOVA of this decision speed shows a significant main effect for the groups and a significant interaction effect between the groups and the repetition. In the normals and the minimally demented, we find a facilitation from the first to the second and certainly to the third presentation, while in the mildly demented it is no longer found (see Table 5). Even though the minimally demented show slight memory difficulties in short and long-term memory as measured in the recognition task, they do manifest facilitation from a previous presentation of a word. The mildly demented do not show this repetition facilitation while associative priming is still intact. We hypothesize that this longer duration repetition priming rests on automatic, episodic memory traces. Research among demented elderly people suggests that this form of facilitation is disturbed. From the research with amnesic patients we know that controlled processes can also play a role in so-called indirect memory tasks, and this could also be the case in the repetition effect of the words in the lexical decision task. Comments by a number of subjects during the execution of the task suggest a conscious recognition of repeated words. This conscious recognition can

Table 5 : Lexical decision task: mean reaction time (msec) of repeated target-words

Repetition	Normals	DAT mimimal	DAT mild	Mean
1	776	955	1335	1022
2	733	902	1319	9843
2	723	799	1440	987
Mean	744	885	1364	988

partially explain the repetition priming in normals and the minimally demented. In the mildly demented, however, we have shown that these controlled memory processes are disturbed.

Conclusion

We can state that these provisional findings support the literature on facilitation effects in amnesia and dementia patients. We are aware of the imperfections of this research, such as the small number of minimally demented patients and particularly mildly demented patients. Further expansion of the number of demented patients is needed to confirm these findings. The mildly demented do show associative but no repetition priming, suggesting that there are several forms of facilitation processes that can be differentially affected in the demented elderly, possibly depending on the severity of the dementia. The findings in repetition priming also suggest that the dichotomy of direct- indirect memory tasks is not automatically equivalent to the opposition of direct-indirect memory processes. Direct and indirect memory tasks help us to understand the many differences between tasks and forms of measurement procedures. The differential effect of dementia on direct and indirect memory processing in demented elderly people in comparison with the normal elderly and amnesic patients will give us a better insight into memory functioning in dementia of the Alzheimer type.

Acknowledgements

We thank Noël Bovens for the development of the computer tests, Rob Stroobants for the statistical processing of the data, Dr. H. Hauman and Dr. P. Bourgeois for the administration of the CAMDEX, the general practitioners for their cooperation and, last but not least, the elderly people for their participation in the research.

References

(1) Roth M, Thym E, Mountjoy CQ, Huppert FA, Hendrie H, Verma S, Goddard R. CAMDEX. A standardized instrument for the diagnosis of mental disorders in the elderly with special reference to the early detection of Alzheimer's disease. *British Journal of Psychiatry* 1986, **149**, 698-709.

(2) Richardson-Klavehn A, Bjork RA. Measures of Memory. *Annual Review of Psychology* 1988, **39**, 475-543.

(3) Jacoby LL, Witherspoon D. Remembering without awareness. *Canadian Journal of Psychology* 1982, **36**(2), 300-324.

(4) Roediger HL, Blaxton TA. Retrieval modes produce dissociations in memory for surface information. In Gorfein DS, Hoffman RR (eds.), *Memory and Cognitive Processes: The Ebbinghaus Centennial Conference*. Hillsdale, NJ: Lawrence Erlbaum, 1987, 349-379.

(5) Schachter DL. Implicit Memory: History and Current Status. *Journal of Experimental Psychology: Learning, Memory and Cognition* 1987, **13**(3), 501-518.

(6) Collins AM, Loftus EF. A spreading activation theory of semantic processing. *Psychological Review* 1975, **82,** 407-428.

(7) Nebes RD, Martin DC, Horn LC. Sparing of semantic memory in Alzheimer's Disease. *Journal of Abnormal Psychology* 1984, **93**(3), 321-330.

(8) Wens L, Baro F, d'Ydewalle G. The information processing approach in clinical memory assessment. *Psych. Rep. 70,* Leuven, Belgium, Laboratory of Experimental Psychology, 1987.

(9) Uit den Bogaert *Woordfrequenties in geschreven en gesproken Nederlands.* Utrecht, Oosthoek, Scheltema & Hoekema, 1974.

(10) De Jong ED. *Spreektaal. Woordfrequenties in gesproken Nederlands.* Utrecht, Bohn, Scheltema & Holkema, 1979.

(11) Van Loorn-Vervoorn WA. *Voorstelbaarheidswaarden van Nederlandse woorden.* Lisse, Swets & Zeitlinger, 1985.

Further references from Dr Wens

Chapter 44

DEMENTIA AND DEPRESSION IN A NURSING HOME POPULATION

D O'Neill, D Bagley, N McCormack, JB Walsh, D Coakley,
Alzheimer Society of Ireland, St John of God Hospital, Stillorgan, Co Dublin and Mercer's Institute for Research on Ageing, St James's Hospital, Dublin 8, Ireland

This paper presents the results of the first research project organized by the Alzheimer Society of Ireland. It is representative of the type of practical research that a national Alzheimer's association can carry out, as outlined elsewhere in this book.[1] This is particularly important in environments where there is limited government funding for health and services research. One of the remits of any Alzheimer's association is to look after the welfare of its patients: an area of particular concern is the nature of extended care, particularly that provided in nursing homes. In the United States one and a quarter million elderly people are in nursing homes as a result of dementing illness: the corresponding figure for Ireland is unknown. The inexorable rise of the private sector nursing home has been a phenomenon in the last ten years in Ireland, the United Kingdom and in many other countries.

There is a mixed public and private health care system in Ireland. Extended care options are catered for in two ways: either in hospitals and welfare homes or in nursing homes. The hospitals and welfare homes (public beds) are based to a great extent on former work houses and large institutions and are administered by local health authorities. Patients usually have a medical assessment at or prior to admission and permanent medical staff are in attendance. However, of the 4.8 per cent of the elderly who are in institutional care in Ireland, 6280 of these are in nursing homes, about 1 per cent of the elderly.[2] With reductions in public spending and with an increased emphasis on the private sector, there has been a dramatic rise in the number of nursing homes in this country. In 1980, there were 2.2 public beds to 1 nursing home bed and this has dropped in 1985 to 1.6 public beds to 1 nursing home bed.

When community care is no longer feasible, admission to a welfare home can be difficult, particularly in the largest health-care region in the country (Eastern Health Board). So there may be pressure for carers to place relatives in a private nursing home. The Department of Health, through the Health Board, partially subsidizes them at a rate which in combination with their pension amounts to somewhere between 40 and 60 per cent of the cost of the nursing home. By and large carers make up the difference in price.

One of the concerns of the Alzheimer Society is that patients may be admitted to nursing homes without proper assessment. Cognitive impairment may not be detected and screened for reversible components. Affective disorders may not be detected and treated: this is particularly important as (i) depression occurs commonly in dementing illness[3] and (ii) treatment of depression may result in improvement of cognitive function.[4]

Methodology

We screened for cognitive impairment and depressive illness in nursing homes in the largest health board in Ireland, the Eastern Health Board. We chose 23 out of 180 nursing homes on the basis of an alphanumeric sort. Of 456 patients approached 51 (11 per cent) refused or were unable to comply with the questionnaire. The mean age of our patients was 82 years and the sex ratio was 92 per cent female, 8 per cent male: these demographic features are shared by nursing home populations throughout the Western world: predominantly elderly and female.

Two survey instruments were used. The Folstein Mini-Mental State Examination (MMSE) was altered in its orientation section to adapt it to an Irish setting:[5, 6] the second instrument was the Geriatric Depression Scale. We have reported its utility in an acute hospital setting.[7] It is a simple 30-item questionnaire with yes/no answers. Although originally proposed by Yesavage to be self-administered by the patients, we feel that a flaw with this methodology is that patients who cannot fill it out on their own should have it administered to them. We have checked the questionnaire as both self-administered and staff-administered with very different outcomes.[8] Therefore we used it administered by health care professionals only and found it to be sensitive and specific in an acute hospital setting.

A question mark hangs over whether depression scales can be used in dementia. Using the approximate categorization of cognitive impairment suggested by Reisberg – MMSE scores under 16 indicating moderate to severe cognitive impairment and scores of 16 to 23 suggesting mild to moderate impairment[9] - we have shown that the Geriatric Depression Scale is effective in mild to moderate cognitive impairment.[10] Therefore, we have applied it to patients scoring from 16–30 on the MMSE. The two researchers were trained over a two-week period in St. James's Hospital and underwent regular feed-back sessions.

Results

The cut-off point for cognitive impairment used for the MMSE was 23/30. 228 out of the 405 scored in the impaired range. This suggests a 58 per cent prevalence of cognitive impairment. The distribution of MMSE score with age demonstrates a slight reduction (Fig. 1), which is considerably less than might be expected in a normal population. Prevalence of cognitive impairment rises from nearly 50 per

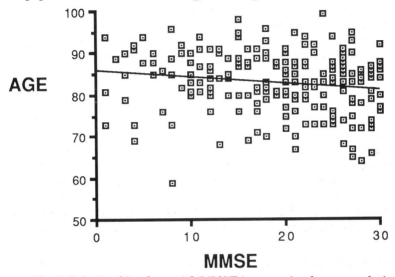

Fig.1. Relationship of age with MMSE in a nursing home population.

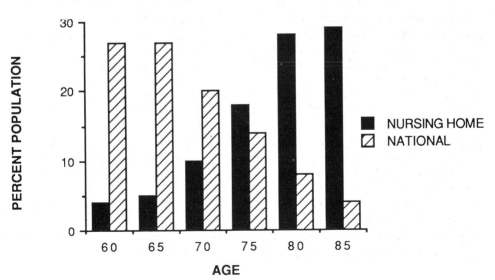

Fig. 2. Relative percentages of age-groups in the over-65 age-group in (a) the nursing-home population, and (b) the elderly in the community.

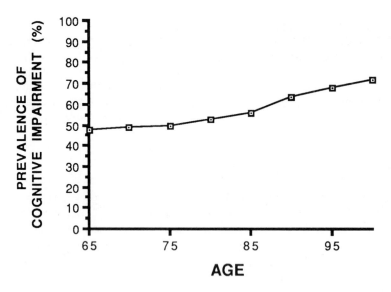

Fig. 3. Prevalence of cognitive impairment with age in a nursing-home population.

cent to over 70 per cent in the nursing home population (Fig. 2), compared with under 10 per cent to nearly 50 per cent between the ages of 65 and 90 in the community: this is despite the population skew in favour of the very elderly (Fig. 3). These facts may suggest that (i) "younger" people admitted to nursing homes are relatively severely handicapped, and (ii) that they may be admitted as a result of their cognitive impairment.

A score of greater than 11 on the Geriatric Depression Scale was considered to be suggestive of depressive illness. 120 out of the 405 scored over 11/30: this represents a 30 per cent positive screening rate for depression. Combined cognitive impairment and depression on the rating score suggested that 66 out of 405 (16 per cent) rated as positive for both cognitive impairment and for depression.

Discussion

The high prevalence of cognitive impairment and depression suggested by this study indicate the need for a medical and multi-disciplinary assessment before admission. One health board, the Eastern Health Board, insists on assessment by a geriatrician before paying the subsidy for nursing home care, but this only extends to a proportion of the nursing home residents. We would suggest that comprehensive multi-disciplinary assessment should be mandatory for all admissions to nursing homes. The high level of depression as noted on this screening is in keeping with figures from acute hospital figures. In the light of the therapeutic implications referred to above, it is important that the assessment schedule should take account of affective illness.

Ongoing assessment for residents should be available from doctors experienced in care of the elderly. Although it is mandatory for nursing homes in the Republic of Ireland to have a doctor in consultation, systematic reassessment is the exception rather than the rule. Full multi-disciplinary services such as physiotherapy, occupational therapy and other resources should be available in these nursing homes commensurate with these patients' significant degree of handicap. Quality control is very important to ensure the suitability of nursing homes for residents with dementia.

Conclusion

This study has confirmed that cognitive impairment and depression are very common in nursing homes in the area served by the Alzheimer Society of Ireland. It has also highlighted a gap in the assessment of those who are most likely to use nursing homes. We hope that it will encourage Alzheimer's associations to pursue research into areas of practical concern to sufferers and their carers.

References

(1) Graham N. The silent epidemic – who cares? In O'Neill D (ed), *Carers, Professionals and Alzheimer's Disease*. London, John Libbey, 1991.

(2) National Council for the Aged. *Institutional Care of the Elderly in Ireland*. Dublin, National Council for the Aged, 1985.

(3) Reifler BV, Larson E, Hanly R. Coexistence of cognitive impairment and depression in geriatric outpatients. *Am J Psychiatry* 1982, **139**, 632.

(4) Reifler BV, Larson E, Teri L, Poulsen M. Dementia of the Alzheimer's type and depression. *J American Geriatrics Society* 1986, **34**, 855-859.

(5) O'Neill D, Condren L, O'Kelly F, King A, Young M, Walsh JB, Coakley D. Cognitive impairment in the elderly. *Irish Medical Journal* 1988, **81**, 11-13.

(6) O'Neill, D, O'Shea B, Walsh JB, Coakley DC. Screening for dementia and delirium using an adapted Folstein Mini-Mental Status Examination. *Irish Medical Journal* 1989, **82**, 24-25.

(7) O'Riordan T, Hayes J, Shelley R, O'Neill D, Walsh JB, Coakley D. The prevalence of depression in an acute geriatric medical unit. *International Journal of Geriatric Psychiatry* 1989, 4, 17-21

(8) O'Neill D, Rice I, Blake P, Walsh JB, Coakley D. Should the Geriatric Depression Scale be self-administered? *J American Geriatrics Society*, 1990, **38**, A19.

(9) Reisberg B, Ferris SH, Anand R, de Leon MJ, Schneck MK, Crook T. Clinical assessment of cognitive decline in normal aging and primary degenerative dementia: concordant ordinal measures. In Pinchot P, Berner R, Thau K (eds), *Psychiatry* 1985, **5**, 333-338.

(10) O'Riordan T, Hayes J, O'Neill D, Shelley R, Walsh JB, Coakley D. The effect of mild to moderate dementia on the Geriatric Depression Scale and on the General Health Questionnaire in the hospitalised elderly. *Age and Ageing* 1990, **19**, 57-61

Carers, Professionals and Alzheimer's Disease. D O'Neill ed © 1991 John Libbey & Company Ltd

Chapter 45

DIFFICULTIES IN DIAGNOSING ALZHEIMER'S DISEASE IN DOWN'S SYNDROME

V Keane[1] *MRCPsych*, D O'Neill[2] *MRCPI*, JB Walsh[2] *MRCP*, D Coakley[2] *FRCPI*, V Coffey[3] *FRCPI*, M Mulcahy[1] *FRCPI Stewart's Hospital[1], Palmerstown, Dublin 20; Mercer's Institute for Research on Ageing[2], St James's Hospital, and Foundation for the Prevention of Childhood Handicaps[3], St James's Hospital, Dublin, Ireland*

Down's syndrome is the largest single cause of mental handicap. In Ireland the condition accounted for almost a quarter of all persons within the moderate, severe and profound range of handicap in 1981.[1] In developed countries one child in every 800 to 1,000 live births has Down's syndrome. Alzheimer's disease is the single most common cause of dementia. The cause is unknown and definitive diagnosis cannot be made during life as it depends ultimately on finding the characteristic neuropathological features. As far back as 1876 an association between Alzheimer's disease and Down's syndrome was noted by Frazer and Mitchell.[2] In 1929, Struwe was the first to describe the characteristic senile plaques of Alzheimer's disease in the brains of individuals with Down's syndrome.[3] By the late 1960s the link between Alzheimer's and Down's was fairly clearly established. In 1977 Heston noted that all people with Down's syndrome over the age of 35 seemed to have neuropathological features of Alzheimer's disease on the basis of post mortem studies.[4]

Clinical discrepancy

Despite over three decades of research into premature ageing in Down's syndrome, a discrepancy remains between the neuropathological and the clinical evidence. Among elderly people in the general population, pathological changes of the same order of magnitude as those found in the Down's syndrome brain over

315

the age of 35 are accompanied by overt clinical signs of dementia: for example, intellectual deterioration, personality change and loss of self-care skills. However, many people with Down's syndrome live healthy lives until death and do not show signs of dementia despite positive post mortem findings.

One of the principal problems in studying the dementia of Down's syndrome is the difficulty in measuring neuropsychological changes in a mentally retarded population, particularly in subjects with little or no language development. Discrepancies between overt behaviour and underlying brain pathology divide investigators. Malamud in 1964 noted that the initially severe grade of mental retardation in Down's syndrome is not conducive to adequate clinical evaluation.[5] On the other hand, Ropper and Williams noted in 1980 that clinical evidence suggests that retarded persons are usually more susceptible to clinical deterioration in response to a second acquired cerebral disorder:[6] on these grounds it is not likely that dementia is masked by pre-existing mental retardation.

As the life expectancy of Down's syndrome individuals increases,[7,8] research into the association between Down's syndrome and Alzheimer's disease has become an important and interesting area. Research into the association between Down's syndrome and Alzheimer's disease is important. If people with Down's syndrome are at risk for dementia there is a need (i) to establish reliable diagnostic methods, and (ii) to develop the appropriate services for this population. An understanding of this association may give some insight into the cause of Alzheimer's disease.

Method and subjects

We conducted a study of all Down's syndrome patients in Stewart's Hospital over the age of 35 to explore the difficulty in making a clinical diagnosis of dementia in this population. Of the 37 resident Down's syndrome patients in Stewarts Hospital, 21 are aged 35 and over. The diagnosis of Down's syndrome is confirmed in all but 3 of the 21 patients by chromosomal analysis.

The case notes of all patients were reviewed in this cross-sectional study. In addition nursing staff who were familiar with the patients for at least 5 years were interviewed. All patients had psychological assessments in the last 3 years, and their cases were discussed with the clinical psychologist. All patients were assessed using a questionnaire, previously used by the Wessex Health Care Evaluation Research Team (Table 1). The physical and psychiatric diagnosis were noted as were each patient's medications. A medical evaluation was conducted in seven areas: vision, hearing, thyroid status, prescribed medication, psychiatric and physical status.

Table 1. Survey form based on the Wessex Health Care Evaluation Research Team form

A. INCAPACITIES

Wetting (nights)	1.Frequently	2.Occasionally	3.Never
Soiling (nights)	1.Frequently	2.Occasionally	3.Never
Wetting (days)	1.Frequently	2.Occasionally	3.Never
Soiling (days)	1.Frequently	2.Occasionally	3.Never
Walk with help	1.Not at all	2.Not upstairs	3.Upstairs & elsewhere
Walk by himself	1.Not at all	2.Not upstairs	3.Upstairs & elsewhere
Feed himself	1.Not at all	2.With help	3.Without help
Dress himself	1.Not at all	2.With help	3.Without help
Wash himself	1.Not at all	2.With help	3.Without help
Vision	1.Blind or almost	2.Poor	3.Normal
Hearing	1.Deaf or almost	2.Poor	3.Normal
Speech	1.Never a word	2.Odd words	3.Normal
Reads	1.Nothing	2.A little	3.Newspapers/books
Writes	1.Nothing	2.A little	3.Own correspondence
Counts	1.Nothing	2.A little	3.Understands money

B. SPEECH

If this person talks in sentences, is the speech? –	1.Difficult to understand even by close acquaintances	2. Easily understood by close acquaintances	3. Clear enough to be understood by anyone

C. BEHAVIOUR PROBLEMS

Hits out or attacks others	1.Marked	2.Lesser	3.No
Tears up papers, clothing or damages furniture	1.Marked	2,Lesser	3.No
Overactive, pacing, does not sit down for a minute	1.Marked	2.Lesser	3.No
Constantly seeking attention, will not leave adults	1.Marked	2.Lesser	3.No
Continuously injures himself, e.g., head banging	1.Marked	2.Lesser	3.No

Results

There were 14 male and 7 female patients. The mean age was 42 years and the mean duration in hospital was 26 years. Mental handicap assessment showed one person to be in the moderate range, 8 in the severe range and 12 in the profound range. The patient of moderate IQ could read, write and count a little. The remaining 20 patients could not read, write or count. Language assessment revealed that 4 patients never spoke a word, 9 spoke odd words only and the remaining 8 could speak in sentences but some of them could be understood only by close acquaintances.

Ophthalmic examination showed 8 patients to have bilateral opacities, either corneal or lens and one patient had a unilateral cataract. 10 patients had normal sight. One patient was myopic and a further patient was blind and had congenital nystagmus. The nursing staff assessed 10 patients without cataracts as having normal vision, excluding the patients with myopia and congenital nystagmus. Of some note is that of the 8 people with bilateral cataracts (as assessed by an ophthalmologist), nursing staff assessed 5 as having normal vision, 1 as having poor vision and 2 as almost blind.

Hearing loss was detected in 15 patients on audiological testing. Five patients had hearing within normal limits and 1 patient could not be assessed as her behaviour would not permit this. Nursing staff assessed the 5 patients whose hearing is within normal limits as having normal hearing. Of the 15 assessed by audiology as having hearing loss, nursing staff felt that 7 had poor hearing, 7 had normal hearing and 1 patient was almost deaf. So, as with vision, there appears to be discrepancies between formal examination and clinical observation in assessing hearing in Down's syndrome patients. Of the 21 patients only 3 had both hearing and vision within normal limits.

Assessment of thyroid function revealed that only 4 patients required replacement therapy. Fourteen of the patients are receiving no medication. As mentioned above, 4 are receiving thyroxine for hypothyroid status, one of whom had been recently commenced on a neuroleptic for apparently unprovoked screaming episodes. Only one other patient was on a neuroleptic agent for a ten year history of self injurious behaviour. Two other patients were on medication: an epileptic of one year's standing was on anti-convulsants and a patient with a ten year history of an affective disorder was on antidepressants.

Just over half the patients had no psychiatric or behavioural problems. The remaining 9 patients present a number of varying problems, for example, self injurious behaviour, affective illness and psychosis. Of note is that two of the psychiatric problems have emerged in the last two years.

Physical status

Excluding loss of vision and hearing, only seven patients were physically healthy. Of the remaining 14 patients, 4 were hypothyroid, 4 had skin conditions, 2 had leucopaenia (secondary to hepatitis vaccination), 3 had varicose veins, and one was a carrier of hepatitis B. If one combines psychiatric and physical status (excluding vision and hearing), 8 patients had both a psychiatric and physical problem, 6 had a physical problem only and 3 had a psychiatric problem only. So only 4 out of 21 patients had neither psychiatric nor physical problems: but of these 4, one had cataracts and hearing loss, and 3 had normal vision but hearing loss. If hearing and vision are assessed as mentioned previously only 3 patients of the 21 were within normal limits. Of these 3 patients each had a further problem: one a physical problem and the other two both physical and psychiatric problems (Table 2).

Table 2. Health problems among 21 adult Down's syndrome patients.

NUMBERS	HEALTH PROBLEMS
3	Psychiatric – nil else
6	Physical – nil else (excluding vision and hearing)
8	Psychiatric and physical (excluding vision and hearing)
1	Visual and hearing impairment – nil else
3	Visual or hearing impairment – nil else

Finally some basic self-care skills were assessed: continence, feeding, washing, dressing and mobility. The self-care skills varied with each individual and could be equated with IQ. Overall, staff felt that 2 patients had deteriorated over the last two to three years. Both have cataracts, hearing loss, are on medication and have a psychiatric and physical problem.

Discussion

As can be seen from these results, not one patient in this group of 21 Down's syndrome individuals over the age of 35 is without some problem, either physical, psychiatric, visual or hearing. This makes the assessment of dementia in this group very difficult.

A deterioration in self-care skills and general motor slowing have been noted in Down's syndrome individuals who have subsequently been diagnosed on post mortem findings as suffering from Alzheimer's disease. The results from this study do not show any consistent pattern within mobility and self-care skills abilities. Long-term follow-up is needed to establish the significance of these observations. As noted from the results, great variability exists in the skills possessed by Down's syndrome individuals. This makes it difficult to infer a previous performance level and therefore to recognize signs of deterioration. Apart from the physical and psychiatric morbidity in our study group, the underlying mental handicap of people with Down's syndrome results in wide inter-individual variation in developmental history and IQ. Normal test procedures are therefore unsatisfactory as failure on test items may be due to either the underlying mental handicap or to dementia.

It is important to clarify clinical symptomatology of dementia in Down's syndrome, its development and possible correlations with histopathology and karyotype. Should a form of treatment and care emerge for Alzheimer's disease, it would be sad if such an advance was not applicable to Down's syndrome individuals due to the absence of a practical system for diagnosis. It is possible that the premature ageing and high incidence of age-related disabilities found in people with Down's syndrome are related to the disturbance in growth and development attributable to the presence of the extra chromosome.[9] The association of Down's syndrome and Alzheimer's disease has major implications for the role of genetics in understanding ageing.

Conclusion

Many questions remain unanswered about Alzheimer's disease and its presence in Down's syndrome persons. In the general public early warning signs tend to be memory loss and confusion: in Down's syndrome these symptoms are extremely difficult to detect reliably. Even if they are noticed they may be attributed to other causes, for example, cataracts or hearing loss. Dementia is a very difficult diagnosis to make in a Down's syndrome population. The criteria for diagnosis of dementia in individuals with Down's syndrome may require modification of current DSM III diagnostic criteria. The ability to make a diagnosis of dementia in Down's syndrome has far reaching effects, not only into giving a better understanding of dementia but perhaps more importantly in being able to plan appropriate and adequate services for the mentally handicapped.

References

(1) Mulcahy M, O'Connor S, Reynolds A. Census of the mentally handicapped in the Republic of Ireland, 1981. *Irish Medical Journal* 1983, **76,** 71-75.

(2) Fraser J, Mitchell A. Kalmuc idiocy: report of case with autopsy, with notes on 62 cases. *J Mental Science* 1876, **22,** 161.

(3) Struwe F. Histopathologische Untersuchungen uber Entstchung und Wesen der senilen Plaques. *Zeitschrift für die gesampte Neurologie und Psychiatrie* 1929, **122,** 291.

(4) Heston LL. Alzheimer's disease, trisomy 21 and myeloproliferative disorders: associations suggesting a genetic diathesis. *Science* 1977, **196,** 322-323.

(5) Malamud N. Neuropathology. In, Stevens HA, Heber R (eds). *Mental Retardation.* Chicago, Chicago University Press, 1964.

(6) Ropper AH, Williams RS. Relationship between plaques, tangles and dementia in Down's syndrome. *Neurology* 1980, **30,** 639-644.

(7) Thase ME. Longevity and mortality in Down's syndrome. *J Mental Deficiency Research* 1982, **26,** 177-192.

(8) Penrose LS. *The Biology of Mental Defect.* New York, Grune and Stratton, 1963.

(9) Zigman WB, Schupf N, Lubin R, Silverman W. Premature regression of adults with Down's syndrome. *American J Mental Deficiency* 1987, **92,**2 161-168.

Carers, Professionals and Alzheimer's Disease. D O'Neill ed © 1991 John Libbey & Company Ltd

Chapter 46

ACTIVITIES OF DAILY LIVING AND MENTAL STATUS IN ELDERLY PATIENTS WITH ORGANIC BRAIN DISORDERS

Fumio Eto MD, *Division of Rehabilitation Medicine, University of Tokyo Hospital, Tokyo. 7-3-1 Hongo, Bunkyo-ku, Tokyo, 113, Japan.*

Improvement of self-care performance and activities of daily living (ADL) is one of the most important goals in treatment and rehabilitation of the elderly patients with chronic organic brain diseases or dementia. ADL performances may partly depend on the mental status of those patients. While the detailed and complicated measurements of ADL as well as mental status have been developed, simple and reliable ways of assessment are needed for everyday assessment and management of elderly patients with cognitive impairment. Of the many instruments available for assessing mental status, the short portable mental status questionnaire (SPMSQ) by Pfeiffer is simple and easily administered.[1] We use a 3-point rating system on four basic items (walking, eating, dressing and toiletting activities) as a measure for ADL. The correlation between mental status examination and ADL scores is of some interest, since each measurement may be considered to indicate different types of problems in the management of the demented patients. This paper presents a comparative study of the SPMSQ and of our simple ADL scoring instrument.

Subjects and methods

Eighty-four subjects from two different groups were involved in this study. The first group consisted of 41 patients who had been long-stay patients for more than 7 years in a psychiatric hospital. Their mean age was 78 years, and their mean period of hospitalization was 9.4 years. This group included 12 patients with cerebrovascular disease whose mean age was 73.5 years. The second group consisted of 43 patients with cerebrovascular disease who had been monitored at the outpatient clinic of geriatric medical department of the University of Tokyo Hospital for more than 5 years. Their mean age was 73.7 years, and the mean period of follow-up there was 8.0 years. This group was divided into two subgroups according to the age of onset of initial stroke, i.e. below or above 60 years of age. There were 11 patients with a mean age of 62.5 years in the early onset subgroup and 32 patients with their mean age of 77.5 years in the late onset subgroup.

The SPMSQ consists of ten items: for cultural reasons, the question asking for the name of the American president was changed to asking for the name of the prime minister of Japan. The question asking for the patient's mother's maiden name is a little more difficult as maiden names are not generally used in Japan. The various ADL items were scored from 0 (total dependency) to 2 (independent) in each activity. Total ADL score thus ranged from 0 to 8 points. Patients with 8 points were usually independent in daily hospital routine. We have been using this simple ADL scoring system for evaluation of the elderly patients with organic brain disease since 1980.[2]

Results

The inpatient group scored an average score of 3.2 on the ADL and 1.8 on the SPMSQ. The correlation coefficient between the scores was 0.57 ($p < 0.01$, t-test). The outpatient group scored an average score of 7.5 on the ADL and 8.6 on the SPMSQ. The correlation coefficient between the two scores was again significant with a value of 0.85. The ADL and SPMSQ scores of both groups together also showed a significant correlation (Fig. 1). Average ADL score was 5.3 and average SPMSQ score was 5.0. Their correlation coefficient was significantly large with the value of 0.81.

The inpatients were divided into three small groups according to their clinical diagnosis on admission; 12 patients with cerebrovascular disease, 14 with senile dementia of the Alzheimer type or Alzheimer's disease, and 15 with other psychiatric disorders. The correlation coefficient of ADL score and SPMSQ score was not significant in the cerebrovascular disease subgroup of the inpatients group and in the early onset cases of the outpatients group. Average scores of both ADL and SPMSQ were a little higher in the early onset group than in the late onset group with cerebrovascular disease, but this was not significant.

Thirty out of forty-one inpatients scored in the cognitively impaired range on the SPMSQ. Among patients with cerebrovascular disease, outpatients scored significantly better scores on ADL and SPMSQ than inpatients. The average follow-up period of the outpatients was 8.0 years and average duration of hospitalisation for inpatients with cerebrovascular disease was 9.0 years. Average duration after the onset of initial stroke was 9.3 years in the outpatients group and 12.5 years in the inpatients group.

ADL score & SPMSQ

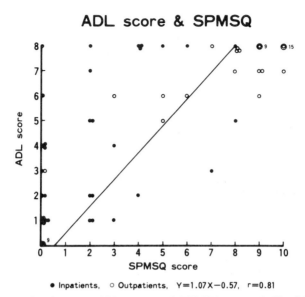

● Inpatients, ○ Outpatients, Y=1.07X−0.57, r=0.81

Fig. 1. Relationship between ADL score and SPMSQ score of all subjects studied.

Discussion

ADL performance is a measure of functional disability, while mental status scores such as the SPMSQ reflect impairment in problem classification by patients. These measures represent different types of disability associated with dementing illness, as shown in our model of disability (Fig. 2). However, we have demonstrated that these two scores are significantly correlated in the elderly patients with chronic organic brain diseases.

We have previously reported a simple evaluation system for demented patients using the Hasegawa Dementia Scale (HDS), the Barthel Index[5] and our simple

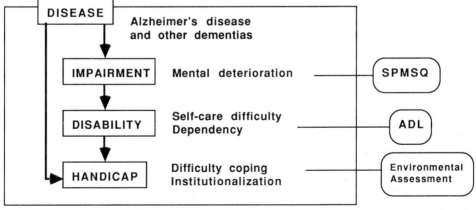

Fig. 2. A model for disability in patients with dementia, illustrating three levels of classification.

325

ADL score.[3] The HDS is the most popular screening test for dementia in Japan. It is very similar to the Folstein Mini-Mental State Examination[4] apart from a visuomotor task. Frontal horn index (FHI) and cella media index (CMI) were also assessed: these have been used for assessment of cerebral atrophy on the brain by computerized tomography.[6] These five assessments were administered to ten patients with a clinical diagnosis of primary degenerative dementia at the Hatsuishi hospital. A very high correlation was found between our ADL score and the Barthel Index: this might be expected because of the common characteristics of both measurements. The HDS score showed also a significant correlation with ADL score. However, FHI and CMI showed no significant correlation with ADL score or with the HDS, suggesting that measures of cerebral atrophy may not relate to the clinical findings in primary degenerative dementia, as has been previously recognized.

Assessment and treatment

One of the important goals when planning treatment for demented patients is to improve the quality of their life: all such decisions should be based on proper evaluation schedules. Evaluation of problems in management of elderly patients with dementia should be carried out in acute as well as long-term care facilities. An assessment of ADL should be routine in elderly patients, not only because it correlates with cognitive status, but also as a useful gauge for progress or deterioration of patients with dementia. This may stimulate more rational management schedules and will presumably improve the quality of care. It is extremely important that evaluation instruments for demented patients should be easily applicable by all levels of health-care worker engaged in the management of dementia. For this purpose the measurement of ADL with a simple scoring system like ours may be rather useful, because it can easily be carried out by non-professional workers during routine care of the severe mentally deteriorated elderly. This kind of simple ADL score may not be as influenced by cognitive status as the instrumental ADL score[7] which is a more complicated psychobehavioural aspect of daily living activities.

A result of emphasis on ADL assessment should be that approaches to enrich daily activities would be encouraged among all health-care workers dealing with dementia. This attitude may not entail a very hi-tech approach, but should still be a priority at all levels of care.

References

(1) Pfeiffer E. A short portable mental status questionnaire for the assessment of organic brain deficit in elderly patients. *J Am Ger Soc* 1975, 433-441.

(2) Eto F. Activities of daily living of the patients with dementia in long-stay psychogeriatric wards. In, Flax HJ, Matta AA, (ed) *New Frontiers that influence disease and rehabilitation.* San Juan: IRMA IV, 1983, 125-129.

(3) Eto F. Problems and medical management of the demented elderly. *Annual Rep Sasakawa Health Sci Found* 1985, **1,** 3-12 (Japanese).

(4) Mahoney FI, Barthel DW. Functional evaluation: The Barthel Index. *Maryland State Med J* 1965, **14,** 61-65.

(5) Folstein MF, Folstein SE, McHugh PR. 'Mini-Mental State': A practical method for grading the cognitive state of patients for the clinician. *J Psychiatr Res* 1975, **12,** 189-198.

(6) Soininen H, Puranen M, Riekkinen PJ. Computed tomography findings in senile dementia and normal aging. *J Neurol Neurosurg Psychiatry* 1982, **45,** 50-54.

(7) Lawton MP, Brody EM. Assessment of older people: Self-maintaining and instrumental activities of daily living. *Gerontologist* 1969, **9,** 179-186.